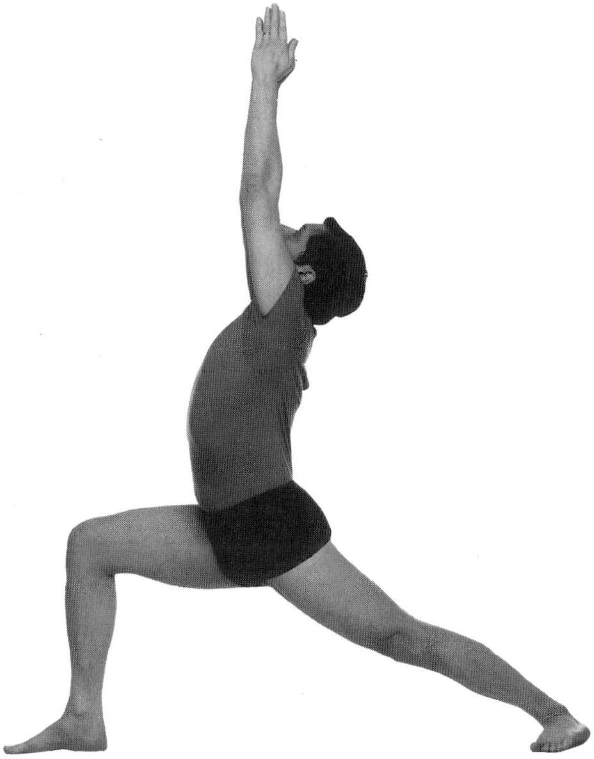

YOGA

THE IYENGAR WAY

To our Guru
Who has taught us this art
And has guided our lives

May the light of his knowledge illumine others
To proceed on the path of Yoga

KNOPF
75
YEARS·OF·PUBLISHING

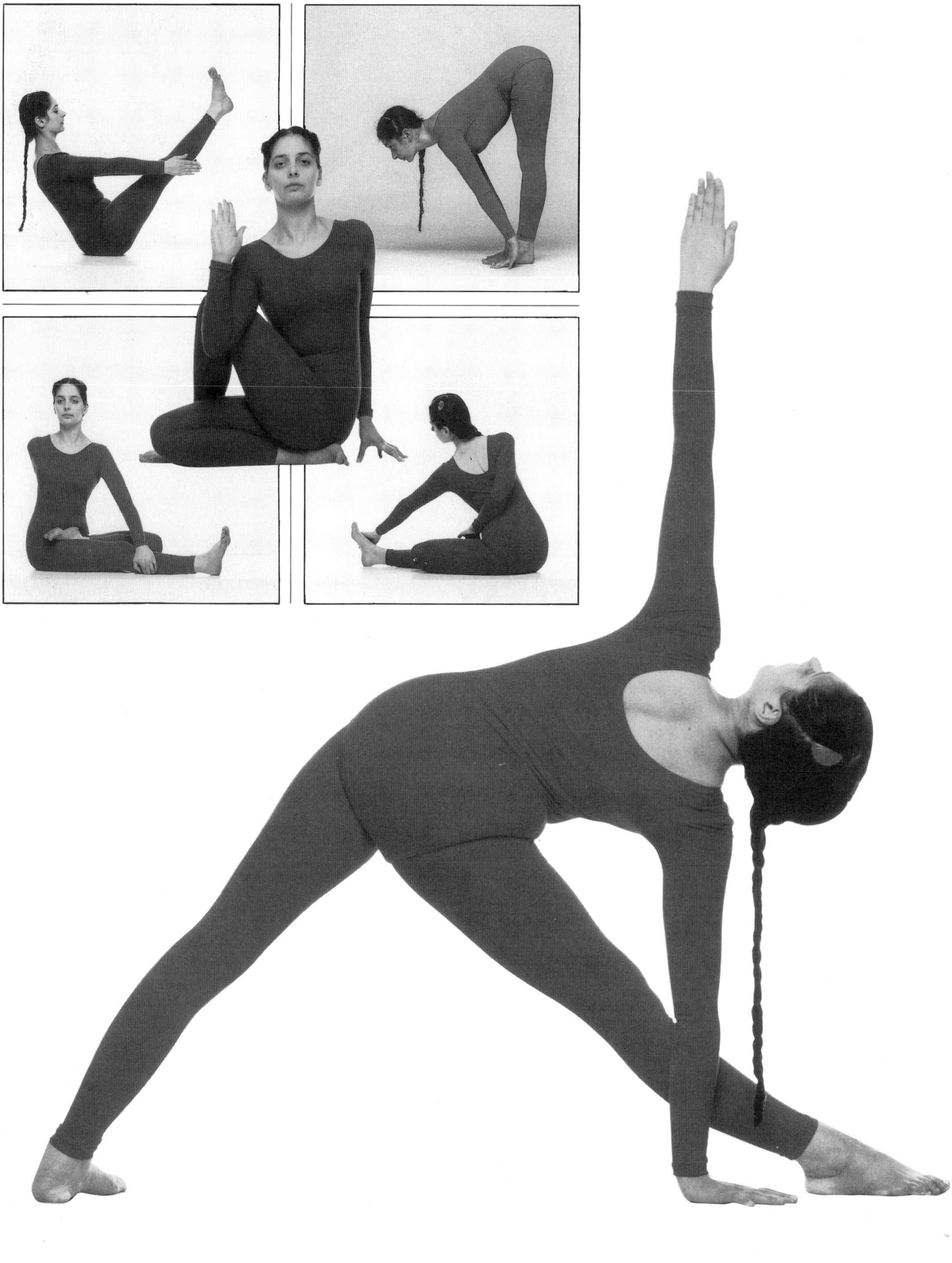

YOGA

THE IYENGAR WAY

Silva, Mira &
Shyam Mehta

ALFRED A. KNOPF · NEW YORK · 1992

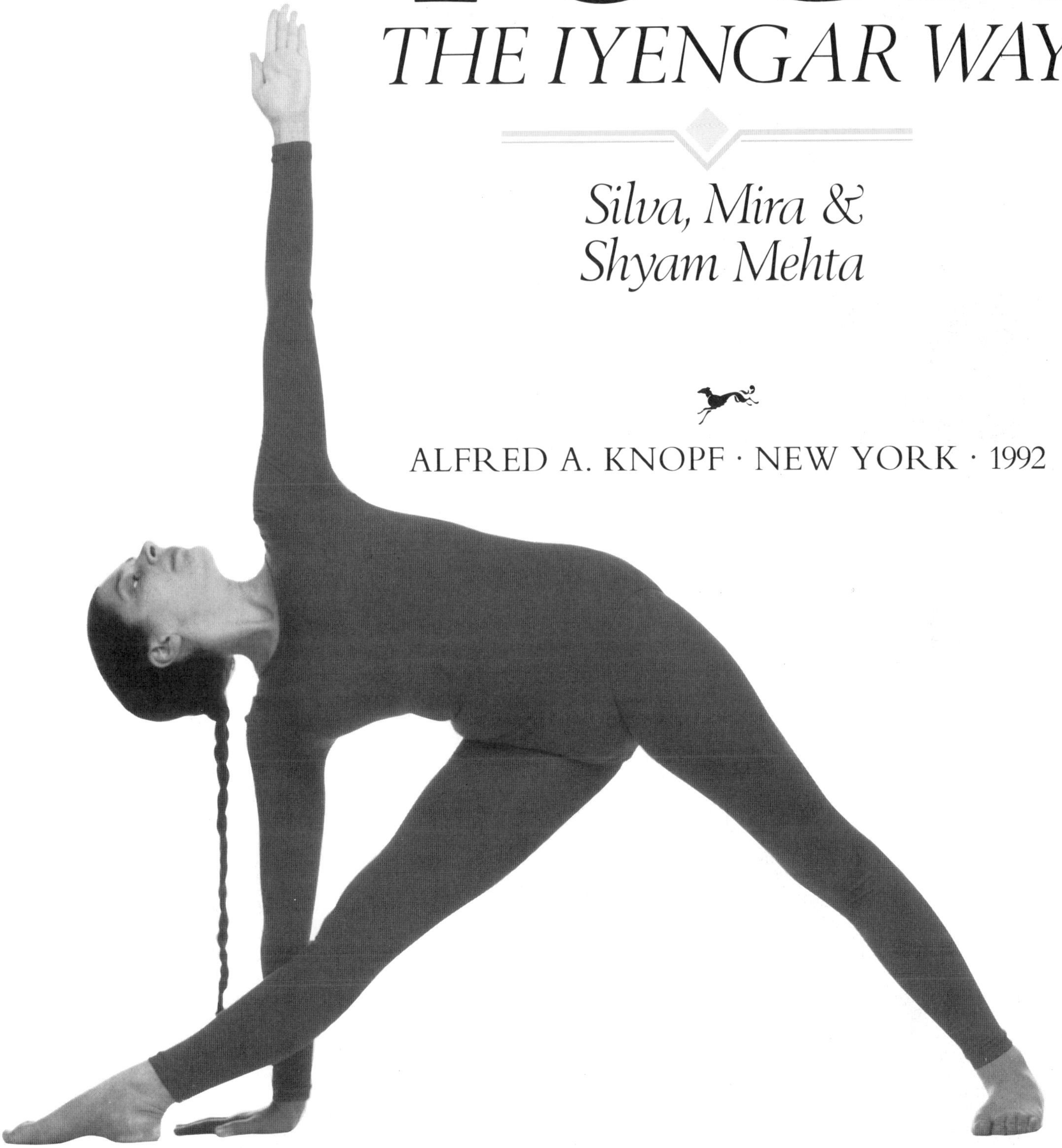

A DORLING KINDERSLEY BOOK

Editor **Susan Berry**
U.S. editor **Toinette Lippe**
Designer **Steven Wooster**

Assistant designer **Claudine Meissner**
Editorial assistant **Sue George**

Managing editor **Daphne Razazan**

Photography **Jeff Veitch**

This is a Borzoi Book published by Alfred A. Knopf, Inc.

First published in Great Britain in 1990 by Dorling Kindersley Limited
9 Henrietta Street, London, WC2 8PS

Library of Congress Cataloging-in-Publication Data
Mehta, Silva, 1926-
Yoga: the Iyengar way/Silva Mehta, Mira Mehta, and Shyam Mehta—1st ed.
p. cm.
Includes bibliographical references.
ISBN 0-679-72287-4 :
1. Yoga, Hatha. 2. Iyengar, B.K.S., 1918-
I. Mehta, Silva, 1926- . II. Mehta, Mira.
III. Title.
RA781.7.M44 1990 89-38785
613.7'046—dc20 CIP

Typeset by Chambers Wallace, London
Printed and bound in Italy
by New Interlitho, Milan
Published May 7, 1990
Reprinted Twice
Fourth Printing, August 1992

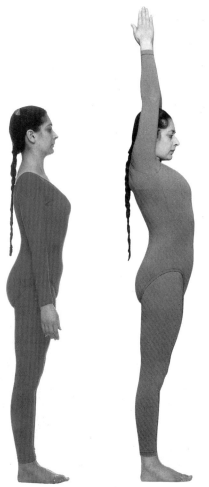

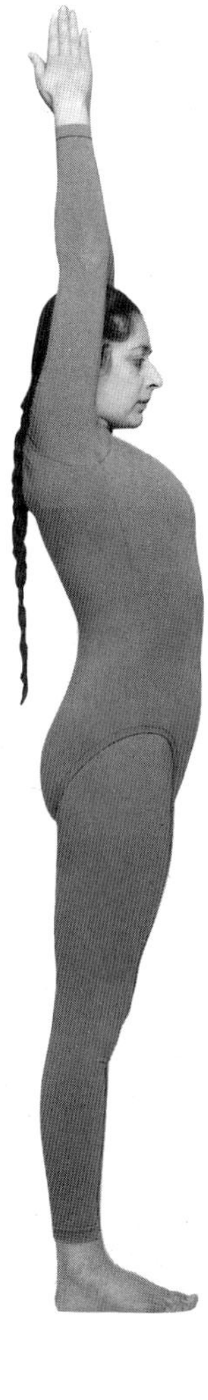

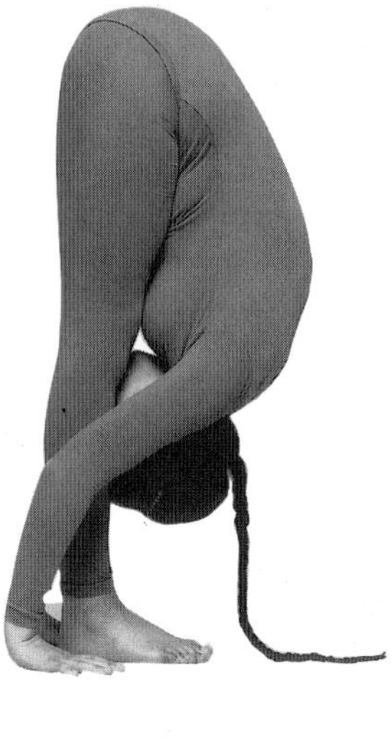

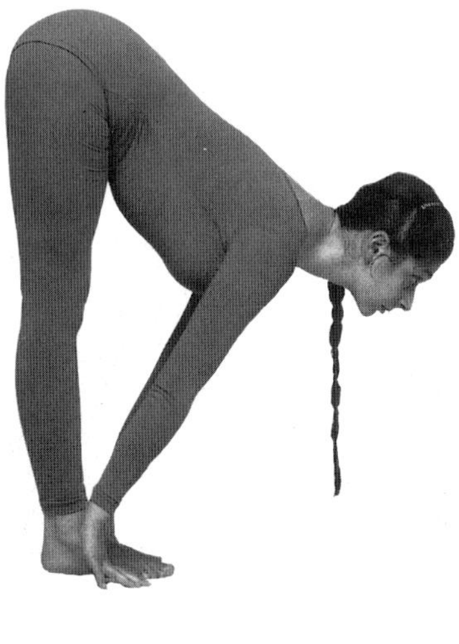

CONTENTS

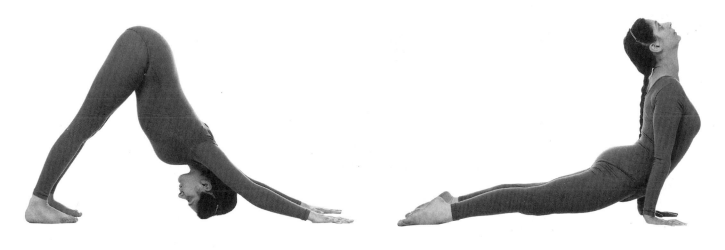

Foreword

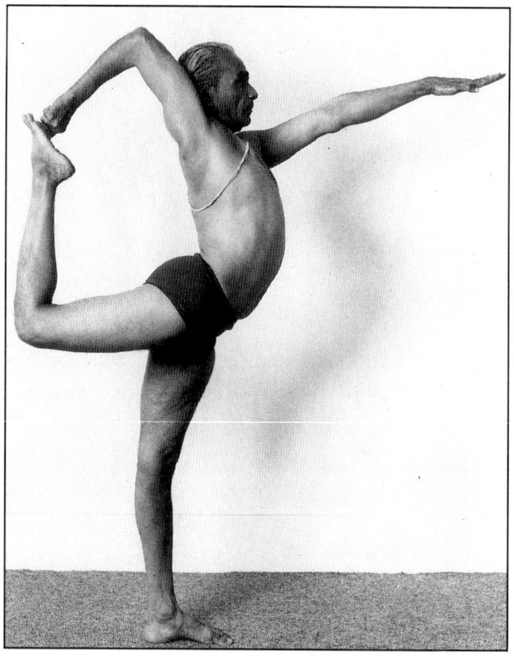

B.K.S. Iyengar in Naṭarājāsana

*I AM INDEED delighted to go through the script of **Yoga: The Iyengar Way** by Silva, Mira, and Shyam Mehta.*

This book is a fine product of eastern thoughts and western minds. The explanations are direct and I am sure that those who read the book will get an insight into Yoga and will enjoy the nectar of health in body, contentment of mind, and spiritual satisfaction.

Yoga is an immortal art, science, and philosophy. It is the best subjective psycho-anatomy of mankind ever conceived for the experience of physical, mental, intellectual, and spiritual well-being. It has stood the test of time from the beginning of civilization and it will remain supreme as a precise psycho-physical science for centuries to come.

*There are many different types of cells in the body, with physical, physiological, emotional, intellectual, and spiritual functions. It is known that each cell has a life of its own. These cells are the pearls of life. In the practice of Yoga every cell is consciously made to absorb a copious supply of fresh blood and life-giving energy, thus satiating the embodied soul. With serenity one then experiences the self by the self, and rests the self in the lap of the soul (*jīvātman*).*

I am pleased to be associated with this work of my pupils. My suggestions have been incorporated in the book. I will be glad if those who read it appreciate and practice the art of Yoga.

B.K.S. IYENGAR

Ramamani Iyengar Memorial Yoga Institute, Pune

Preface

Remaining in the midst of the family, always doing the duties of the householder, he who is free from merits and demerits, and has restrained his senses, attains salvation. The householder practicing Yoga is not touched by sins; if to protect mankind he does any sin, he is not polluted by it.

ŚIVA SAṀHITĀ, V.187

Yoga gives the energy to lead life fully and with enjoyment. Time spent alone in practice puts mundane issues in perspective and builds a fund of inner strength. Family, friends, and work all benefit.

We illustrate the value of Yoga in everyday life by giving a brief outline about ourselves.

SILVA MEHTA

I had an accident when I was 25 in which I sustained a crush fracture of the spine. I was in tremendous pain. Doctors, surgeons, naturopaths, and osteopaths predicted I would be in a wheelchair by the time I was fifty. A few years later I developed osteoarthritis.

I was living in India at the time. A naturopath friend told me: "There is only one thing for your arthritis – Yoga and Mr. Iyengar." I knew very little about Yoga, but within three weeks I was in B.K.S. Iyengar's class and have been ever since, whenever the opportunity presented itself, and so have my children. In India there is a saying, "When the pupil is ready, the Guru appears." We must have been ready.

Starting Yoga gave me periodic, almost miraculous, lifting of pain, and the feeling of excitement and euphoria. I began to shake off the depression caused by physical agony. Over the years Yoga has improved my physical health, and has given me a new outlook and optimism. Far from being in a wheelchair, I am able to help others surmount their physical problems. Teaching Yoga has been rewarding and satisfying.

SHYAM MEHTA

My sister and I have enjoyed a mixture of Yoga and fun in Mr. Iyengar's classes from a young age.

In my case, practice became more intense and dedicated during my college years. Hard work was rewarded by mastery of new postures and less discomfort in others. I began to extend my knowledge of Yoga philosophy from the base gained during Mr. Iyengar's many lectures. I also began teaching.

After my degree, I became an actuary. My Yoga training enables me to concentrate for hours at a stretch and cope with the pressures of work.

For me, the benefits of Yoga are more moral or spiritual than physical. True, if I have a headache or other minor pain, or have missed a night's sleep, I can recover through *āsana* practice. More important, Yoga keeps my mind calm and clear, enabling me to tackle problems at work and at home, to think for the long term, and to evaluate a situation dispassionately.

My Yoga practice has given me determination and the ability to accept the ups and downs of life with an equal mind. It gives me the direction for improvement – how to become more human, understanding, tolerant, and ethical. I can stand back and question my life and yet provide the steady influence required for a stable home life and a successful career. My interest in Yoga is shared by my wife, Rukmini.

MIRA MEHTA

I was brought up with Yoga and classes with Mr. Iyengar from early childhood. As a child I was stiff and weak, suffering from a curvature of the spine and painful neckaches and legaches. In my late teens I developed chronic backache, which in turn affected my stamina and concentration.

I began to take my practice seriously from adulthood. Gradually, helped by frequent visits to India to study at the Institute there, I gained health and strength, as well as flexibility. My early problems have virtually disappeared and the postures are no longer unattainable.

Apart from bringing an equable frame of mind, I feel that Yoga has developed my strength of character. It has also given me the ability to listen to others and understand their point of view, and to think in terms of the common good.

Yoga helped me throughout my university studies. As my interest deepened, I chose a course which gave me a background knowledge of Indian philosophy. While preparing for a research degree, I found Yoga took up more and more time and I turned my whole attention to it, with no regrets.

Introduction

Disciplined action, study of the self, and surrender to the Lord constitute the practice of Yoga.

"Tapas svādhyāya īśvarapraṇidhānāni kriyāyogaḥ." Yoga Sūtra II.1

In Indian philosophy there are always three strands of thought – work (*karma*), knowledge (*jñāna*), and devotion (*bhakti*). The three strands go together.

The above quotation from the Yoga aphorisms (*Yoga Sūtra*) of Patañjali points to this division, and we have taken it as the theme underlying the three parts of this book. *Tapas* relates to energetic practice, *svādhyāya* signifies the study of the self and of Yoga philosophy, and *Īśvarapraṇidhāna* shows the way of devotion, without which practice is not complete.

The Value of Yoga

Human beings are made up of three components: body, mind, and soul. Corresponding to these are three needs that must be satisfied for a contented life: the physical need is health; the psychological need is knowledge; and the spiritual need is inner peace. When all three are present there is harmony.

Modern society faces problems which affect all these aspects. Today's lifestyle with its technological wonders is a mixed blessing. Convenience and speed are obtained at some cost to physical health. Labor-saving devices minimize physical exertion, resulting in stiffness and muscular weakness. A sedentary life causes backache, neck problems, heaviness in the limbs, and difficulty in walking. The extensive use of visual media leads to headaches and eye strain.

The mental anxieties of a competitive world deplete inner resources, inviting stress-related problems such as insomnia and digestive, respiratory, and nervous disorders. If pressures are not balanced with time for quiet reflection, the quality of life is impaired.

Modern trends of thought are a melting pot of old and new ideas. Artificial values stemming from acquisitiveness and self-interest lead to alienation from the spiritual purpose of life. The loss of belief can bring a sense of loss of one's own true identity.

Yoga helps in all these problems. At the physical level, it gives relief from countless ailments. The practice of the postures strengthens the body and creates a feeling of well-being.

From the psychological viewpoint, Yoga sharpens the intellect and aids concentration. It steadies the emotions and encourages a caring concern for others. Above all, it gives hope. The practice of breathing techniques calms the mind. Its philosophy sets life in perspective. In the realm of the spiritual, Yoga brings awareness and the ability to be still. Through meditation, inner peace is experienced.

Thus Yoga is a practical philosophy involving every aspect of a person's being. It teaches the evolution of the individual by the development of self-discipline and self-awareness.

Anyone, irrespective of age, health, circumstance of life, and religion, can practice Yoga.

The Disciplines of Yoga

Yoga is a classical Indian science dealing with the search for the soul. The word "Yoga" signifies both the way to discovery of the soul and union with it.

Yoga philosophy was systematized some 2,000 years ago by sage Patañjali in a single treatise, *Yoga Sūtra*. The work is still acknowledged by all Yoga practitioners as the authoritative text on Yoga.

Yoga comprises eight limbs. These are:

1 Universal ethical principles (*Yama*)
2 Rules of personal conduct (*Niyama*)
3 The practice of Yoga postures (*Āsana*)
4 The practice of Yoga breathing techniques (*Prāṇāyāma*)
5 Control of the senses (*Pratyāhāra*)
6 Concentration of the mind (*Dhāraṇā*)
7 Meditation (*Dhyāna*)
8 Absorption in the Infinite (*Samādhi*)

Glimpses of the latter may come at any stage of practice, elevating it beyond the realms of physical and mental endeavor.

Yoga is built on a foundation of ethics (*yama*) and personal discipline (*niyama*). These are universal precepts found in all societies. Thus from the practical point of view, Yoga can be considered to begin at the level of postures (*āsanas*).

Each limb forms part of the whole, and tradition teaches that, even after attaining great heights in Yoga, the practice of *āsana* and *prāṇāyāma* should be continued, for the health of the body.

Yogācharya B.K.S. Iyengar

Traditionally in India sacred knowledge is passed on by a spiritual leader who is a teacher, guide, and example. This is the Gūru, meaning one who removes the darkness of ignorance, replacing it with the light of intelligence. The Guru guides the student on the spiritual path. He has wisdom, benevolence, tolerance, and the energy and ability to help others. His knowledge is authoritative.

In this century such a teacher is found in Yogācharya B.K.S. Iyengar. He is the world's foremost exponent of Yoga, having devoted a lifetime to its study. He lives his life according to the philosophical precepts of Yoga. Both he and his family set examples of morality, tolerance, and social conscience.

B.K.S. Iyengar began teaching in 1936 at the age of 18 and today, even though over 70, he still continues to teach and inspire students. Perfectionism, observation of scientific detail, and religiosity of practice characterize his teaching and the school of Yoga he has developed.

His system of teaching helps people to progress gradually from beginner to proficient advanced level, taking account of their weaknesses. This progression is educationally sound and brings lasting benefits; it has made his system widely accepted by education authorities.

He has several million students all over the world following his method. There are Iyengar Institutes and centers in the US, the UK, Europe, Australia, Canada, Israel, Japan, New Zealand, and South Africa, as well as India.

He has his own Institute in Pune, India, where his eldest daughter, Geeta, and son, Prashant, carry on the teaching tradition. Geeta Iyengar is much respected as the author of *Yoga: A Gem for Women*. Prashant Iyengar is involved in researching Yoga philosophy.

B.K.S. Iyengar has taught many world-famous figures, but his greatest achievement is in bringing Yoga to ordinary people so that all can benefit.

B.K.S. Iyengar's Contribution to Yoga

Though he has popularized Yoga, he has not sacrificed the purity of its original teachings. Yoga is a philosophy, a science, and an art. It is also a therapy. B.K.S. Iyengar has seen all these aspects and developed them, making an immense contribution to the knowledge and understanding of Yoga. He has written exhaustively on all major aspects of Yoga and his books are regarded as modern classics, used both for reference and as practical guides. They are *Light on Yoga, The Concise Light on Yoga, Light on Prāṇāyāma, The Art of Yoga,* and *The Tree of Yoga.* These books have been translated into many languages. He is currently working on a definitive translation and interpretation of Patañjali's aphorisms (a short version, *Yoga Sūtra* of Patañjali, is already available). The book *Iyengar: His Life and Work* gives a brief autobiography and narrations of his students' own experiences.

B.K.S. Iyengar has systematized over two hundred *āsana* and *prāṇāyāma* techniques and has discovered the anatomical principles on which they are based. He shows how, in the *āsanas,* the various parts of the body have to be positioned in their correct places, so that each individual part as well as the various physiological systems may function to their best potential. Minutiae of the postures are explored to penetrate remote anatomical layers of the body.

This makes Yoga a challenge to the intelligence. Body and mind are stretched beyond their everyday limits and are made to act in unison.

B.K.S. Iyengar has evolved the therapeutic application of the postures. He has devised methods of modifying the postures for maximum benefit of patients with disabilities. Leading members of the medical profession in India and elsewhere recognize his intimate knowledge of the body and his explanations of pathology from a Yogic point of view. He is known as an expert in treating complex medical problems.

B.K.S. Iyengar has matched new thinking in the therapeutic field with fresh insights on meditation. The concept of meditation in action is a keynote of his work. Being totally aware and absorbed in the postures as they are being done is meditation. Body and mind communicate at a subtle level and are harmonized. There is a continuous interchange between the two about every movement and action taking place. The awareness gained by meditation in action translates itself into everyday life.

Finally, B.K.S. Iyengar sees Yoga as an art. The body is shaped into postures that are graceful, and he has perfected and taught their artistic presentation. Through finding the aesthetic in the postures, he has made the subject visually appealing and inspired countless people to take up Yoga.

About this Book

This book explains the basic principles and practices of Yoga. It is based on the authors' thirty years' study with Yogācharya B.K.S. Iyengar and as teachers of his method. The explanations give help to beginners and expand on some of the finer points which are the hallmark of his teaching.

The book is in three parts. Although this division has been made for clarity and convenience, the three parts are integrated. Side by side with the techniques, the book reflects on various philosophical and practical topics. ***Part I: The Body*** deals with postures (*āsanas*), giving general guidelines and step-by-step instructions and photographs for 108 postures. A few important ones have been omitted owing to lack of space, but will be found in *Light on Yoga* and *Yoga: A Gem for Women*. The sequence of the *āsanas* in this book follows that in *Light on Yoga*.

Part II: The Mind gives guidelines and instructions for breathing techniques (*prāṇāyāma*). It introduces the reader to the concept and technique of control of the senses (*pratyāhāra*). This is followed by an outline of Yoga philosophy.

Part III: The Soul discusses the goal of Yoga and how it relates to practice.

Courses, remedial programs, and a selected bibliography are provided at the end of the book.

THE USE OF SANSKRIT

The Iyengar system follows the classical Yoga method in which Sanskrit is used for the names of *āsanas, prāṇāyāma* techniques, and philosophical concepts. The terminology is in worldwide usage. B.K.S. Iyengar has himself named many of the postures. The names symbolize the inner meaning of the *āsanas* – some describe their shape or function; others recall Indian gods and sages or animals and birds.

Learning the Sanskrit names of the postures helps to understand the subject. The following is a brief outline of the pronunciation used in Sanskrit.

Guide to Sanskrit pronunciation

NOTE The stress is always on the first syllable. A superscript over a vowel indicates that it is lengthened. The vowels are pronounced as follows:

a as in about; **ā** as in father
i as in ink; **ī** as in fee
u as in put; **ū** as in food
e as in pay; **ai** as in I
o as in corn; **au** as in loud

c	is pronounced **ch** (e.g. Ardha Candrāsana is pronounced Ardha **Ch**andrāsana, Paścimottānāsana is pronounced Pas**chi**mottānāsana)
ṭ ṭh ḍ ḍh ṇ	are all pronounced with the tongue retroflexed (curled back) and hitting the upper palate
t th d dh n	belong to the dental group where the tip of the tongue touches the teeth. Thus **th** is pronounced as in "penthouse" (not as in "thing"); **dh** is pronounced as in "childhood"
ś ṣ	are both pronounced **sh**, the former as in fish, the latter as in harsh, with the tongue retroflexed. (E.g., Śīrṣāsana is pronounced **Shirsh**āsana, Parśvakoṇāsana is pronounced Par**sh**vakoṇāsana)
ṛ	is pronounced **ru** or **ri**
ḥ	is pronounced with the light repetition of the preceding vowel (e.g. **aḥ**=**aha**; **iḥ**=**ihi**; **uḥ**=**uhu**)
jñ	is pronounced **gnya**
ṅ	the nasal preceding **k** or **g**
ñ	the nasal preceding **c** or **j**
ṁ	the nasal preceding **p**, **b**, or **h** consonant

These spellings and accents are in accordance with the conventions of Sanskrit transliteration.

PART I
THE BODY

Āsana & Practice

Grace, beauty, strength, energy, and firmness
adorn the body through Yoga.
YOGA SŪTRA, III.47

The Āsanas

If you look after the root of the tree, the fragrance and flowering will come by itself. If you look after the body, the fragrance of the mind and spirit will come of itself.

B.K.S. IYENGAR

By their wide-ranging effects, Yoga *āsanas* and relaxation techniques make efficient use of all physical and mental resources. This brings about better adjustment in various life situations and paves the way for the health of future generations.

SEEKING HEALTH

Health is a balanced state of bodily elements and of all anatomical and physiological systems, where each part of the body functions at full potential. All these complex systems must work smoothly and without interruption, but in ordinary life they do not. Mental, moral, and emotional aspects, too, must be sound. Spirituality completes full health and puts human affairs in the perspective of the universal. Striving toward this goal is the main aim of Yoga.

The Patañjali *Yoga Sūtras* (I, 30-31) enumerate the various physical and psychological defects that hamper progress in any undertaking. They are disease, sluggishness, doubt, carelessness, idleness, sensual indulgence, living in the world of illusion, inability to progress and to consolidate progress. In addition, there are other psychophysical disturbances. These are sorrow, despair, shakiness of the body, and labored breathing.

Yoga is a means by which to gain an increasing measure of control over these problems.

To this end, Patañjali lays down the three duties of *tapas, svādhyāya,* and *Īśvarapraṇidhāna.* These are the three cornerstones of the practice of Yoga. Here we deal with the first of these – *tapas* (self-discipline and fervor). It fires the practice of Yoga with zeal. Without it, nothing can be attained. This disciplined approach carries over into other areas of life.

Tapas means warmth, heat, fire. It is the heat and energy gained by devoting one's thoughts and actions toward a particular goal, without dissipating them elsewhere. These thoughts and actions themselves generate energy because they are so concentrated.

Good health cannot be taken for granted but must be striven for. Yoga teaches that this is achieved through the practice of *āsanas*. *Āsanas* need to be practised with *tapas* in order to achieve maximum benefit.

Āsanas are an integral part of Yoga. They are not mere physical exercise as they involve both psychological and physiological processes. They are linked to all the other aspects of Yoga, rooted in ethics and ending in spirituality. Yoga uses the body to exercise and control the mind, so that at a later stage the body and mind together may harmonize with the soul.,

The Yoga *āsanas* affect and penetrate every single cell and tissue, making them come to life.

The wide variety of postures offers a training capable of creating a vigorous body, well-functioning inner organs, and an alert mind.

The *āsanas* each have a distinct form and shape. To execute them, exact stretches, counter-stretches, and resistances are needed. These align the skin, flesh, and muscular structure of the body with the skeleton.

There are postures and cycles of postures that give a variety of different effects: stimulating, calming, energizing, building stamina or concentration, promoting sleep, internally soothing, and so on. These benefits come as a side effect of Yoga through correct practice. Thus the standing poses give vitality, the sitting poses are calming, twists are cleansing, supine poses are restful, prone poses are energizing, the inverted poses develop mental strength, balancings bring a feeling of lightness, backbends are exhilarating and the jumpings develop agility.

Relaxation is a separate art. The quality of relaxation depends on the intensity of the postures that precede it.

Many common physical ailments and defects, including chronic disorders, can be improved by the practice of Yoga postures. They work on specific areas of the body such as the joints, the liver, kidneys and heart. The movements and extensions in the postures, including the positioning of the inner organs in the inverted sequences, have a profound effect on how they function. The body is oxygenated and filled with healthy blood, decongested and rested. Stamina, lung capacity, heart performance, muscle tone, circulation and respiration all improve.

It is on such principles that therapeutic Yoga is founded.

The Importance of Practice

Great emphasis needs to be laid on practice. Practice changes the physical as well as the mental state of the practitioner.

One of the principles of Yoga is not to seek the fruit of actions. Thus practice should be for its own sake, without regard to success or failure. This is the way to gain equanimity.

Practice should be systematic, starting with simple postures. Progress is made by becoming stronger in these before proceeding to more difficult *āsanas*. Gradually the understanding and level of involvement deepens. The basic postures are repeated over and over again throughout, because they are the foundation of knowledge.

Practice is cumulative. First one set of postures is learned. When the second set is learned, it is repeated together with the first. The third set is repeated together with the second and first, and so on.

In the beginning progress is fast. After some time a plateau is reached where improvement seems minimal. With time, this will be overcome. It takes about two years to settle into the postures, to understand them, and to move the various parts of the body in an inter-related fashion. First each posture has to be analyzed and studied.

Diligence and effort are required in practice. Initially, the labor seems greater than the result, and failures are frequent; with perseverance, gains come with less effort. According to Patañjali, the mastery of *āsanas* occurs when practice becomes effortless.

Attention to accuracy is needed. At first alignment is approximate; gradually it becomes more precise. When the posture is aligned correctly, there is no break in the energy flow.

Finally, a devoted attitude to practice is necessary. This involves, in the first place, adhering to a regular routine. Secondly, it involves belief in the efficacy of Yoga. Thirdly, it involves a sensitive, inquiring approach, constantly striving toward perfection. This frame of mind, coupled with the discipline of habitual practice, helps in the various ups and downs of life.

Progress brings satisfaction as health improves, the details of the postures become clear and understanding deepens. When Yoga is practiced with devotion, the spiritual goal will come into sight.

Guidelines for Practice

The amount of time and effort put into practice brings corresponding results. Some students are satisfied with the benefits of a 20- to 30-minute weekly practice. Two or three times a week suits others while very keen students may practice every day.

Āsanas can be done at any time. In the morning the body is stiff, but the mind is fresh; in the evening the body is supple, but the mind is not so alert.

Practice should be enjoyable and stimulating. It should be used constructively in life to tap the enormous diversity of possible effects of the *āsanas*.

The *āsanas* take time to perfect. It is often necessary to work on the intermediate stages until these come with ease, as well as on the complete pose. It is usual to repeat each posture two or three times. The amount of detail given in the book will gradually fall into place and be understood.

Breathing in the postures is important. Where no special instructions are given, normal breathing should be done. Between the stages in a posture, one or two breaths should be taken to quieten the mind.

The postures are not static. Adjustments should be made and then stabilized. Further actions to improve the posture can then be added.

The sequences should be learned (see Courses, p. 175). *Āsanas* from several sections are normally done in one session. Each group of *āsanas* develops the body in a different, complementary way.

It is best to learn the *āsanas* of one grade of difficulty before attempting those of the next grade (see p. 14). This is a safeguard against injury.

It is often helpful to use whatever equipment or furniture is available to improve the postures. This also helps in understanding them.

It is best to go to classes, if possible, to get individual correction from a teacher.

The eyes should be kept open and the mouth closed throughout (unless otherwise instructed).

Some cautions

- The stomach and bowels should be empty. Allow four hours after a heavy meal, two hours after a light one.
- Do not wear tight clothes that restrict breathing, digestion, or circulation.
- Do not practice in direct sunlight or in a cold room.

• Do not hold the breath during the postures as this will cause strain. The eyes, ears, throat, and abdomen should be relaxed.
• To avoid injury, do not force the body beyond its capacity.
• Backaches and various weaknesses come to the fore during practice. If this happens, try the remedial programs or consult a teacher.
• Any pain felt in a posture should be temporary. Persistent pain is a sign of incorrect practice or of a physical problem.
• If exhaustion is felt, the practice has been too long or the wrong postures have been attempted. It may also indicate a weak physical condition or some ailment.

Menstruation and Pregnancy

• During menstruation it is not advisable to follow an ordinary *āsana* session, as this may be injurious. There is heat in the body and cooling postures are done to counteract this. Programs which are physiologically suitable are given at the end of the book.
• During pregnancy two lives are involved. It is not advisable to begin Yoga at this time as so many physiological changes are taking place.
• If already attending a class, inform the teacher as soon as pregnancy has been confirmed.
• Do not attend class in the 11th, 12th and 13th weeks of pregnancy.
• Do not do *āsanas* that constrict the abdomen.
• On no account become fatigued or breathless.
• In case of complications or previous history of miscarriage, seek advice.

Grading of the Postures

The postures are grouped into nine sections: standing poses, sitting poses, twists, prone and supine poses, inverted poses, balancings, backbends, jumpings, and relaxation. The sections broadly follow an order of difficulty, as do the *āsanas* within each section.

The *āsanas* are graded into four levels of difficulty, indicated by diamond symbols at the end of the descriptive heading to each, as follows:

♦ Beginners
♦♦ General – for most students
♦♦♦ Intermediate – for keen practitioners
♦♦♦♦ Advanced – for intense practitioners

Instructions for the Postures

Intermediate steps as well as the final posture are explained and illustrated, as far as space allows.

Work in the Posture gives further instructions aimed at refining the *āsanas*.

The illustrations are annotated with key points.

Ways of Practicing indicates alternative methods, or methods for achieving the postures using props.

Scattered throughout are *Focuses* explaining specific actions, and *Reflections* on various philosophical or practical topics. While they apply particularly to the posture on the page where they appear, they are of general relevance to the practice of Yoga.

Where possible nontechnical terms have been used to describe parts of the body. The terms used are given on the annotated figures, below and right.

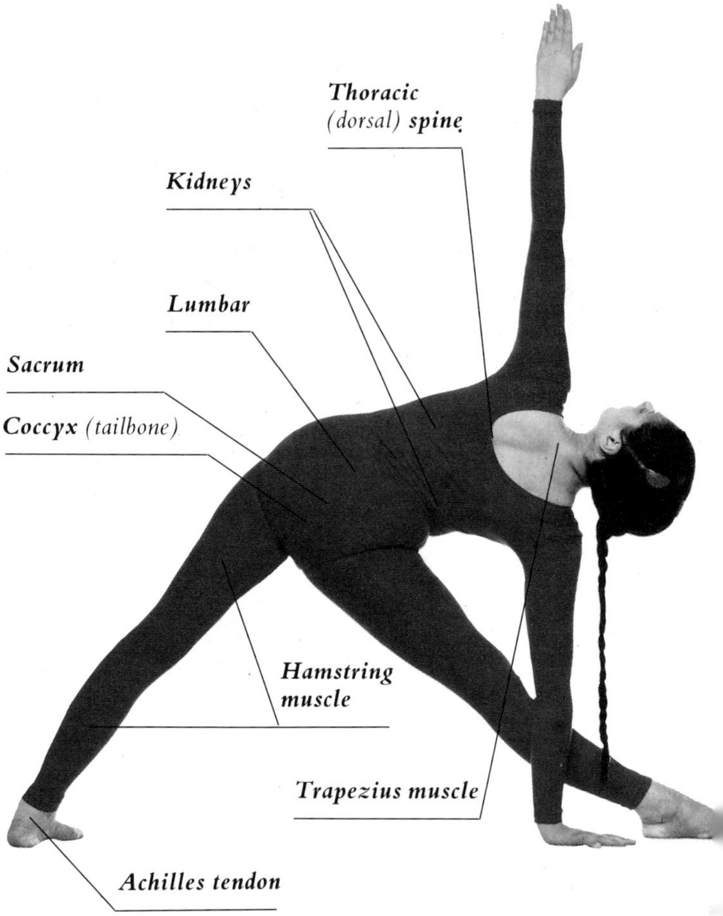
Thoracic (dorsal) spine
Kidneys
Lumbar
Sacrum
Coccyx (tailbone)
Hamstring muscle
Trapezius muscle
Achilles tendon

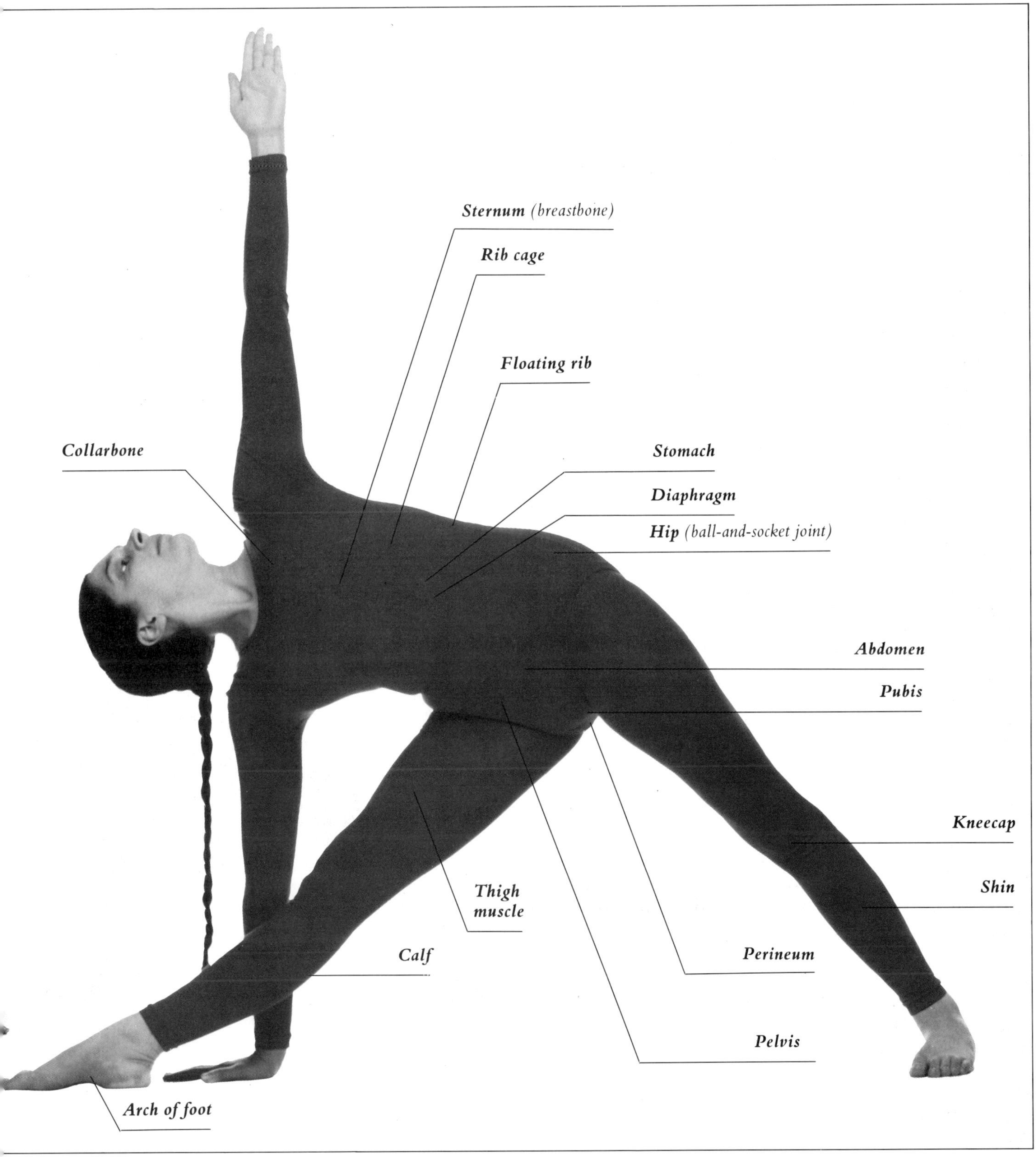
Sternum (breastbone)
Rib cage
Floating rib
Collarbone
Stomach
Diaphragm
Hip (ball-and-socket joint)
Abdomen
Pubis
Kneecap
Shin
Thigh muscle
Calf
Perineum
Pelvis
Arch of foot

A balanced practice session incorporates *āsanas* from several sections, in various combinations. For this reason courses containing *āsanas* of progressive levels of difficulty have been given on pp. 175-184 to guide the student towards systematic practice.

Anyone suffering from a minor ailment should follow the remedial program specified on pp. 183-7, until relief is gained. Those with a serious medical problem need a specially qualified teacher.

The Philosophy of Āsana Practice

The practice of *āsanas* is integrated with Yoga philosophy and the two cannot be separated. Many details are given in the postures which gradually need to be introduced into practice. Making the shapes of the postures is a physical activity; understanding and implementing the finer details is necessary to develop complete involvement.

The body contains millions of cells which have to gain nourishment. Actions must pervade the whole body to improve cellular metabolism and circulation. In order to penetrate them, freedom has to be created. Movement starts with joints, bones, and muscles, and finer actions terminate with the skin, where microscopic muscles are involved.

The skin is a sense organ. By developing the sensitivity of the skin new messages are sent to the brain, which explores new avenues of awareness.

In order to carry out these adjustments and to discover subtle areas of the body, mental effort is required. The mind must be sharply focused toward the part concerned. The mental force is internalized. When an action is performed it is imprinted on the brain, creating a reflective attitude. The brain becomes like a mirror receiving the impressions of actions, but the brain itself does not act.

This reflective attitude refines the intelligence. Practicing in this way refreshes both the mind and the body, and gives a sense of accomplishment. There are always new goals to be achieved and new perceptions to be experienced. This makes Yoga a lifetime interest.

GLOSSARY OF TERMS

In Yoga practice precise terms are used to describe the actions performed. These occur again and again, relating to different parts of the body. Some of the key terms relating to muscle and bone movement are given below.

Aligning; keeping in line
The limbs and trunk are placed evenly on either side of the median line of the posture.

Drawing up
Muscles are firmly pulled up, to lie parallel to the bones and to lift them.

Extending/stretching
Muscles are stretched along their whole length evenly. Stretching is done without tension.

Gripping
An action is maintained by a muscular grip.

Hardening
Muscles are held firm against the bone.

Hitting
The movement of muscle toward bone is done with a strong, swift action, to move the bone in the direction stated.

Keeping lively; full of life
Energy and awareness are maintained in an area.

Lifting/raising
Keeping a firm base, each part of the body is lifted away from the part below. This creates space for a proper extension and internal opening.

Locking
Joints are held firm as part of an extension.

Opening
Space is created within an area.

Relaxing
Tension in the head and body is released consciously. During Yoga practice the brain should be quietly watchful. Actions should be experienced directly in the part of the body involved. In this way measurably better extensions are obtained.

Revolving/turning
The relevant part of the body is turned along its full length, with adjacent parts turning in the same direction.

Softening
Tension is removed from an area.

Tucking in
The relevant part is taken deeper into the body.

STANDING POSES

You should do the āsanas with vigor and at the same time be relaxed and composed.
B.K.S. IYENGAR

The standing poses are invigorating. They refresh the body and mind by removing tension, aches, and pains. They stimulate digestion, regulate the kidneys, and relieve constipation. They improve circulation and breathing. The back, hips, knees, neck, and shoulders all gain strength and mobility through practice.

The standing poses also teach the principles of correct movement. This is fundamental for the postures and also in everyday life, where they develop awareness of the right way to sit, stand, and walk.

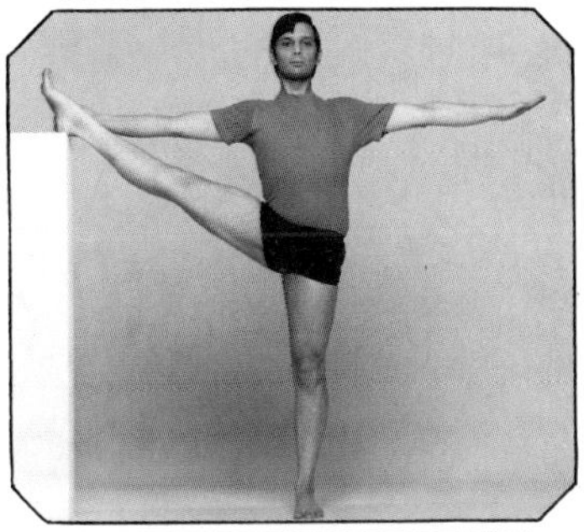

GUIDELINES FOR PRACTICE

It is best to work on a non-slip surface. Precision is essential. Even small inaccuracies in lining up create distortions in the posture. For this reason the body and feet should be aligned with the walls of the room, and the body centered before starting. Accuracy in the postures is developed through working carefully.

To develop energy and to combat laziness, the postures should be done dynamically, with full extension of the limbs and trunk. Working with effort does not mean working with tension, and it is important to learn how to stay relaxed.

Jumping into the postures makes the body and mind alert and teaches coordination. In jumping, the feet should land equidistant from the center and in line, and the arms should move out to the sides simultaneously with the legs.

It is sometimes useful to practice the standing poses with the back against a wall for support and to check alignment. They may also be practiced at right angles to a wall, pressing the back foot against it and extending the trunk away from it. This helps to keep the back leg strong.

Vīrāsana (p. 50) may be done during and after standing poses to recover from fatigue or if the legs are tired.

CAUTIONS: Do not do standing poses if suffering from medical conditions such as high blood pressure, heart problems, or nervous disorders.

Do not practice them during menstruation, in the first three months of pregnancy or if problems arise in pregnancy, as they are strenuous.

Do not jump into the poses if suffering from knee or back injuries, or if pregnant. Instead, walk the feet to the sides, one at a time.

तडासन

Tāḍāsana

TĀḌA = mountain; *ĀSANA* = posture

THE BODY extends upward, with the base as firm as a rock; the mind is steady and attentive. Tāḍāsana teaches balance, centering, and evenness and direction of extensions. These principles apply in all the postures.♦

Feet

Stand straight, facing forward. Keep the feet together, the toes and heels in line, big toes and centers of the inner ankles touching.

For a moment lift the soles of the feet, stretch them forward from the centers of the arches, then put them down. Now raise the heels, extend them back from the centers of the arches and put them down again. The soles of the feet are now extended. Keep all the toes down and stretch them forward, not forgetting the little toes.

Keep the weight even on the inner and outer edges of both feet, and on the heels and soles. Be light on the feet and keep the arches lifted.

Legs

Extend the legs up vertically; lift the inner and outer ankles and stretch the Achilles tendons up. Lift the shin bones. Extend the calf muscles and the skin of the front legs up. Keep the legs facing forward and join the inner knees.

Lock the knees by drawing the kneecaps into the joints and draw the inner and outer knees back. Open and stretch the backs of the knees without straining them.

Lift the thigh bones and pull the thigh muscles up, right to the tops of the thighs. Compress the thighs and draw the muscles toward the bones. Normally the skin and flesh of the thighs sag; when they are drawn up they become parallel to the bones. This happens in other parts of the body also.

Finally tuck in the skin and flesh at the top of the backs of the thighs.

Lower Trunk

Create space between the thighs and the trunk at the front, sides, and back. Lift the hips. Move the coccyx and sacrum forward and up, then lengthen the spine and the trunk. Keeping the pubis tucked back, move the lower abdomen and the abdominal organs up and back without tensing them.

Lightly compress the muscles around the anus to raise the coccyx and sacrum. Draw the buttock muscles up.

Tuck in the waist from all sides and stretch it up to create space between the pelvis and the rib cage. Move the kidney area further into the body.

Upper Trunk

Lift the diaphragm and the rib cage. Open the diaphragm and the floating ribs outward.

Move the thoracic spine and the back ribs in. Lift the collarbones and open the chest by widening the front ribs away from the sternum. Feel the internal opening of the chest.

Raise the upper chest and the collarbones. Draw the skin of the shoulders toward the shoulder blades. Press the shoulder blades into the back and take them down, without collapsing the back ribs.

Relax the shoulders and keep them down. Widen them horizontally at the front, away from the neck.

Arms

Turn the upper arms out and stretch the arms down, palms facing the thighs. Then relax the arms and hands, letting them hang naturally.

Side view
Keep the crown of the head, center of the top of the ear, and center of the ankle in one line.
Stand against a wall to see whether the body is in line.

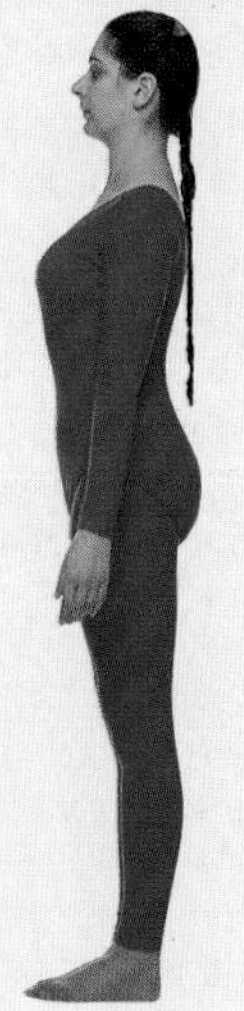

ताडासन

Alignment
This is a sensitive way of adjusting the body. The two sides and the front and back of the body should be exactly in line and parallel. If one little finger is crooked and the other straight, precision is lost.

Balance
This is a delicate concept, bringing equilibrium of gravity, lightness, centering, and alignment.

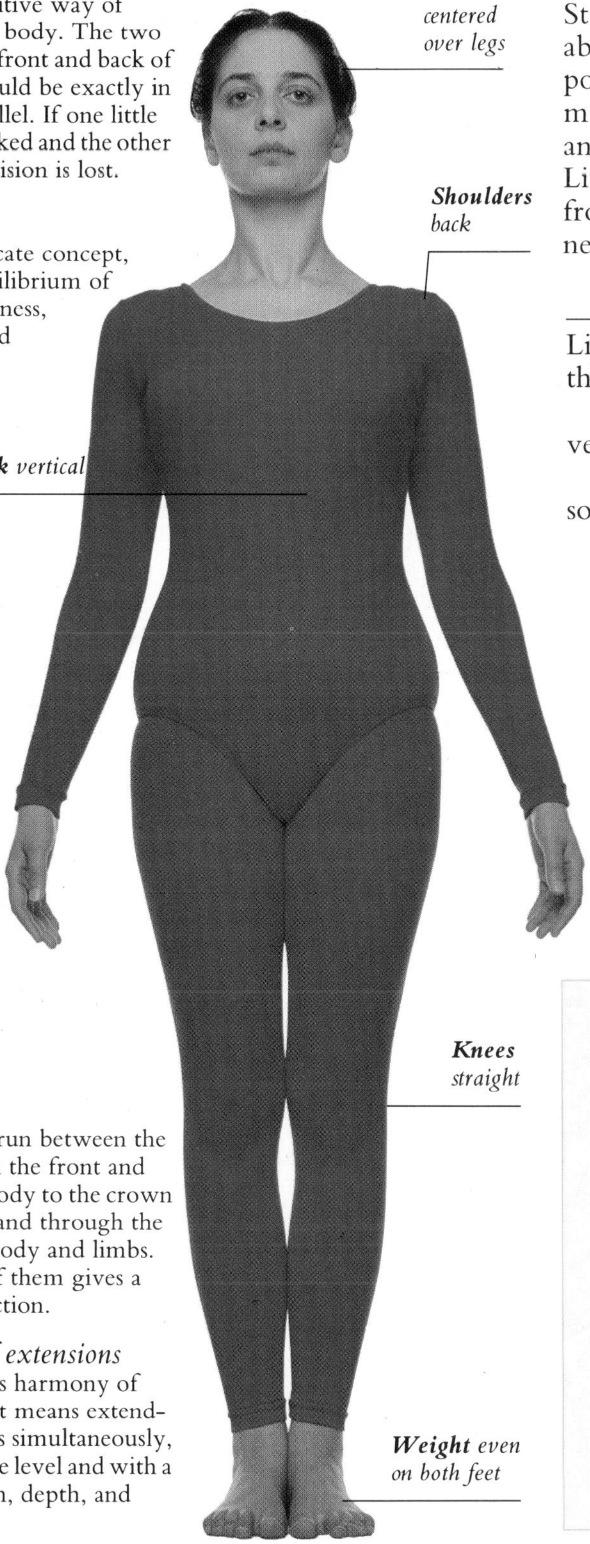

Centering
Center lines run between the legs, through the front and back of the body to the crown of the head, and through the sides of the body and limbs. Awareness of them gives a sense of direction.

Evenness of extensions
This develops harmony of movement. It means extending both sides simultaneously, from the same level and with a similar length, depth, and intensity.

NECK

Stretch the neck up. (The neck becomes supple and able to stretch when it is trained by doing other postures.) If the back is humped, the neck automatically shortens. So, move the dorsal spine inward and extend the neck from below the shoulder blades. Lift the sternum and extend the front of the neck from the jugular notch. Do not tense the throat or the neck.

HEAD

Lift the back of the skull away from the neck to make the head light.

Keep the head straight, the chin level, and the ears vertical.

Relax the face and look ahead, keeping the eyes soft. Stay for 30 to 40 seconds, breathing evenly.

Reflection
Settling into the posture brings repose. It follows precise placement of the limbs, correct extensions, and balance. There is peace and unity within. The mind fills every particle of the body, bringing harmony. This is Yoga.

ŪRDHVA HASTĀSANA

ŪRDHVA = upward, above; *HASTA* = hand
Stretch the arms forward and up. Lock the elbows (see Focus, p. 21). Open the palms, keep the fingers together. Stay for 20 to 30 seconds, then bring the arms back down.♦

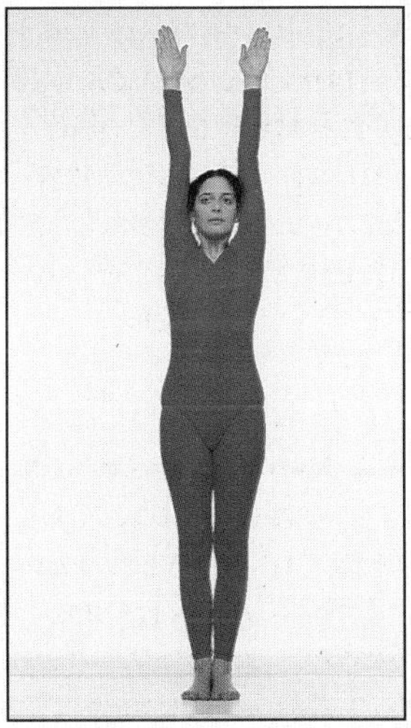

उत्थित हस्त पादांगुष्ठासन

Utthita Hasta Pādāṅguṣṭhāsana I

UTTHITA = extended; *HASTA* = hand; *PĀDA* = foot; *PADĀṄGUṢṬHA* = thumb or toe

THESE TWO postures strengthen the legs and the lower back.♦

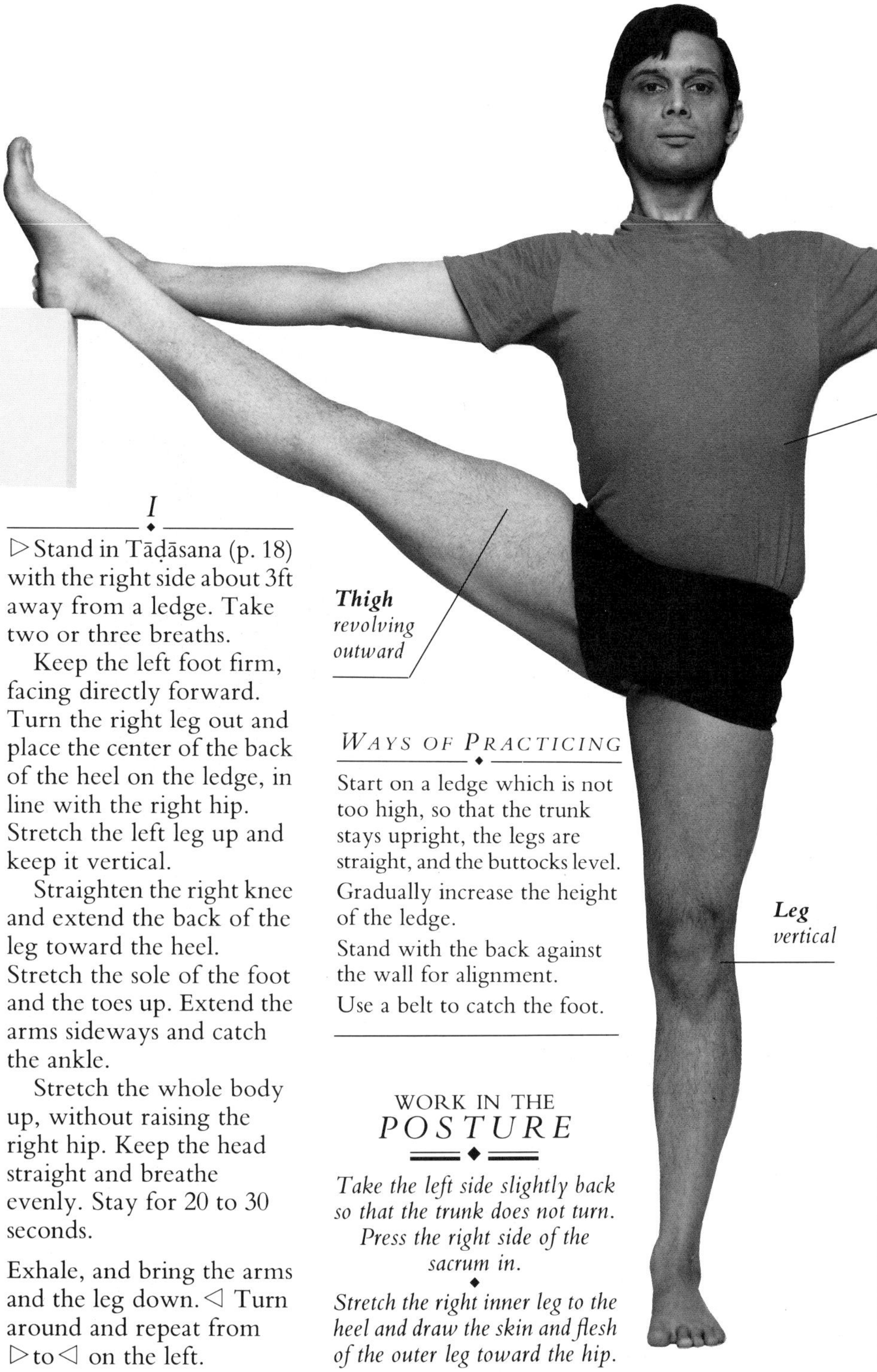
Trunk *upright*
Thigh *revolving outward*
Leg *vertical*

I

▷ Stand in Tāḍāsana (p. 18) with the right side about 3ft away from a ledge. Take two or three breaths.

Keep the left foot firm, facing directly forward. Turn the right leg out and place the center of the back of the heel on the ledge, in line with the right hip. Stretch the left leg up and keep it vertical.

Straighten the right knee and extend the back of the leg toward the heel. Stretch the sole of the foot and the toes up. Extend the arms sideways and catch the ankle.

Stretch the whole body up, without raising the right hip. Keep the head straight and breathe evenly. Stay for 20 to 30 seconds.

Exhale, and bring the arms and the leg down. ◁ Turn around and repeat from ▷ to ◁ on the left.

WAYS OF PRACTICING

Start on a ledge which is not too high, so that the trunk stays upright, the legs are straight, and the buttocks level.

Gradually increase the height of the ledge.

Stand with the back against the wall for alignment.

Use a belt to catch the foot.

WORK IN THE POSTURE

Take the left side slightly back so that the trunk does not turn. Press the right side of the sacrum in.

♦

Stretch the right inner leg to the heel and draw the skin and flesh of the outer leg toward the hip.

II

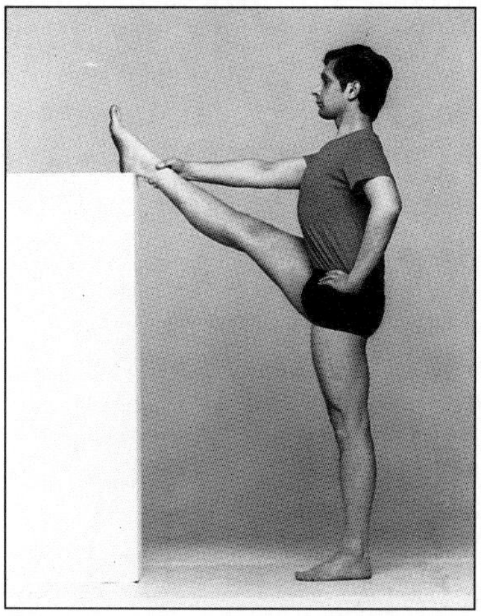

Stand facing a ledge. ▷ Keep the left leg firm. Place the right heel on the ledge directly ahead. Do not let the feet or legs turn outward. Stretch both legs straight. Pull the trunk up, keeping both sides parallel. Do not lean forward. Keep the right hip down and pulled slightly back. Catch the right foot; keep the left hand on the hip. Stay for 20 to 30 seconds. ◁ Repeat from ▷ to ◁ on the left.

वृक्षासन

Vṛkṣāsana

VṚKṢA = tree

THE TREE pose gives a beautiful upward stretch and a sense of balance.♦

1 Stand in Tāḍāsana (p. 18). ▷ Be firm on the left leg. Make the foot steady and stretch the leg up. Place the left hand on the hip. Bend the right leg out to the side, hold the foot and press the sole into the top of the left inner thigh. Do not push the thigh or hip out of line. Harden the left inner thigh. Straighten the left knee and take the right knee back, in line with the right hip. Lift the hips and stretch the waist and chest up.

WAYS OF PRACTICING

Stand near a wall for support.

If you cannot join the palms with the elbows straight, keep the arms parallel.

2 Extend the arms to the sides, turn the palms up, then stretch the arms over the head. Join the palms, keeping the elbows straight. Extend the sides of the body. Keep the head straight. Breathe evenly and balance for 20 to 30 seconds. With an exhalation, bring the arms and leg down. ◁ Repeat from ▷ to ◁ on the left.

Focus *Stretching the arms up*
Stretch the arms and fingers vertically up; lift the sides of the body. Do not hunch the shoulders; keep the shoulder blades in.

Locking the elbows
Press the backs of the elbows into the elbow joints and stretch the inner elbows.

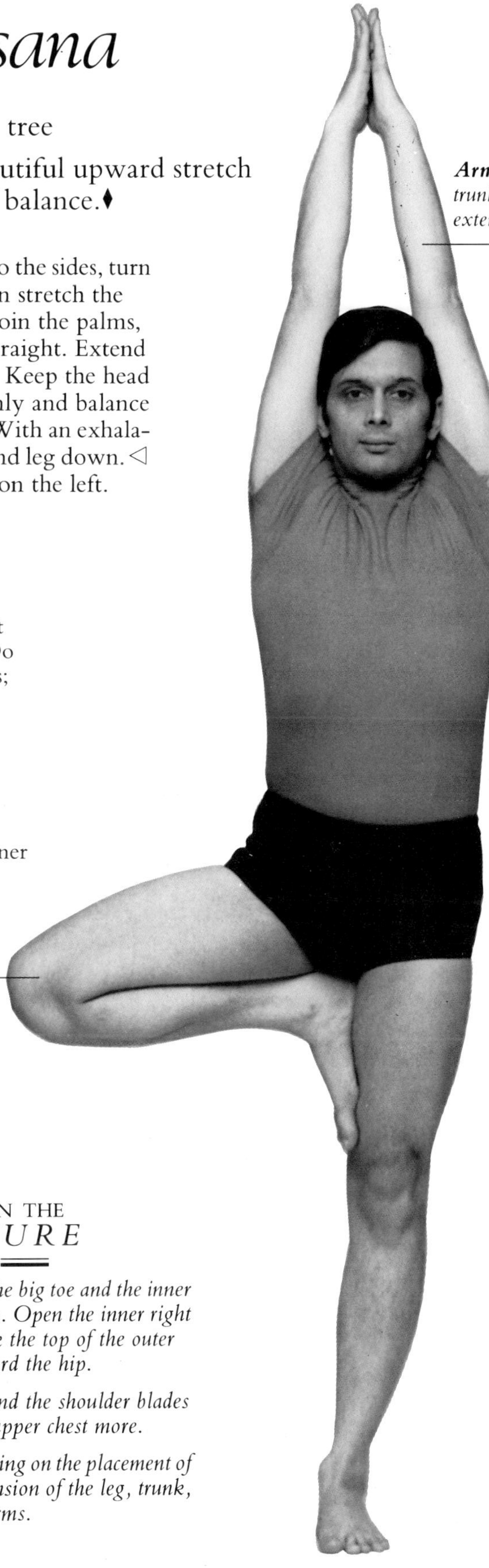

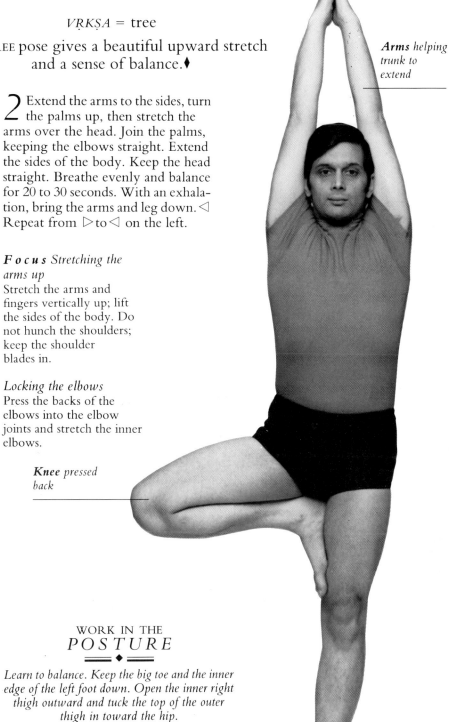

***Arms** helping trunk to extend*

***Knee** pressed back*

WORK IN THE POSTURE

Learn to balance. Keep the big toe and the inner edge of the left foot down. Open the inner right thigh outward and tuck the top of the outer thigh in toward the hip.

♦

Move the dorsal spine and the shoulder blades in and extend the upper chest more.

♦

Stay steady by concentrating on the placement of the left foot and the extension of the leg, trunk, and arms.

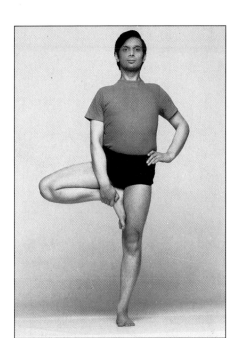

उत्थित त्रिकोणासन

Utthita Trikoṇāsana

UTTHITA = extended; *TRIKOṆA* = triangle

THE EXTENSION of the limbs and trunk to form several triangles teaches alignment and a sense of direction.

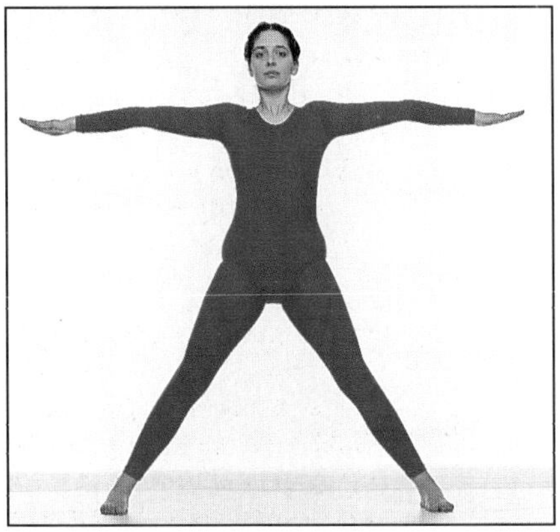

1 Stand in Tāḍāsana (p. 18). With a deep inhalation jump the legs $3\frac{1}{2}$ to 4ft apart. As you jump, stretch the arms to the sides at shoulder level, palms down.

Keep the feet in line, pointing forward. Extend the soles and lift the arches. Straighten the knees and stretch the shins, knees, and thighs up. Hit the inner thighs away from each other (see Focus, p. 43). Raise the hips, extend the trunk up, and open the chest. Keep the head straight. Elongate the arms from the sternum to the thumbs, and from the spine to the little fingers. Lock the elbows (see Focus, p. 21). Open the palms, stretch the fingers, and keep them together.

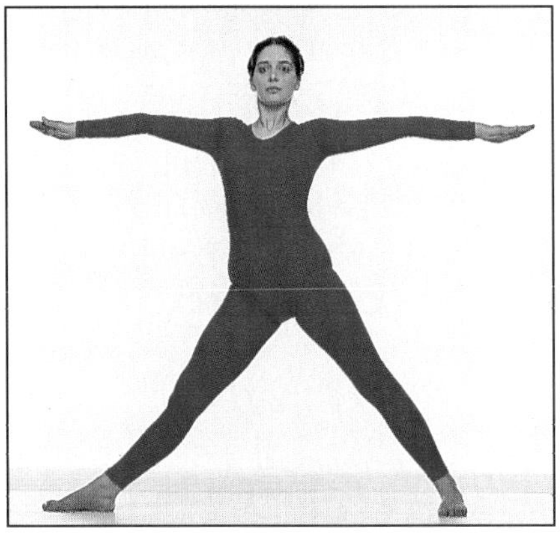

2 ▷Turn the left foot 15° in and turn the right leg in its socket 90° out so that the centers of the thigh, knee, and big toe point directly to the right (see Focus, below).

In turning the feet, extend them forward. Adjust them so that the right heel is in line with the left arch. Stretch the legs up, pressing down the outer edge of the left foot and the right inner heel and big toe. Lift the ankles. Lock the knees (see Tāḍāsana, Legs, p. 18). Draw the thigh muscles up. Keep the arms extended. Do not hold the breath.

Focus *Turning the back foot in*
Lift the front of the foot and turn it in, then raise the heel and turn it out. Do not bring the back hip forward in turning the foot.

Turning the front leg out
Lift the front of the foot, turning on the heel; then take the heel in. Rotate the leg from the inner to the outer thigh, otherwise it will turn the wrong way.

Lining up the feet
Line up the front heel with the center of the arch of the back foot. Keep the foot pointing straight ahead. Lift the arch of the back foot. Extend both feet forward.

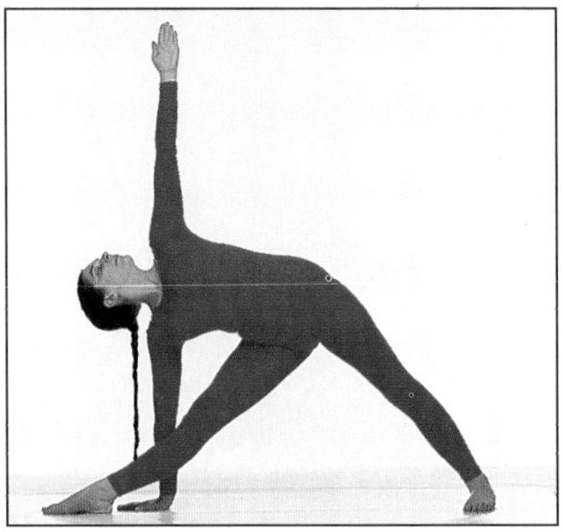

3 Exhale, and bend sideways toward the right leg, placing the right palm or fingertips by the outer heel, fingers pointing the same way as the toes. Stretch the left arm up, palm face forward.

In going down, move the hips to the left. Revolve the trunk up and extend it toward the head. Take the head slightly back, turn it, and look up. If the neck is tense, keep the head facing forward. Stay for 20 to 30 seconds, breathing normally.◁

Inhale, come up. Turn to the center. Repeat from ▷ to ◁ on the left. Jump the legs together and bring the arms down.

WAYS OF PRACTICING

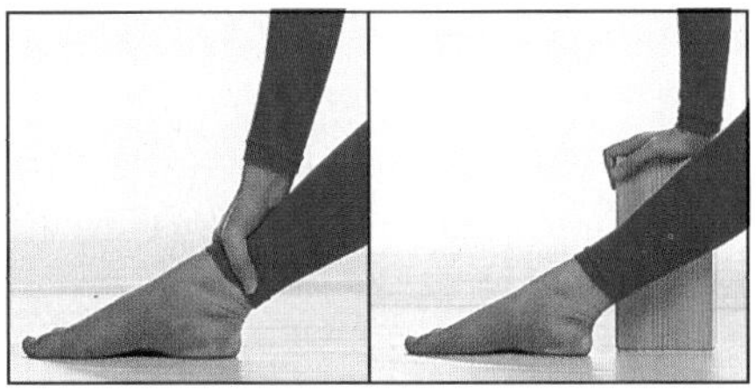

Hold the ankle or place the hand on a brick.

Back view
Keep the back of the body in one plane. Open the backs of the knees. Press the right buttock and the right side of the sacrum forward, lift the left hip, and take it back. Take the shoulders back, the shoulder blades and the back ribs in.

WORK IN THE
POSTURE

Hit the left inner ankle and inner leg to the left.

◆

Tuck the top of the right thigh and the bottom of the hip into the hip joint to increase the bend.

◆

Stretch the spine vertebra by vertebra from the coccyx to the head. Extend the back of the neck away from the trunk, and the skull away from the neck, keeping the head in line with the spine.

◆

Stretch the right arm from the wrist up. Raise the right rib cage and bring it forward. Stretch the left arm from the trunk up and turn the left rib cage back. Keep the left side directly over the right.

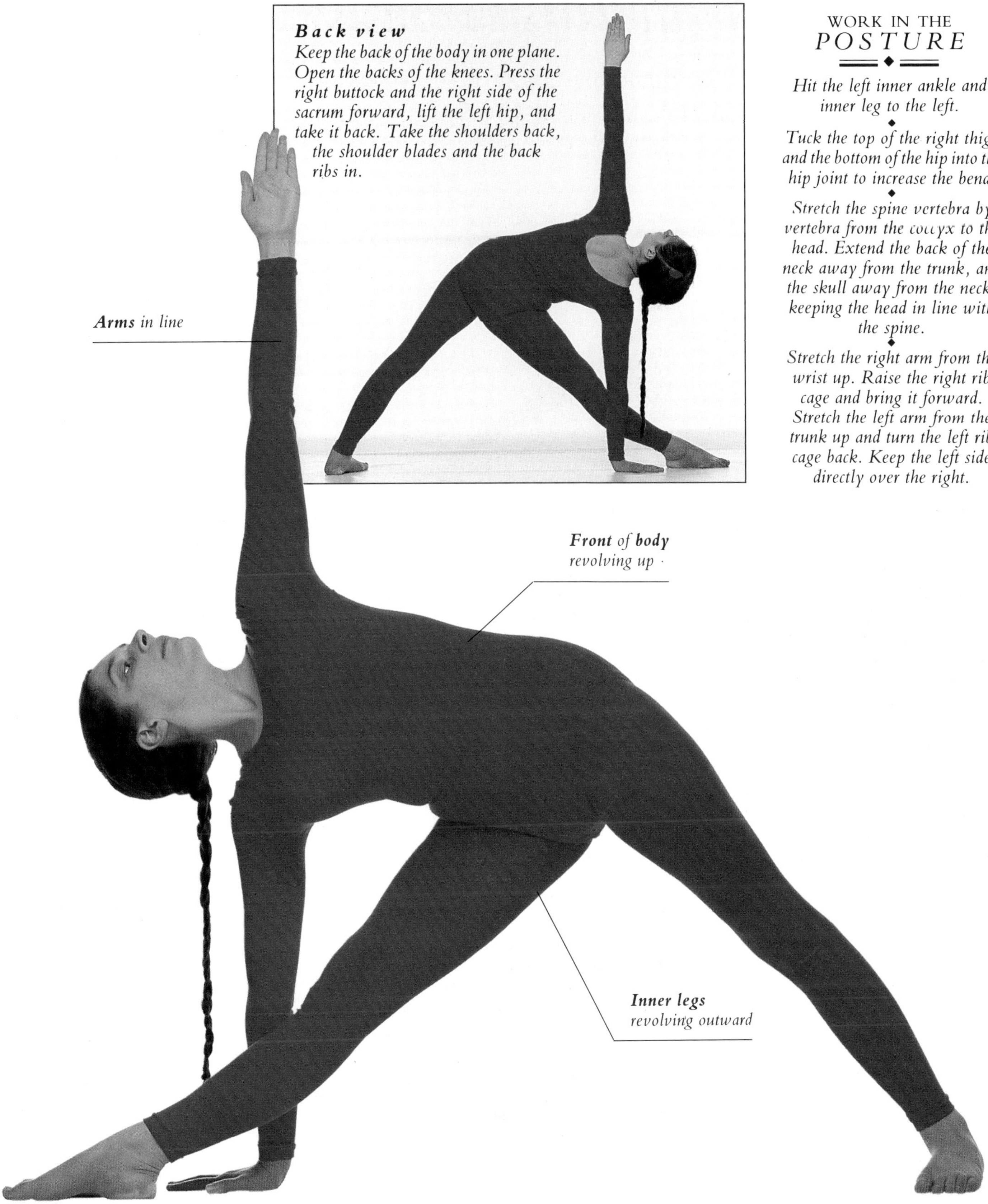
Arms *in line*
Front *of* **body** *revolving up*
Inner legs *revolving outward*

उत्थित पार्श्वकोणासन

Utthita Pārśvakoṇāsana

UTTHITA = extended; *PĀRŚVA* = sideways; *KOṆA* = angle

In this pose the trunk extends sideways into space, over a leg bent to a right angle. There is a single stretch from back foot to fingertips.♦

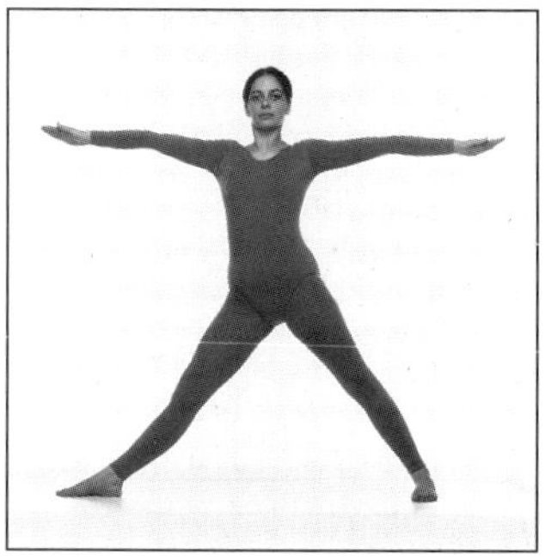

1 Stand in Tāḍāsana (p. 18). Inhale and jump the legs 4 to $4\frac{1}{2}$ft apart, arms stretched sideways as in Trikoṇāsana (p. 22). ▷Turn the left foot about 15° in, the right leg 90° out. Line up the feet.

Ways of Practicing

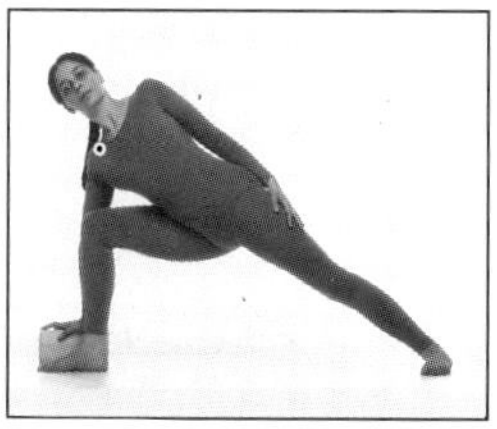

Place the hand on a brick.

Rest the top arm on the hip.

Stand with the back to a wall, feet a little away from it.

Move the right hip away from the wall and the right knee and left hip toward it.

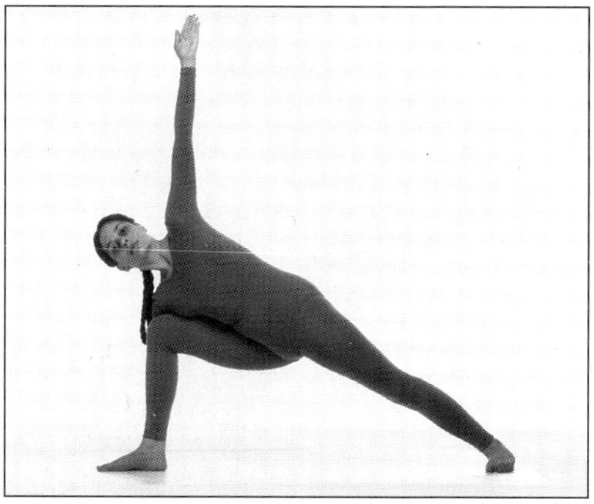

2 With an exhalation bend the right leg to a right angle (see Focus, p. 28); bend the trunk sideways toward the leg and place the right hand beside the outer edge of the right foot, pointing the fingers in the same direction as the toes. Straighten the right arm and keep the left arm stretched up.

In going down, keep the weight on the outer edge of the left foot and the heel of the right foot. Press the right thigh and upper arm against each other to turn the chest up and to keep the knee in line with the hip and pointing straight ahead. Make the right shin perpendicular, with the knee directly over the ankle. Stretch the calf muscle up. Drop the top of the right thigh until it is parallel to the ground, keeping the thigh muscles soft. Take two or three breaths.

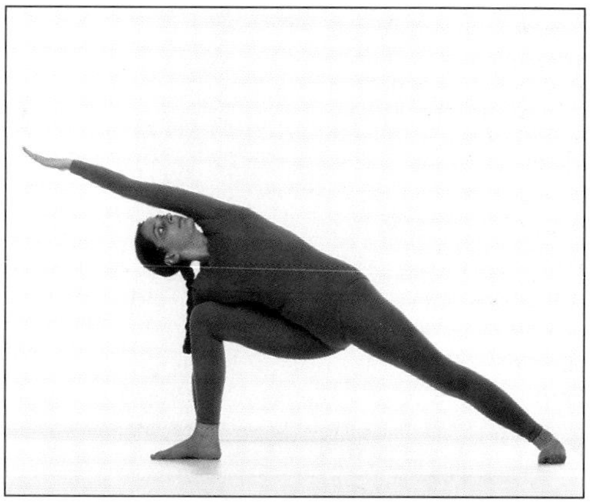

3 Stretch the left arm over the head, palm face down and upper arm over the left ear. Extend the trunk and take it closer to the bent leg, moving the top of the thigh and the bottom of the hip deep into the hip joint.

Bring the whole right side of the trunk forward and take the left side back. Extend the hips, waist, and chest as much as you can to the right. Feel the extension in one line from the left outer ankle to the fingertips of the left hand. Keep the head in line with the spine and take it slightly back. Turn the head and look up. Stay for 20 to 30 seconds, breathing evenly.

Inhale, straighten the right leg, and come up. Turn to the center. Rest the arms if necessary.◁ Repeat from ▷to◁ on the left. Exhale, bring the legs together and the arms down.

उत्थित पार्श्वकोणासन

Focus *Turning and extending the top arm*

Take the arm over the head, turn it in its socket from the outer (little finger) side in, with the inner upper arm facing the ear and the palm face down.

Stretch the upper arm from the armpit and lock the elbow (see p. 21); continue extending the inner forearm, wrist and hand; open the palm horizontally and extend the fingers, keeping them together, all the knuckles tucked in. Keep the hand in line with the arm.

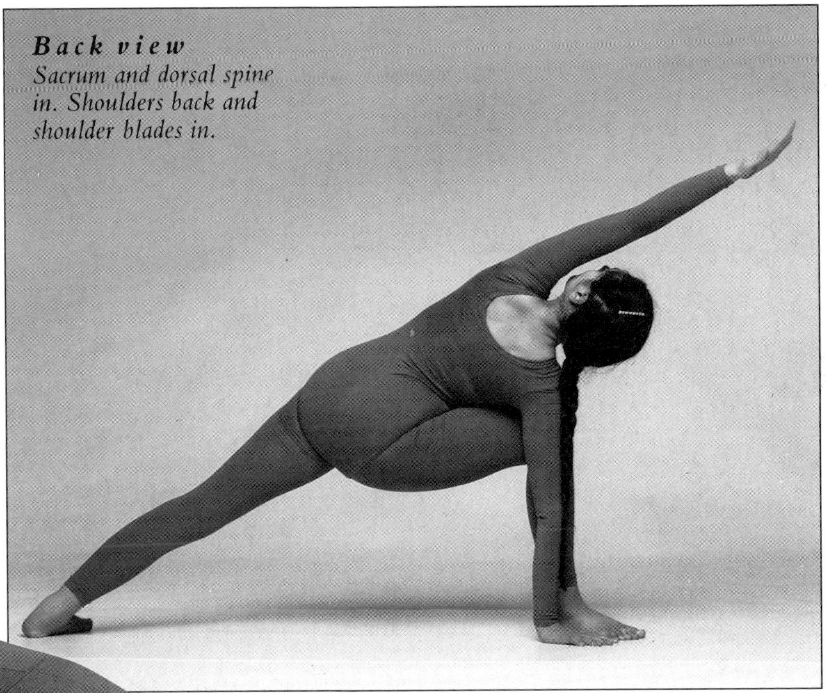

Back view
Sacrum and dorsal spine in. Shoulders back and shoulder blades in.

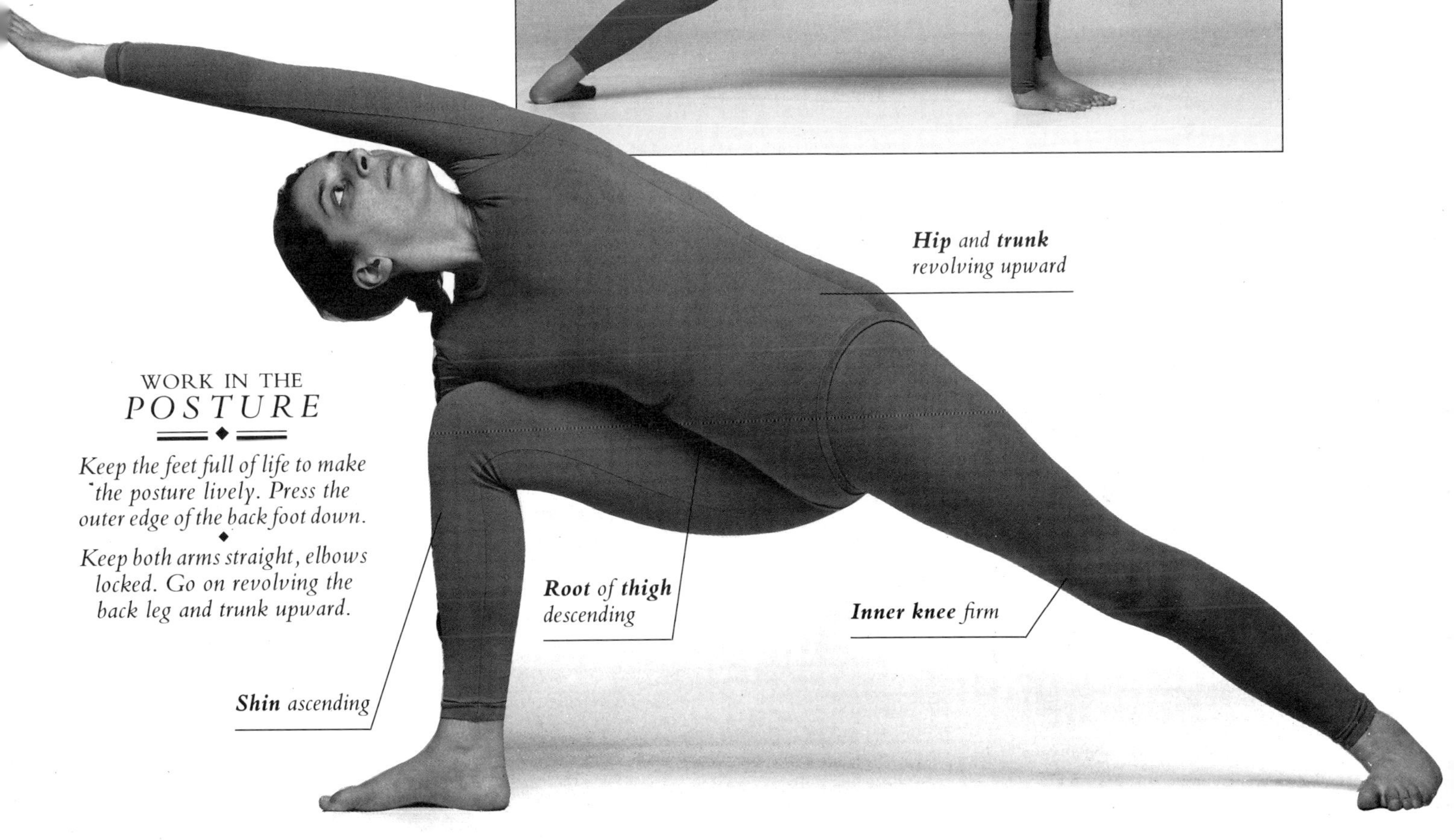
Hip and trunk revolving upward
Root of thigh descending
Inner knee firm
Shin ascending

WORK IN THE
POSTURE

Keep the feet full of life to make the posture lively. Press the outer edge of the back foot down.

◆

Keep both arms straight, elbows locked. Go on revolving the back leg and trunk upward.

वीरभद्रासन १

Vīrabhadrāsana I

VĪRABHADRA = a warrior from Indian mythology

THIS IS a vigorous posture which fills the body with strength.♦
It should not be done by those suffering from heart problems or high blood pressure.

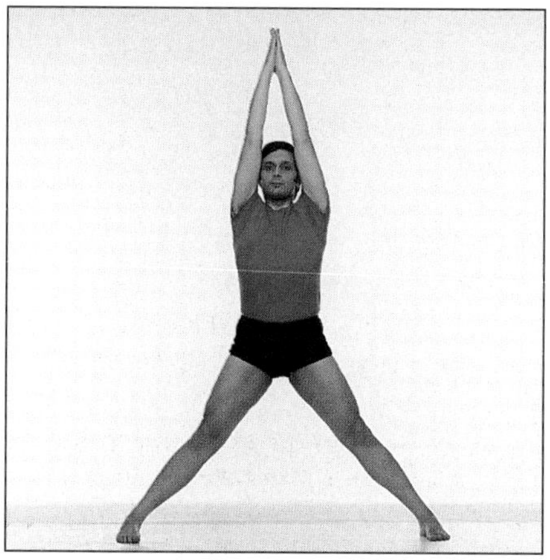

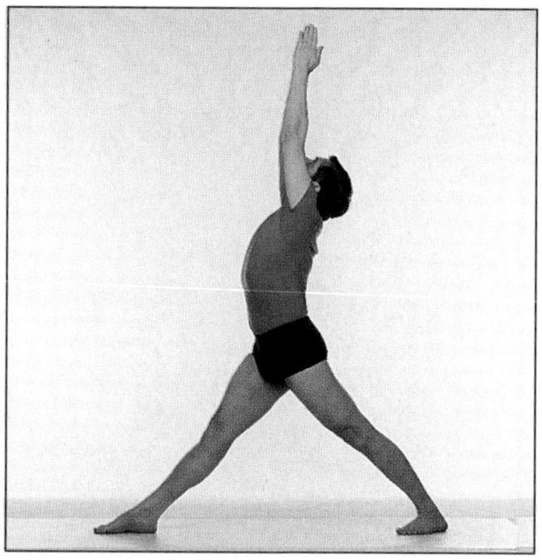

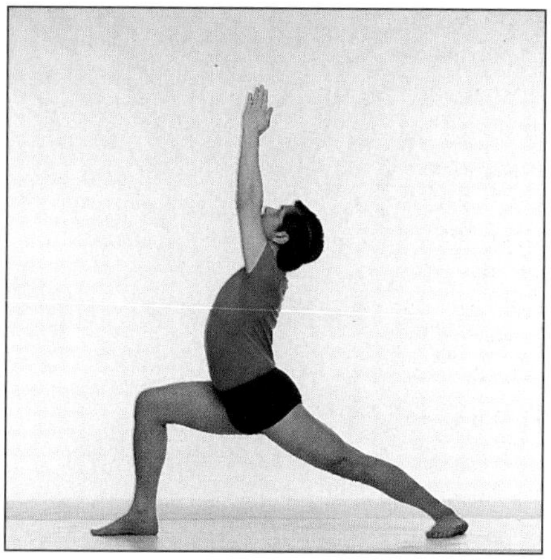

1 Stand in Tāḍāsana (p. 18). Inhale and jump the legs 4 to $4\frac{1}{2}$ft apart with the arms stretched sideways. Turn the arms circularly in their sockets so that the palms face the ceiling. Keeping the arms straight, take them up over the head until they are parallel. As the arms go up, stretch the sides of the chest and the armpits. Take the arms back, bring them close together, and join the palms with the fingers stretching up. Lock the elbows (see Focus, p. 21).

WAYS OF PRACTICING

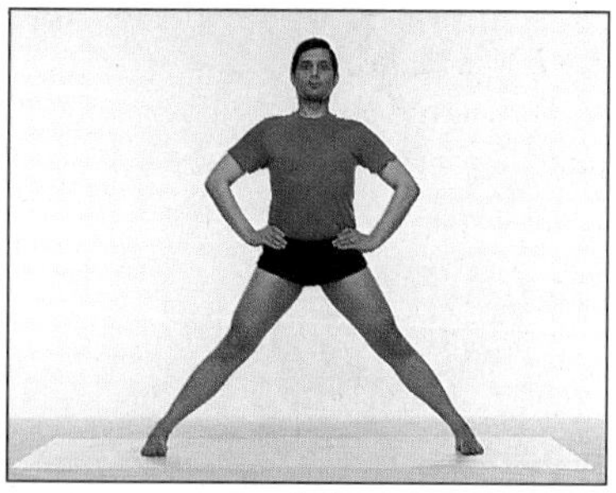

Keep the arms parallel.

To avoid strain in the lumbar, do the posture with the hands on the hips. Pressing the hands lightly, stretch the trunk up.

2 ▷Turn the left foot 45 to 60° in, the right foot 90° out and turn the trunk to the right so that it faces in the same direction as the right leg. Turn the back of the leg and the hip together with the foot (otherwise the knee may strain). Line up the feet (see Focus, p. 21).

Keep both sides of the body parallel and take the right hip slightly back. Keep the pubis, navel, sternum, and bridge of the nose centered and facing directly ahead, and look up. Take the waist back. Extend the trunk and arms up vertically.

3 With an exhalation, and keeping the left leg firm, bend the right leg to a right angle, with the shin perpendicular and the thigh parallel to the ground (see Focus, p. 29). Keep the knee facing directly forward. Keep the coccyx and sacrum vertical.

In going down, maintain the turn of the trunk and the lift of the hips. Finally extend the whole trunk up; lift the chest, and throw the head further back. Do not strain the throat or constrict the back of the neck. Stay for 20 to 30 seconds, breathing evenly.

Inhale, straighten the right knee, and come up. Turn to the center.◁ If necessary, rest the arms. Repeat from ▷to◁ on the left. Exhale, jump the legs together, take the arms to the sides, and bring them down. Rest in Uttānāsana I (p. 44).

वीरभद्रासन १

Focus *Avoiding strain*
Do not be tense when doing the postures. Keep the face, throat, and abdomen soft. Before starting, take two or three breaths to calm the mind. Even when stretching to the maximum, breathe normally and do not hold the breath. Keep the brain passive. Tension causes strain, which blocks energy; correct practice generates it.

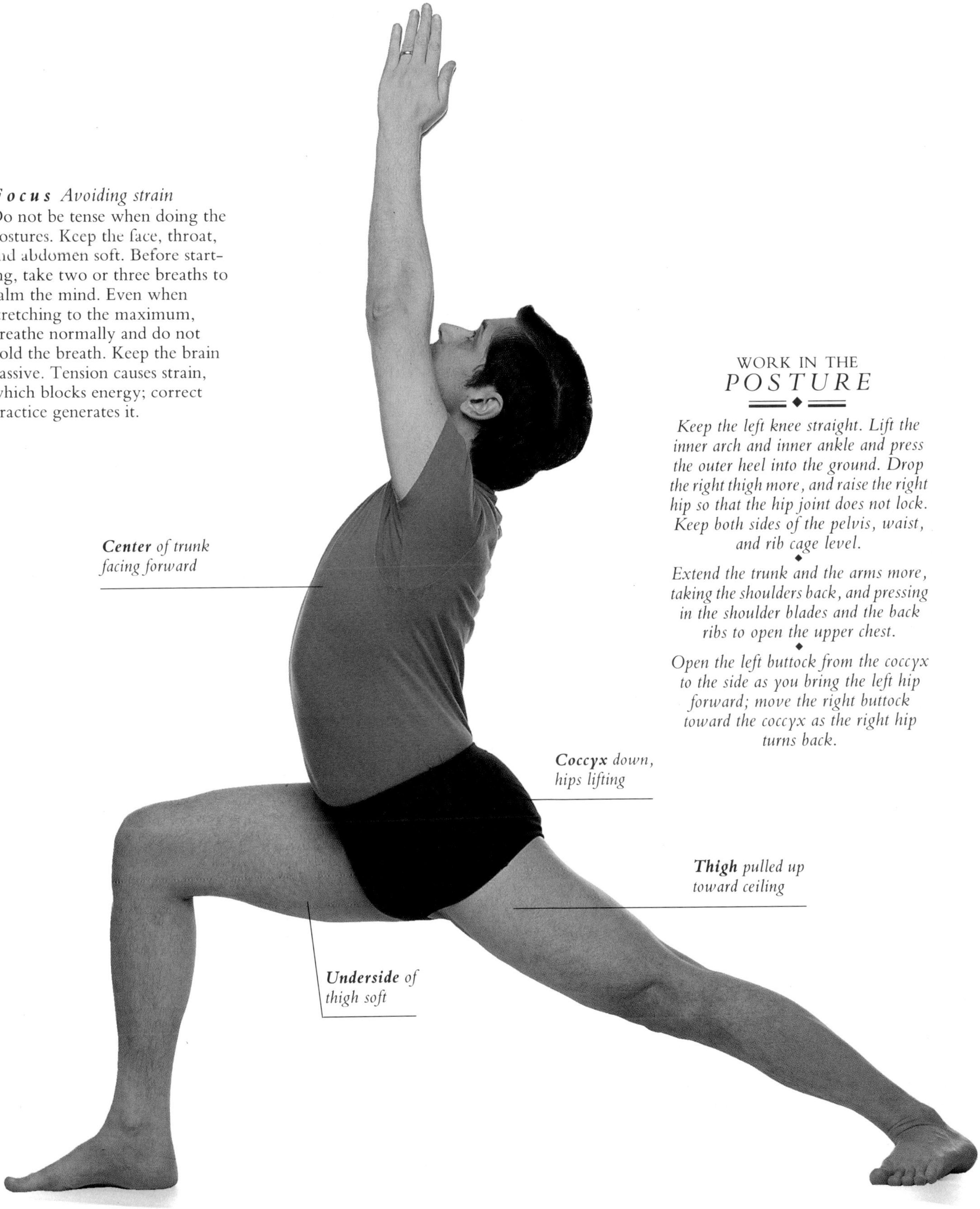

Center *of trunk facing forward*
Coccyx *down, hips lifting*
Thigh *pulled up toward ceiling*
Underside *of thigh soft*

WORK IN THE POSTURE

Keep the left knee straight. Lift the inner arch and inner ankle and press the outer heel into the ground. Drop the right thigh more, and raise the right hip so that the hip joint does not lock. Keep both sides of the pelvis, waist, and rib cage level.

◆

Extend the trunk and the arms more, taking the shoulders back, and pressing in the shoulder blades and the back ribs to open the upper chest.

◆

Open the left buttock from the coccyx to the side as you bring the left hip forward; move the right buttock toward the coccyx as the right hip turns back.

वीरभद्रासन २

Vīrabhadrāsana II

VĪRABHADRA = a warrior from Indian mythology

THIS IS the second warrior pose. The body rises erect over the legs, while the arms reach out to opposite sides.♦

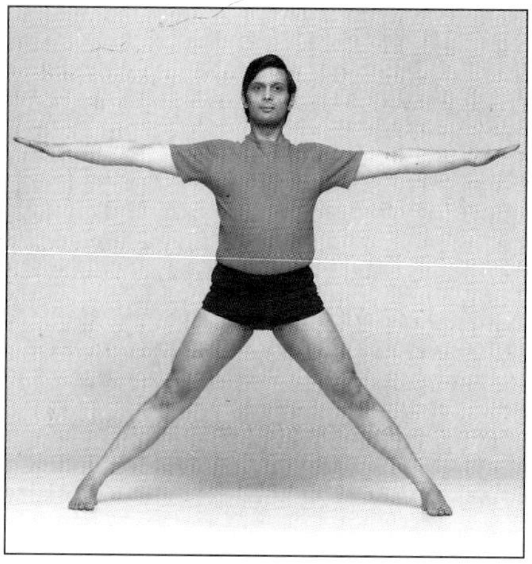

1 Stand in Tāḍāsana (p. 18). Inhale and jump the legs 4 to $4\frac{1}{2}$ft apart, arms stretched sideways.

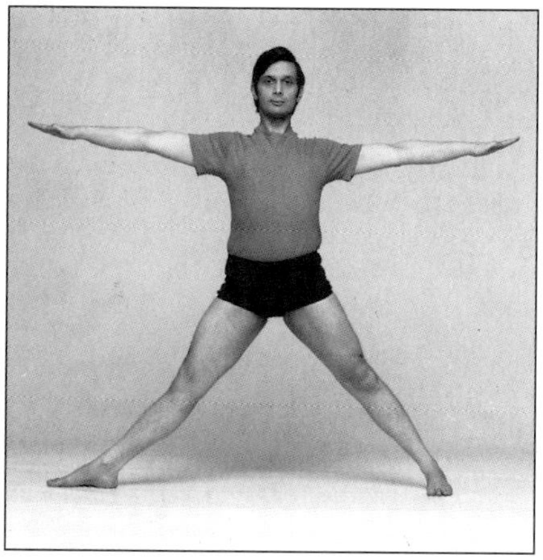

2 ▷Turn the left foot 15° in and the right leg 90° out. Lock the left knee (see Tāḍāsana, Knees, p. 18). Extend the trunk up.

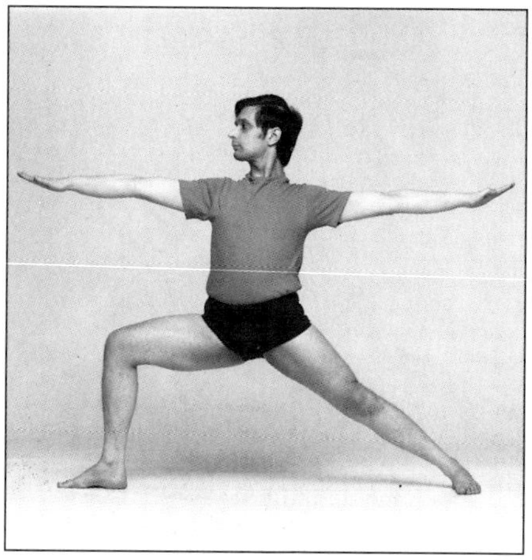

3 Exhale and bend the right leg to a right angle. Bend in the left hip joint between the hip and thigh to keep the trunk vertical. Raise the hips and keep the trunk facing forward.

Press the outer edge of the left foot down, keeping the leg firm. Press the right heel down and bring the right hip, right side of the trunk, and spine forward. Stretch the right inner thigh toward the knee and turn the knee to the right so that it faces directly ahead (see Focus, right). Tuck the top of the outer thigh into the right hip joint. Relax the shoulders and extend the arms further away from the trunk, stretching from the sternum and spine to the fingertips of both hands. Look over both arms to see that they are level. Finally harden the left arm, turn the head and look over the right arm. Stay for 20 to 30 seconds, breathing normally.

Inhale, come up and turn to the center.◁ Repeat from ▷ to ◁ on the left. Jump the feet together, lower the arms.

***Focus** Ankles and feet*

The feet should keep their natural shape. Extend the soles, toes, and arches, then lift the arches. Lift the inner and outer ankles from under the ankle bones. Draw the skin of the top of the feet toward the legs.

Bending the leg to a right angle

Be firm on the heel. Keep the shin perpendicular, with the bent knee directly over the ankle. Stretch the calf muscles up. Keep the thigh parallel to the floor, with the underside of the thigh relaxed and moving toward the back of the knee. Take the skin and flesh at the back of the knee into the knee joint.

Shoulders and arms

Drop the backs of the shoulders. Dip the tops of the upper arms slightly, but keep the arms horizontal. Extend the inner arms and the undersides more. Harden the skin and flesh of the outer arms. Lock the elbows and extend the arms in one line to the fingertips, keeping the wrists down. Point the middle fingers directly out to the sides.

वीरभद्रासन २

WORK IN THE
POSTURE

Lift the left inner ankle. Open the left hip outward and keep the left inner leg pulled to the left.

◆

Lift the sternum and the back ribs. Open the right side of the trunk to the right and the left side to the left.

◆

Move the coccyx, lumbar, and kidneys in. Extend the spine and the sides of the body up. Take the shoulder blades in and keep the back straight.

Reflection

There is a constant challenge and response in practicing the āsanas. Thus, the heel presses into the floor and the foot responds by stretching forward, or the leg replies by stretching up. When one side is working well, it challenges the other side to work with the same intensity. This interplay brings awareness and sensitivity to the whole body.

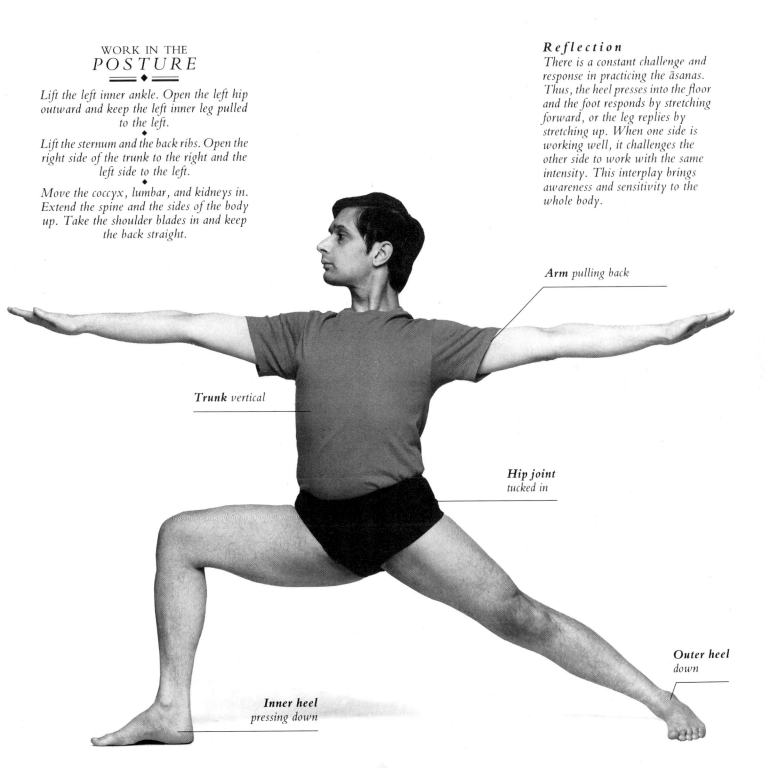

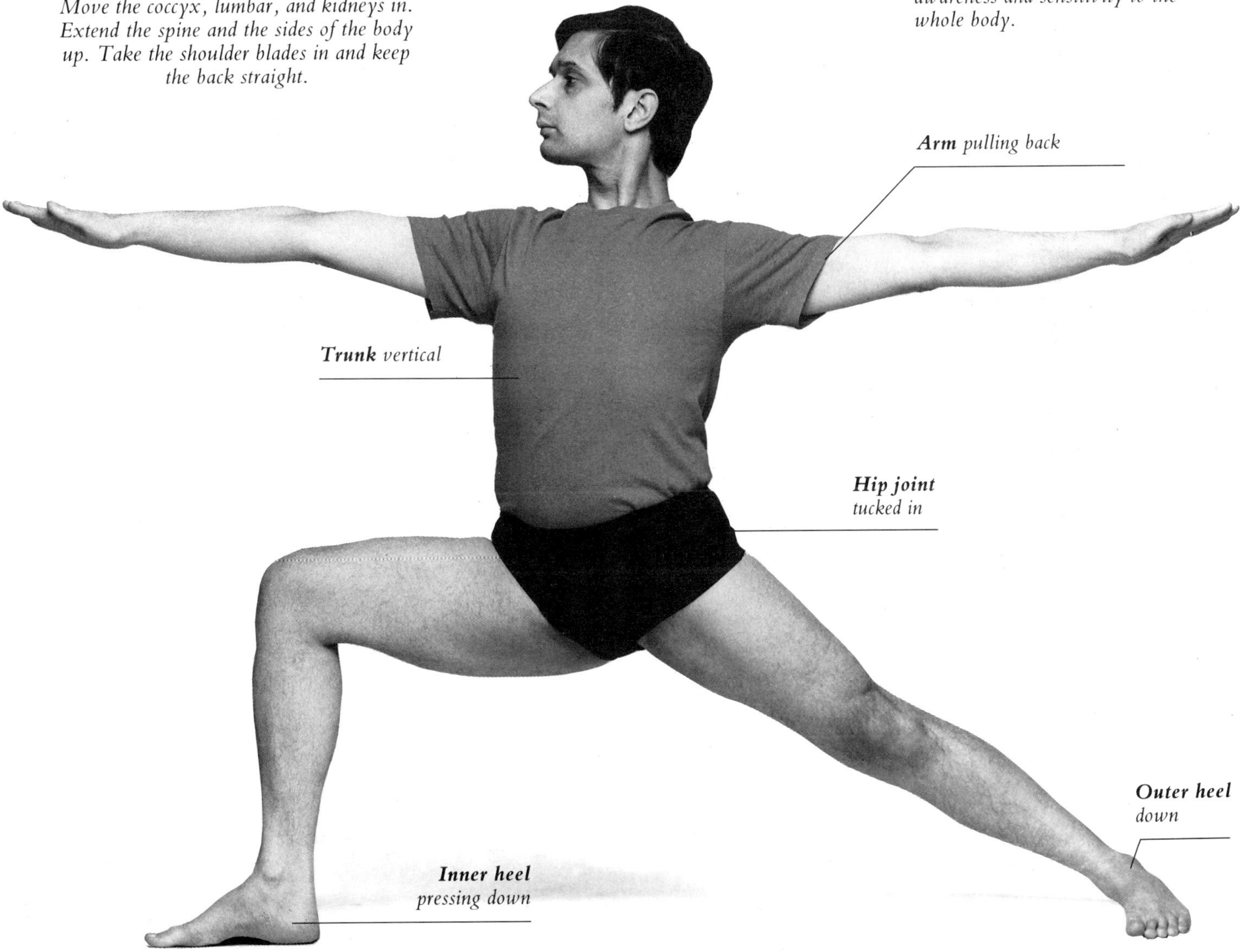

Arm pulling back
Trunk vertical
Hip joint tucked in
Outer heel down
Inner heel pressing down

अर्ध चन्द्रासन

Ardha Chandrāsana

ARDHA = half; *CHANDRA* = moon

THE EXTENDED trunk, poised over a finely balanced leg, is reminiscent of the Indian moon floating in space.♦

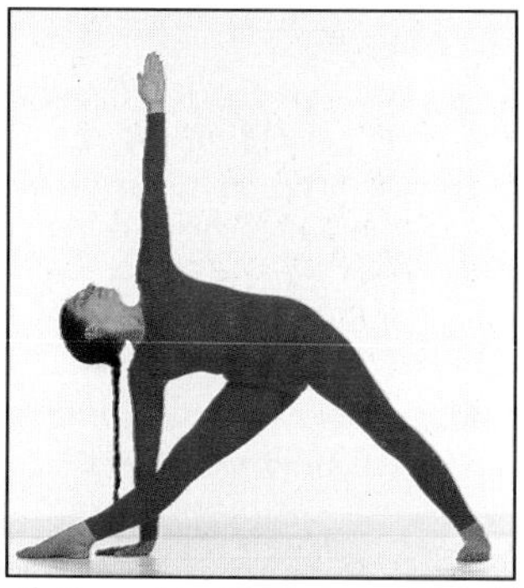

1 Stand in Tāḍāsana (p. 18). Inhale and jump the legs $3\frac{1}{2}$ to 4ft apart, arms stretched sideways. ▷Take the left foot 15° in, the right leg 90° out. With an exhalation bend the trunk sideways to the right, and go into Trikoṇāsana (p. 22), turning and extending well. Stay for two or three breaths.

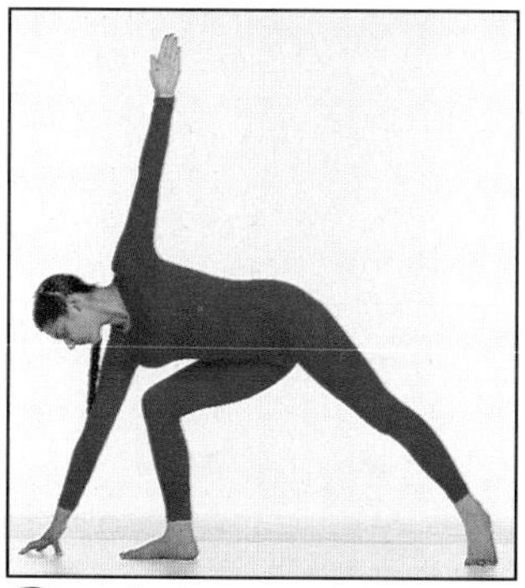

2 Exhale, bend the right knee, and bring the left foot slightly in toward the right foot. Place the fingertips of the right hand on the floor, making them into a cup shape (see Focus, opposite). The hand should be about 1ft in front of the right leg, in line with it or a little to the side.

WAYS OF PRACTICING

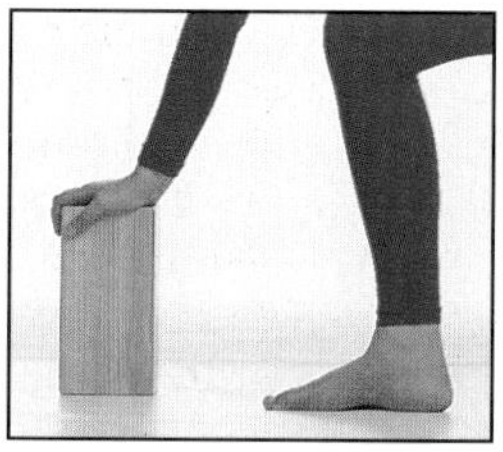

To help with balance, do the posture with the back against a wall. Rest the left hip, left foot, and the head on it.

To keep the back leg up, rest the foot on a ledge.

Place the right hand on a brick. Keep the left arm extended along the trunk.

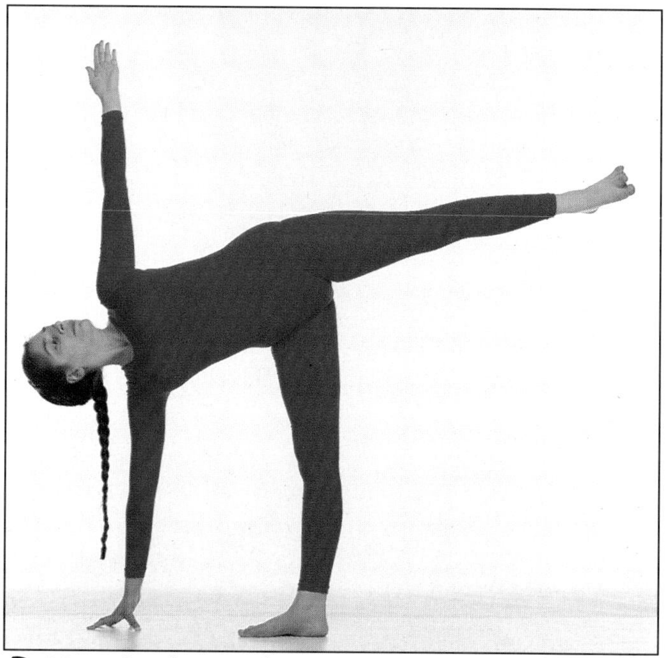

3 Now simultaneously raise the left leg, keeping it extended, straighten the right knee, and stretch the right leg up. Straighten the right arm and stretch the left arm in line with it.

Be firm on the right foot, especially on the heel, the big toe, and the second toe. Lock the right knee (see Tāḍāsana, Legs, p. 18) and pull the thigh muscles up. Draw the flesh of the outer thigh toward the bone and up. Move the back of the thigh forward so that the leg is vertical, not leaning back.

Revolve the lower abdomen up; lift the left hip and take it back, so that it rests over the right hip.

Extend the trunk from the pubis toward the head, and stretch the left leg and inner heel away from the trunk. Keep the leg and the side of the body in line, and the toes facing forward. Stretch the sole of the foot and the toes.

Turn the head and look up. Stay, breathing evenly, for 20 to 30 seconds.

Exhale, bend the right knee, and lower the left leg. Straighten the right leg and go into Trikoṇāsana. See that the feet are in line and the correct distance apart. Take two or three breaths.

Inhale and come up. Turn to the front.◁ Repeat from ▷to◁ on the left. Exhale and jump the legs together; bring the arms down.

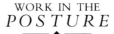

अर्ध चन्द्रासन

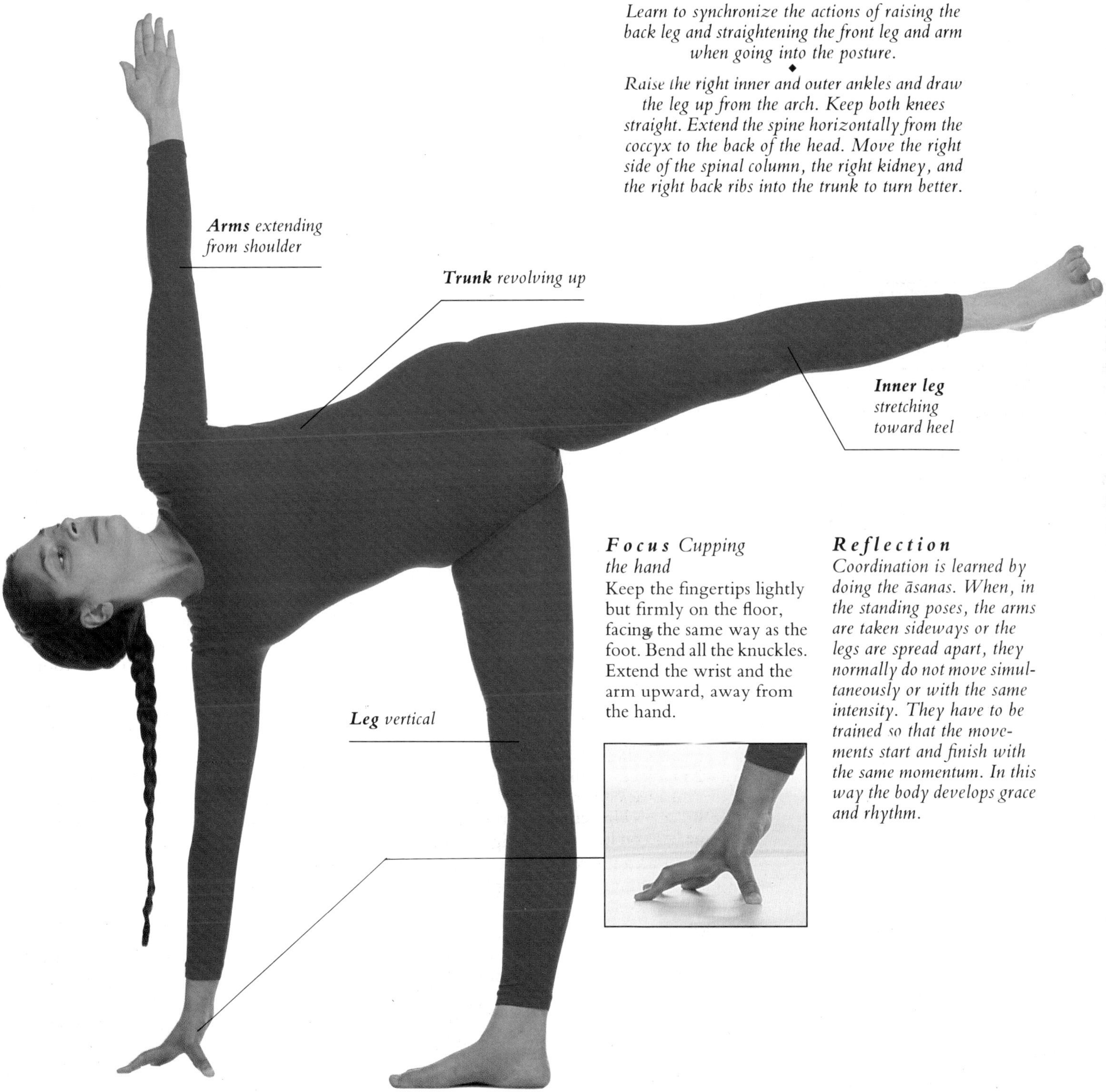
Arms *extending from shoulder*
Trunk *revolving up*
Inner leg *stretching toward heel*
Leg *vertical*

WORK IN THE *POSTURE*

Learn to synchronize the actions of raising the back leg and straightening the front leg and arm when going into the posture.

◆

Raise the right inner and outer ankles and draw the leg up from the arch. Keep both knees straight. Extend the spine horizontally from the coccyx to the back of the head. Move the right side of the spinal column, the right kidney, and the right back ribs into the trunk to turn better.

Focus *Cupping the hand*

Keep the fingertips lightly but firmly on the floor, facing the same way as the foot. Bend all the knuckles. Extend the wrist and the arm upward, away from the hand.

Reflection

Coordination is learned by doing the āsanas. When, in the standing poses, the arms are taken sideways or the legs are spread apart, they normally do not move simultaneously or with the same intensity. They have to be trained so that the movements start and finish with the same momentum. In this way the body develops grace and rhythm.

वीरभद्रासन ३

Vīrabhadrāsana III

VĪRABHADRA = a warrior from Indian mythology•

THIS IS the third and most difficult warrior pose. It combines strength and dynamism with firm balance.♦

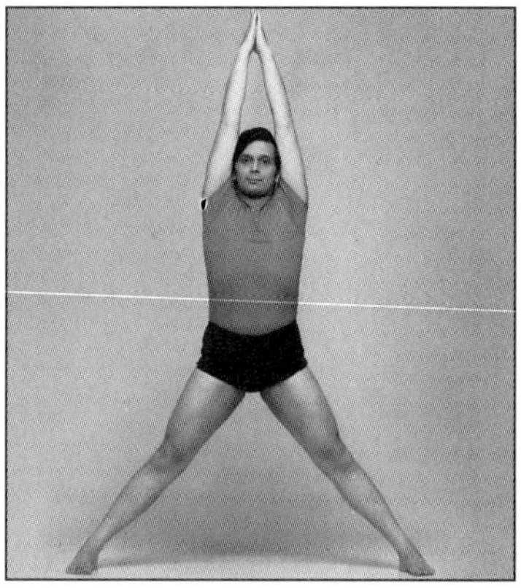

1 Stand in Tāḍāsana (p. 18). Inhale and jump the legs 4 to $4\frac{1}{2}$ft apart, arms stretched sideways. Stretch the arms and the trunk up as in Vīrabhadrāsana I (p. 26).

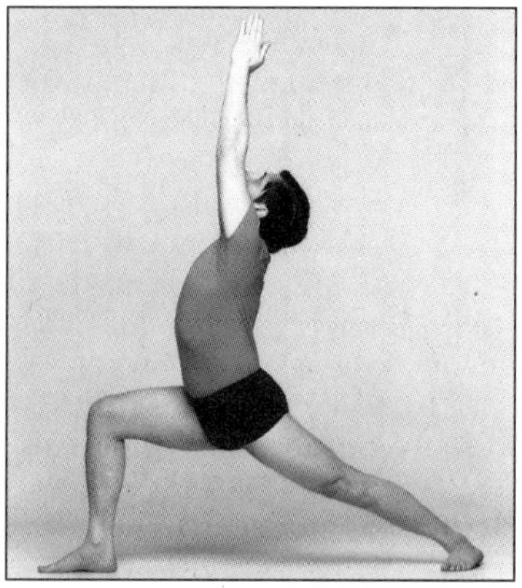

2 ▷Turn the left leg and foot 45° in, the right foot 90° out, and the trunk completely to the right. Exhale, bend the right knee, and go into Vīrabhadrāsana I.

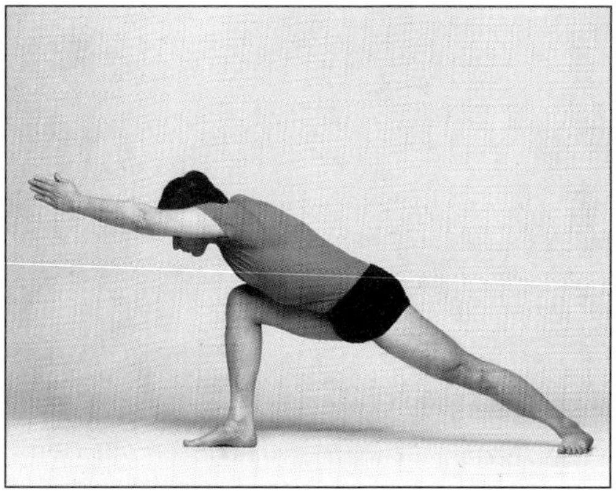

3 Exhale; bend the trunk over the right leg, going deep into the right hip joint. Rest the chest on the thigh. Keep the right foot firm, and extend the trunk and the arms forward. Lift the left heel and turn the leg with the back of it facing the ceiling.

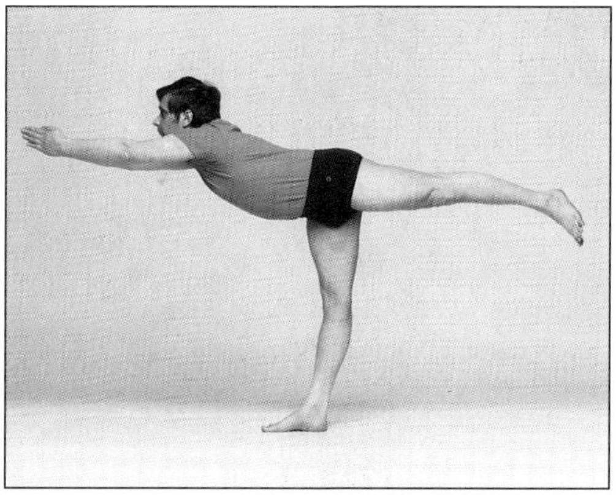

4 Simultaneously (a) bring the hips and the body weight forward onto the right leg, (b) straighten the leg, and (c) bring the left leg in and raise it to the level of the left hip while (d) keeping the left hip down.

Balance on the right leg, make the hips level, and extend the left leg back. Keep the knee pointing down and the heel and toes stretching. At the same time stretch the arms and the trunk forward and the left leg back. Keep the trunk, arms, and leg parallel to the ground. Keep the chest down. Lower the head for a moment to relax the neck, then raise the head, and gaze forward. Balance, maintaining the horizontal stretch, for 20 to 30 seconds. Do not hold the breath.

With an exhalation bend the right leg, lower the left leg, and go into Vīrabhadrāsana I.

Come up, straighten the leg, and turn to the front.◁ Rest the arms if necessary. Repeat from ▷to◁ on the left. Finally take the arms to the sides, jump the legs together, and bring the arms down. Rest in Uttānāsana I (p. 44).

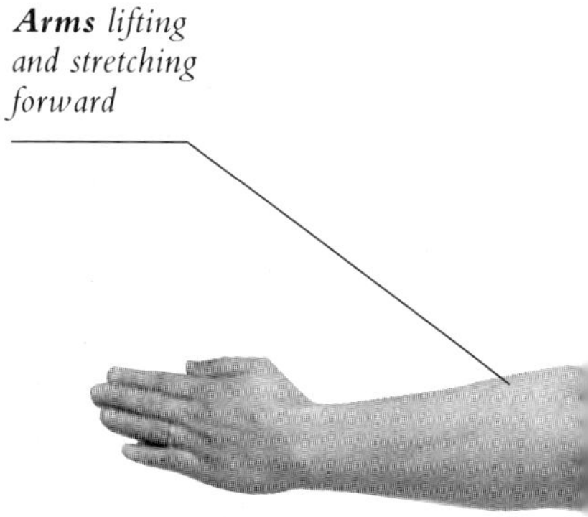

वीरभद्रासन ३

WORK IN THE POSTURE

Keep the right heel and toes firmly down, the kneecap tucked in, and the thigh muscles pulled up. Stretch the inner and outer leg right to the top of the thigh. Keep the left leg strong.

Do not collapse the chest but stretch the front of the body toward the head. Press the shoulder blades into the back and stretch the armpits and upper arms forward while extending the left leg back. Keep the elbows locked.

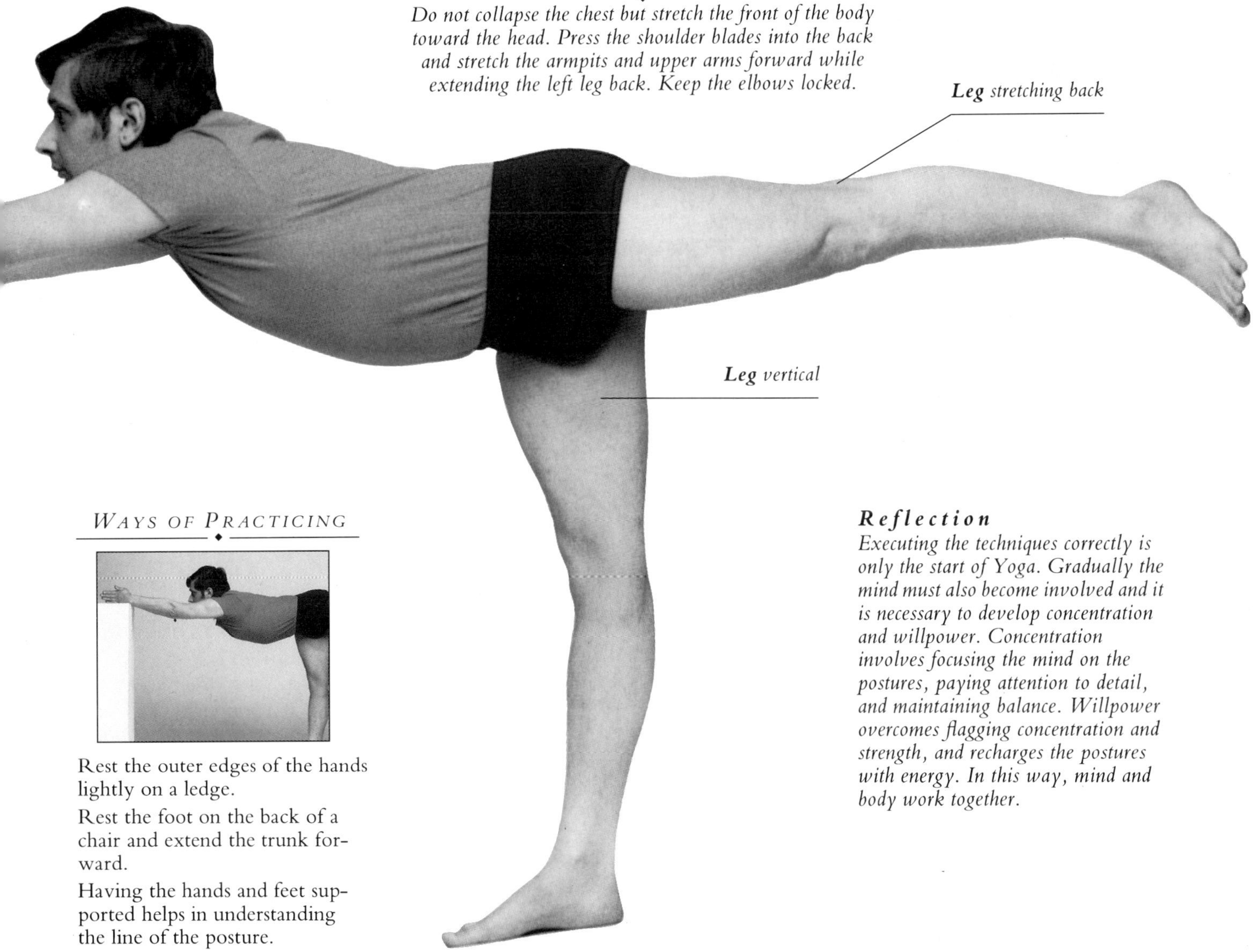

WAYS OF PRACTICING

Rest the outer edges of the hands lightly on a ledge.

Rest the foot on the back of a chair and extend the trunk forward.

Having the hands and feet supported helps in understanding the line of the posture.

Reflection

Executing the techniques correctly is only the start of Yoga. Gradually the mind must also become involved and it is necessary to develop concentration and willpower. Concentration involves focusing the mind on the postures, paying attention to detail, and maintaining balance. Willpower overcomes flagging concentration and strength, and recharges the postures with energy. In this way, mind and body work together.

परिवृत्त त्रिकोणासन

Parivṛtta Trikoṇāsana

PARIVṚTTA = reverse, revolved; *TRIKOṆA* = triangle

IN THIS pose, the trunk revolves a full 180° backward. ♦♦

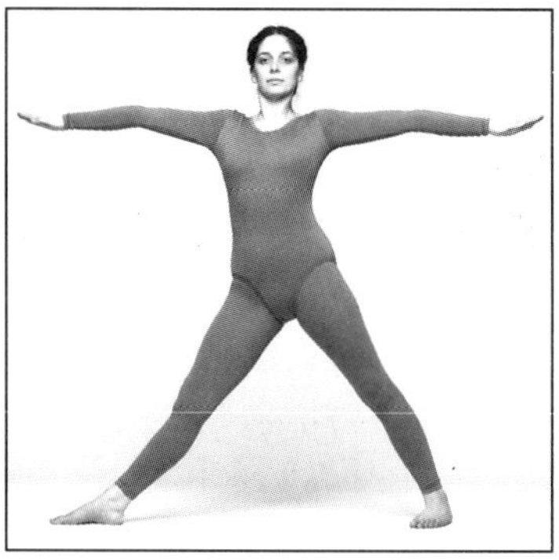

1 Stand in Tāḍāsana (p. 18). Inhale and jump the legs $3\frac{1}{2}$ to 4ft apart, arms stretched sideways. ▷ Turn the left leg and foot 45 to 60° in and the right leg 90° out. Line up the right heel with the left instep.

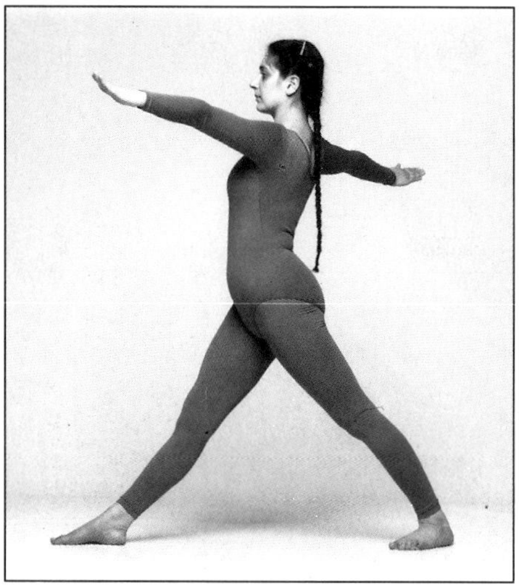

2 Stretch the right leg up and hit the left leg back, revolving it inward to the maximum. Simultaneously bring the left hip and the left side of the trunk forward and take the right side slightly back until both sides of the body are parallel. Extend the trunk up and keep the arms extended.

(The front of the body – the pubis, navel, and sternum – now faces completely forward [to the right] and the back of the body and the spine face directly back [to the left].)

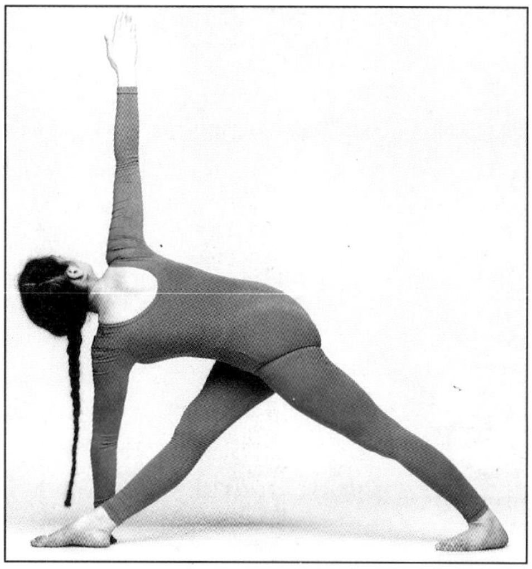

3 Press the left heel down and, with an exhalation, swing the left side of the trunk down toward the right foot, and turn the right side up. Extend the left arm from the shoulder until the hand rests on the floor beside the outer edge of the foot. Use the pressure of the fingers to turn the trunk more. Bear the direction of the spine in mind: keep it centered and turning on its own axis; let the trunk follow the movement of the spine. Do not sway the hips to one side.

Extend the whole back from the coccyx to the head. Revolve the hips, waist, and chest. Move the left kidney, the left back ribs, and the shoulder blades in to bring the chest over the right leg. Then lengthen the front of the body from pubis to abdomen, abdomen to chest, chest to shoulders. Extend the right arm up, turn the head, and look up. Stay for 20 to 30 seconds, breathing evenly.

Inhale and come up. Turn to the center. ◁ Repeat from ▷ to ◁ on the left, then jump the legs together and bring the arms down.

WAYS OF PRACTICING

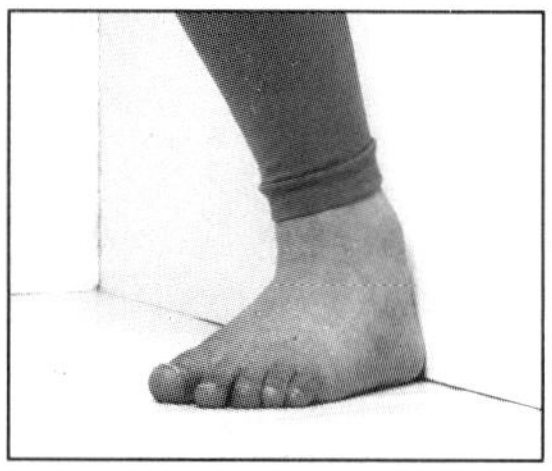

To learn alignment, do the posture at right angles to the wall. Press the back heel into the wall (above), with the back of the trunk parallel to the wall. Center the trunk, bend forward, and then turn to the right.

Place the hand on a brick.

Keep the top hand down on the hip.

If you are stiff, keep the lower hand beside the inner edge of the foot.

परिवृत्त त्रिकोणासन

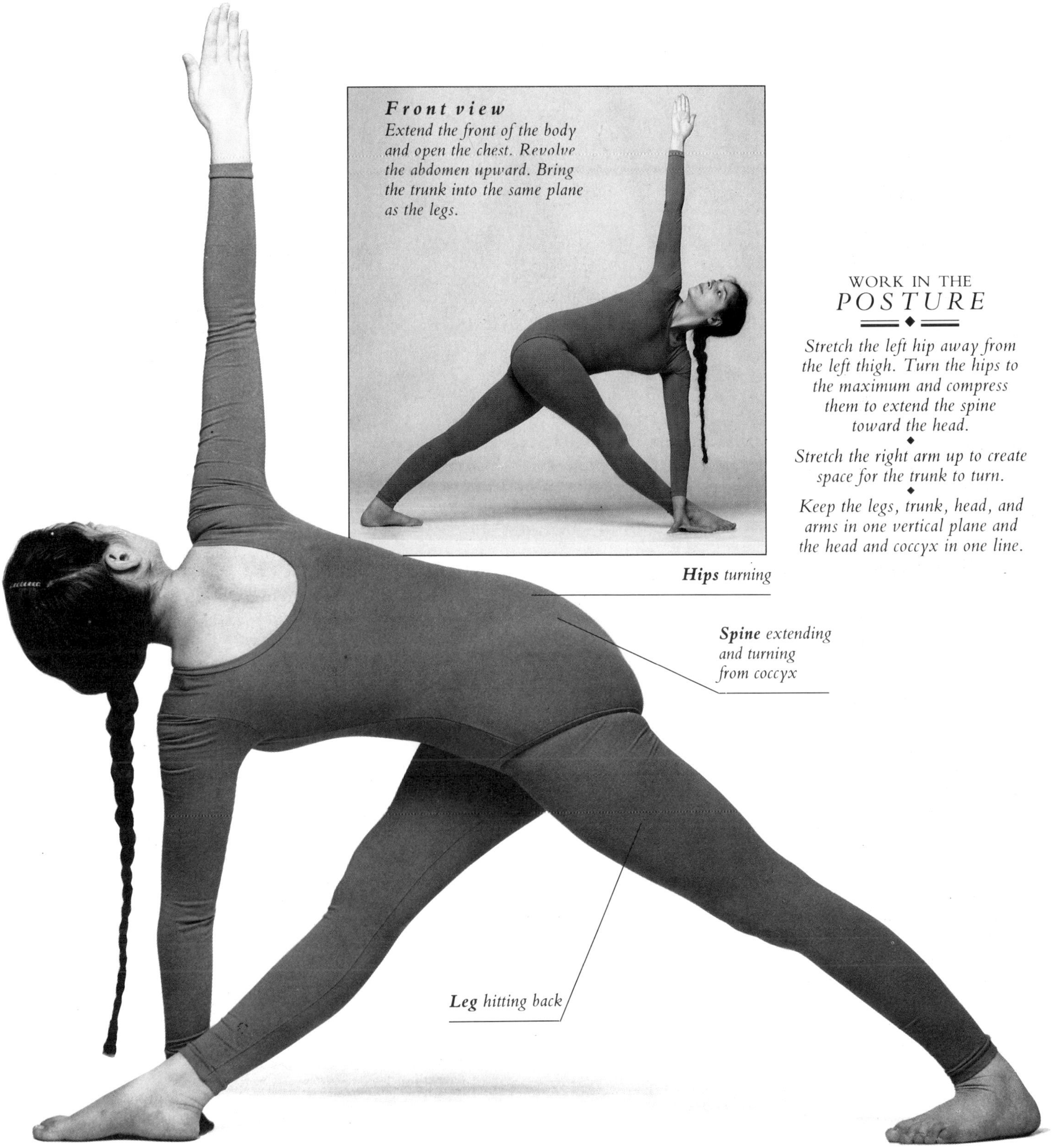
Hips turning
Spine extending and turning from coccyx
Leg hitting back

Front view
Extend the front of the body and open the chest. Revolve the abdomen upward. Bring the trunk into the same plane as the legs.

WORK IN THE POSTURE

Stretch the left hip away from the left thigh. Turn the hips to the maximum and compress them to extend the spine toward the head.

◆

Stretch the right arm up to create space for the trunk to turn.

◆

Keep the legs, trunk, head, and arms in one vertical plane and the head and coccyx in one line.

परिवृत्त पार्श्वकोणासन

Parivṛtta Pārśvakoṇāsana

PARIVṚTTA = revolved; *PĀRŚVAKOṆA* = lateral angle

WITH THE opposite arm locked against the bent leg, the trunk turns 180° away from the front.♦♦

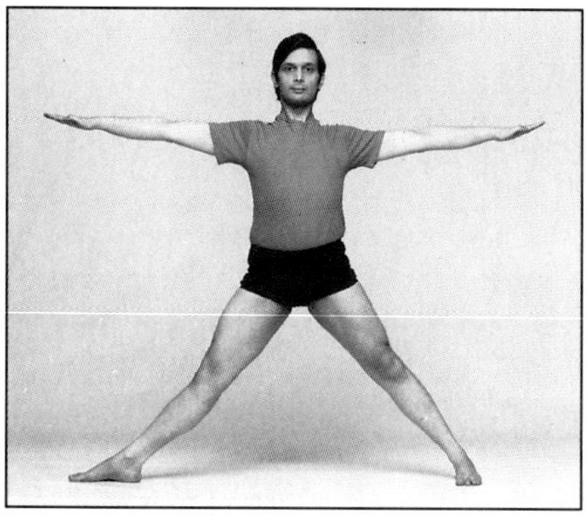

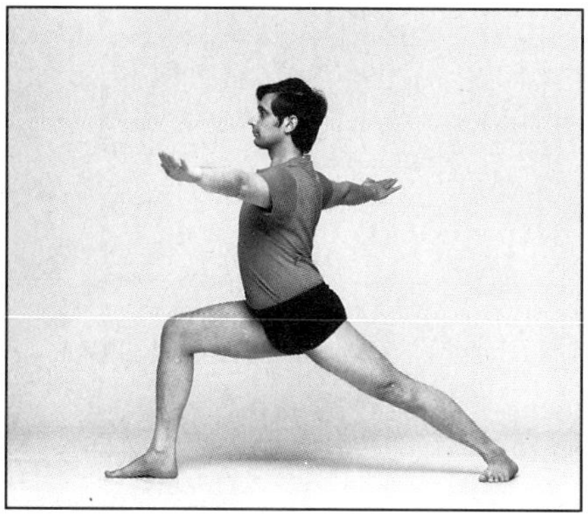

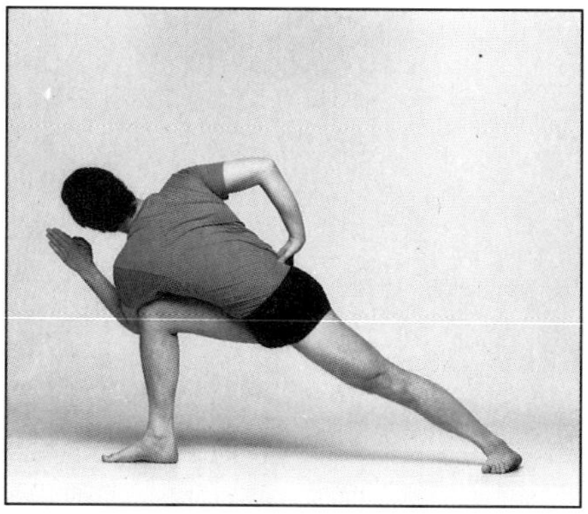

1 Stand in Tāḍāsana (p. 18). Inhale and jump the legs 4 to 4½ft apart, arms stretched sideways. ▷Turn the left leg and foot about 60° in and the right leg 90° out; line up the feet. Extend the trunk up.

2 Turn the left hip well in, bend the right leg to a right angle, and turn the trunk to face the right leg. Keep the coccyx facing directly back and the middle of the pubis and sternum facing directly ahead.

Keep the outer edge of the left heel down on the floor.

Ways of Practicing

Raise the left heel and turn the leg, with the front of the thigh and the knee facing the floor. Stand on the tips of the toes with the sole vertical and the heel facing the ceiling. Keep the knee straight.

Use a wall for stability, keeping the heel on the wall, toes on the floor.

Keep the top hand on the hip.

3 With an exhalation turn and bend the left side of the body toward the right leg. Bend the left arm and place it against the right outer knee with the forearm and hand stretched. Place the right hand on the right hip and tuck the hip in toward the coccyx to keep the coccyx centered.

Press the left upper arm against the thigh to bring the left side of the chest to the right. Squeeze the abdomen up, away from the right thigh. Extend the front of the body from the pubis to the head. Revolve the right side of the trunk up and back.

परिवृत्त पार्श्वकोणासन

4 Now straighten the left arm and place the hand on the floor, without losing the lift and turn of the trunk.

Take the right shoulder back, stretch the right arm up and then over the ear, with the palm face down. Take the head back, turn it, and look up. Stay for 20 to 30 seconds, breathing evenly.

Inhale and come up; turn to the front. Straighten the knees and stretch the arms sideways. ◁ If necessary, rest the arms for a moment, then raise them again.

Repeat from ▷ to ◁ on the left. Bring the legs together and the arms down to the sides.

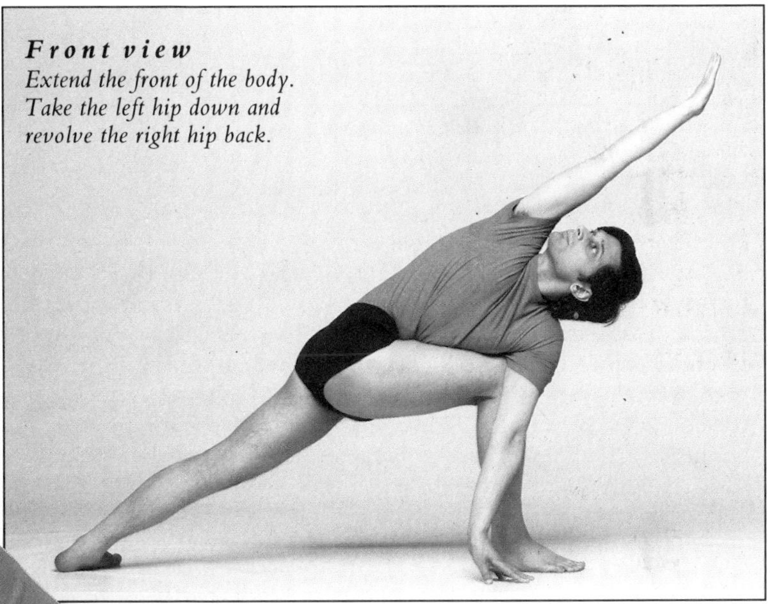

Front view
Extend the front of the body. Take the left hip down and revolve the right hip back.

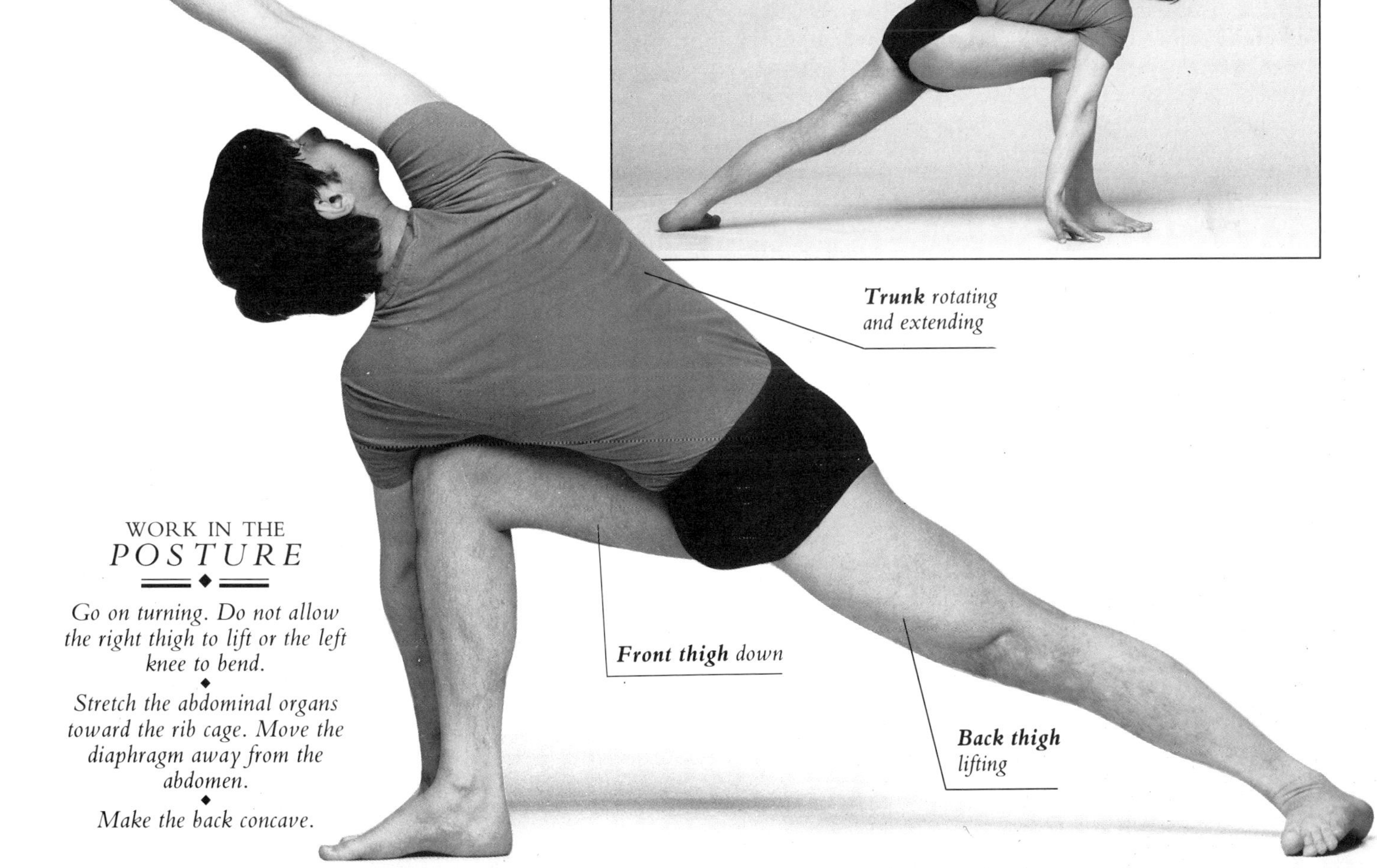
Trunk rotating and extending
Front thigh down
Back thigh lifting

WORK IN THE
POSTURE

Go on turning. Do not allow the right thigh to lift or the left knee to bend.

◆

Stretch the abdominal organs toward the rib cage. Move the diaphragm away from the abdomen.

◆

Make the back concave.

परिवृत्त अर्ध चन्द्रासन

Parivṛtta Ardha Chandrāsana

PARIVṚTTA = reverse; *ARDHA* = half; *CHANDRA* = moon

THIS IS the reverse half-moon pose in which the trunk turns 180° backward while balancing on one leg.♦♦

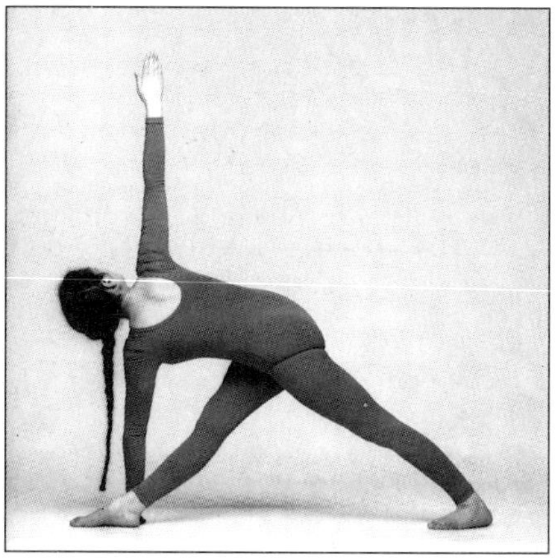

1 Stand in Tāḍāsana (p. 18). Inhale and jump the legs $3\frac{1}{2}$ to 4ft apart, arms stretched sideways. ▷ Turn the left leg and foot about 60° in, the right foot 90° out. Line up the feet (see Focus, p. 22). The line between the feet is the center over which the trunk extends and turns. Exhale and go into Parivṛtta Trikoṇāsana (p. 34), with the left hand beside the outer edge of the right foot, the right arm stretched up, and the trunk turned back. Stay for two or three breaths.

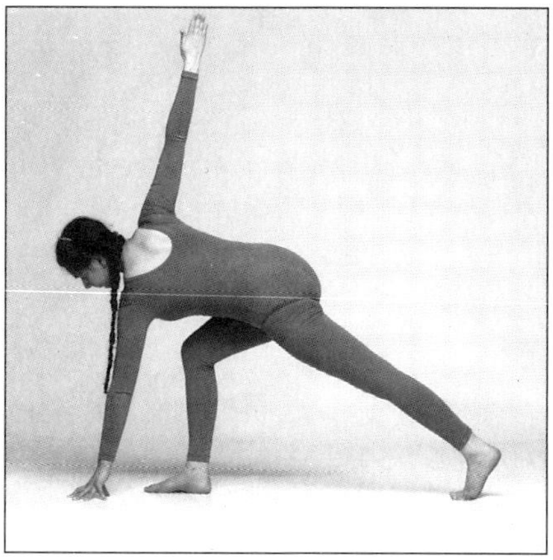

2 Bend the right knee, place the left hand about 1ft forward, in line with the right foot, and take the left foot slightly in.

Ways of Practicing

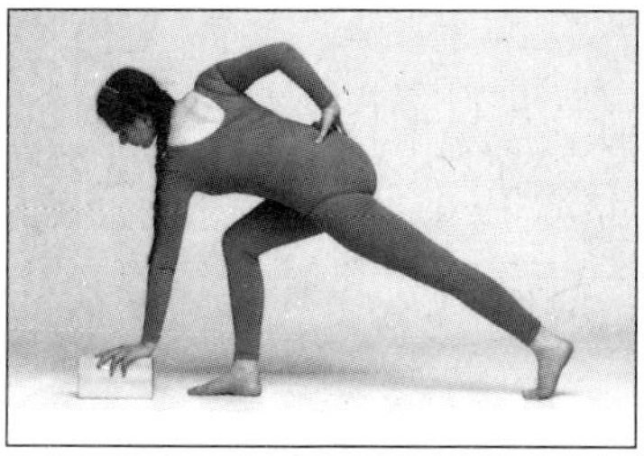

Rest the right hand on the right hip.
If you are stiff, keep the left hand on the inner side of the right foot.

Place the hand on a brick beside the right foot.

Rest the foot on a ledge.

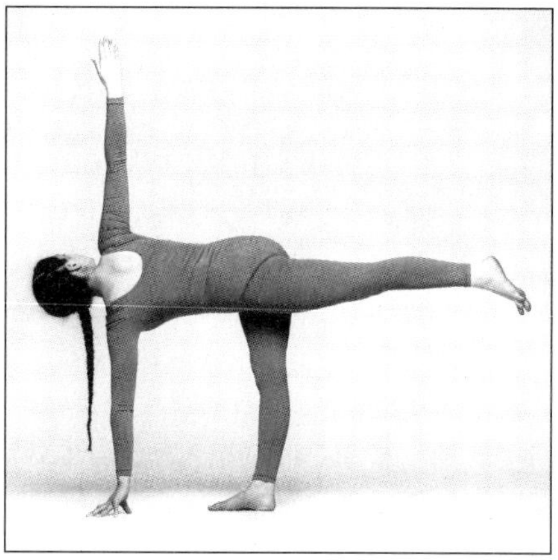

3 Take the body weight and the hips forward; straighten the right leg and raise the left leg to hip level, turning it so that the knee and big toe point down and the back of the leg faces the ceiling.

Stretch the right leg up, keeping the heel and toes steady and the arch lifted. Stretch the left leg back, extending the heel, the sole of the foot, and the toes. Turn the trunk, lowering the left hip and left side of the trunk and moving them to the right; raise the right side and revolve it back. (The front of the body now faces completely backward.) Extend the spine from the coccyx. Keep the left leg firm. Press the fingertips of the left hand into the floor, revolve the arm outward, and bring the left side of the trunk forward. Finally stretch the right arm up strongly, turn the head and look up. Balance for 20 or 30 seconds.

Exhale, bend the right leg, and take the left leg back and down. Do Parivṛtta Trikoṇāsana (p. 34).

Inhale, come up, and turn to the front. ◁ Repeat from ▷ to ◁ on the left. Jump the legs together and bring the arms down.

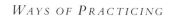

परिवृत्त अर्ध चन्द्रासन

WORK IN THE POSTURE

Extend the trunk and left leg away from each other. Keep the left thigh and knee strongly gripped.

◆

Move the left side of the spine into the trunk. Bring the left side of the chest over the right leg to keep the posture in line.

◆

Flatten the back ribs and turn the rib cage more. Revolve the chest and abdomen upward.

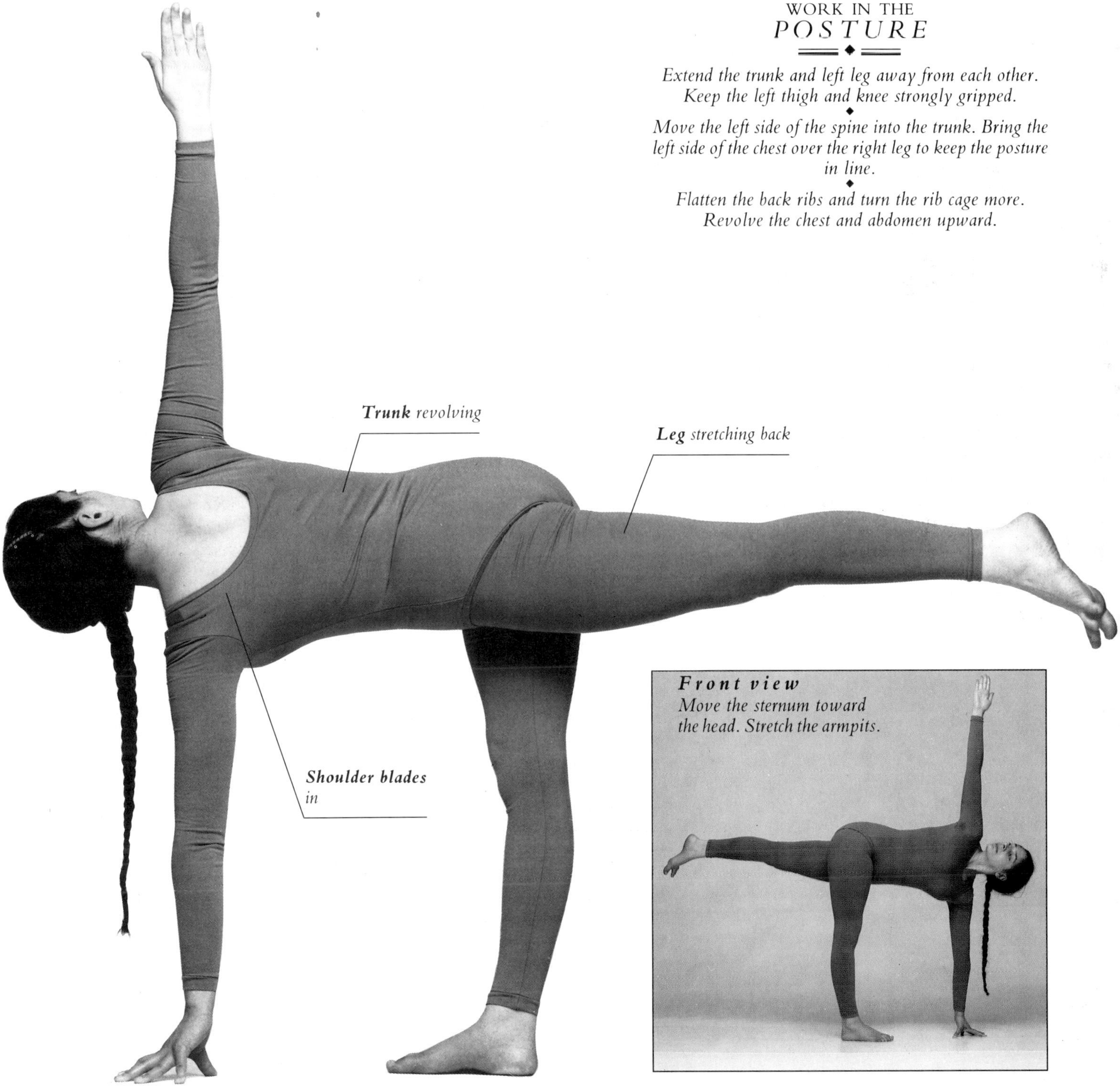
Trunk revolving
Leg stretching back
Shoulder blades in

Front view
Move the sternum toward the head. Stretch the armpits.

पार्श्वोत्तानासन

Pārśvottānāsana

PĀRŚVA = sideways; *UTTĀN* = extended

THE TRUNK stretches first up and then down over the legs, with the hands joined in prayer position behind the back.♦

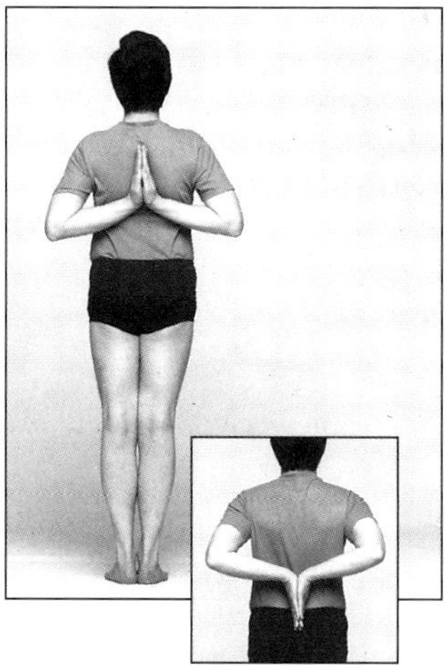

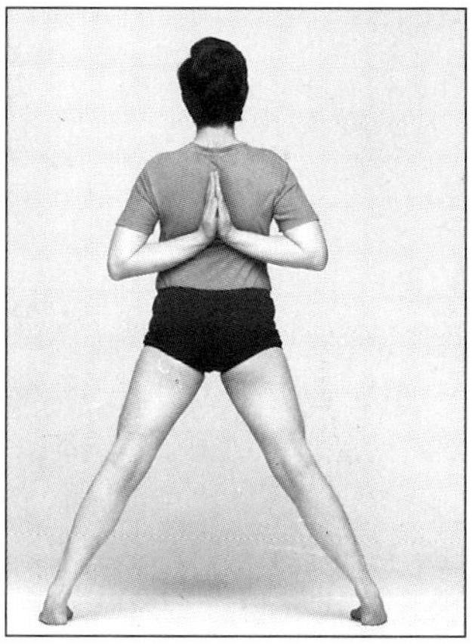

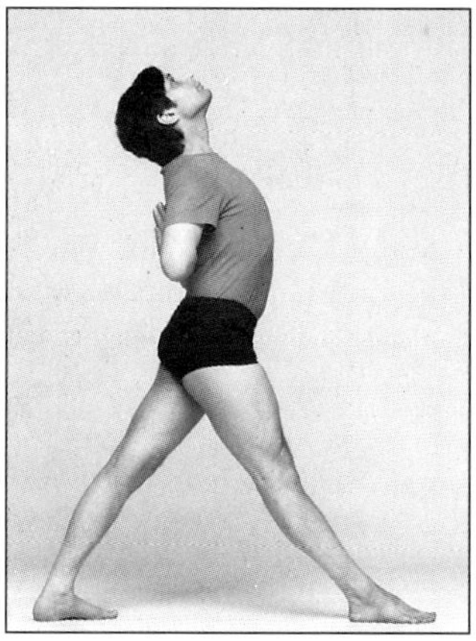

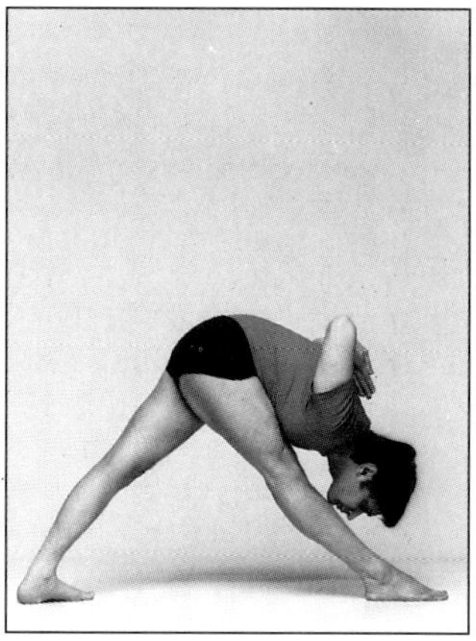

1 Stand in Tāḍāsana (p. 18). Join the palms behind the back, fingers pointing down and in line. Turn the hands toward the trunk and then up. Take them as high as possible between the shoulder blades. Join the heels of the hands and press the little fingers into the dorsal spine. Stretch the fingers up, tucking in all the knuckles. Turn the upper arms outward and take the shoulders and elbows back and down.

2 Inhale and jump the legs $3\frac{1}{2}$ to 4ft apart. Do not collapse the lower back but keep the coccyx and sacrum pressed in. Extend the trunk up and open the chest.

WAYS OF PRACTICING

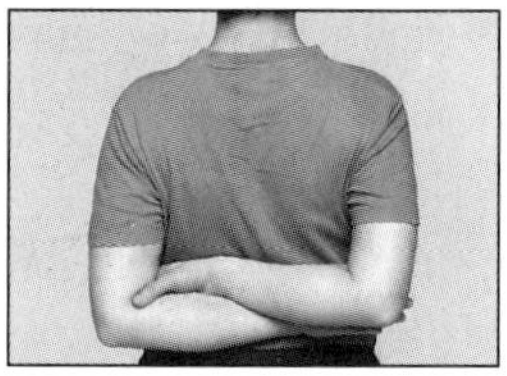

If you cannot join the palms behind the back, catch the elbows.

If you are stiff or have a bad back, place the hands on a ledge and bend halfway down as in Uttanāsana (p. 44).

Keep the hands on the floor on either side of the foot. For stability, keep the back foot against a wall (see Parivṛtta Trikoṇāsana, p. 34).

3 ▷Turn the left leg and foot about 60° in and the right leg 90° out, revolving the hips and trunk to the right so that the pubis, the navel, and the sternum face forward (to the right) and the spine faces directly back.

Keep the legs strong. Revolve the left leg and the left side of the body forward. Tuck the right leg and right side of the trunk slightly back.

Extend the hips, waist, and chest up, stretching both sides of the body evenly. Take the sacrum, lumbar, and kidneys inwards and up; make the dorsal spine concave. Curve the chest and move the sternum toward the chin. Take the head back and look up, without straining the throat.

Stay for a moment, breathing evenly.

4 With an exhalation extend the trunk down over the right leg; widen the buttock bones and move the tops of the thighs back, stretching the left side diagonally toward the right foot. Synchronize the downward movement with the exhalation. Move the hips, lower abdomen, and chest closer to the leg, placing the sternum over the center of the leg. Rest the head on the shin. Relax the head and neck. Stay for 20 to 30 seconds, breathing evenly.

Inhale and come up, stretch the trunk up, and straighten the head. Turn to the front.◁ Repeat from ▷to◁ on the left, then jump the legs together and release the hands.

पार्श्वोत्तानासन

Alternative method
Instead of coming up in step 4, turn to the center with the head and trunk down; stay down. Turn the feet and trunk to the left (trunk bending over the left leg) and stay. Inhale, come up, stretch up, and throw the head back. Bend down again over the left leg, stay down; then come to the center, raise the trunk, jump the feet together, and release the hands.

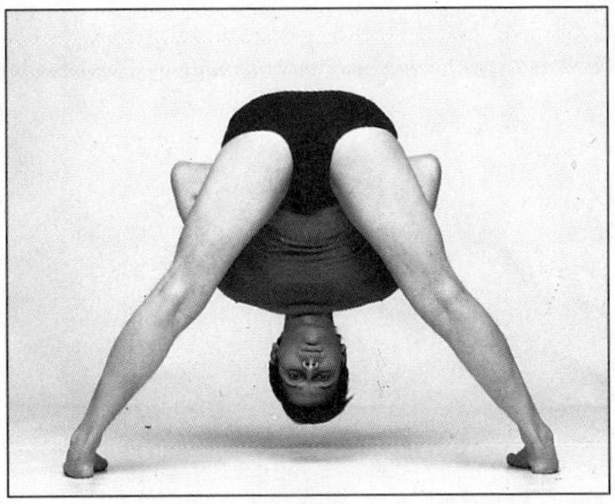

WORK IN THE
POSTURE

Go on pressing the outer edge of the back foot into the ground in order not to lean too much on the front leg. Keep the hips level and the buttock bones lifting as the trunk descends.

◆

Take the elbows up.

◆

Hit the front leg away from the head and the back leg away from the front leg.

Focus *Turning the legs when the back foot is turned deep in*
Turn the back foot 60° in, turning the leg and hip together with the foot. Keep the top of the thigh pulled back so that the weight goes onto the back of the leg and the heel presses down. Turn the front foot out (see Focus, p. 22); tuck the hip back so that the trunk faces directly forward (to the right). Synchronize the movements of the hips and legs.

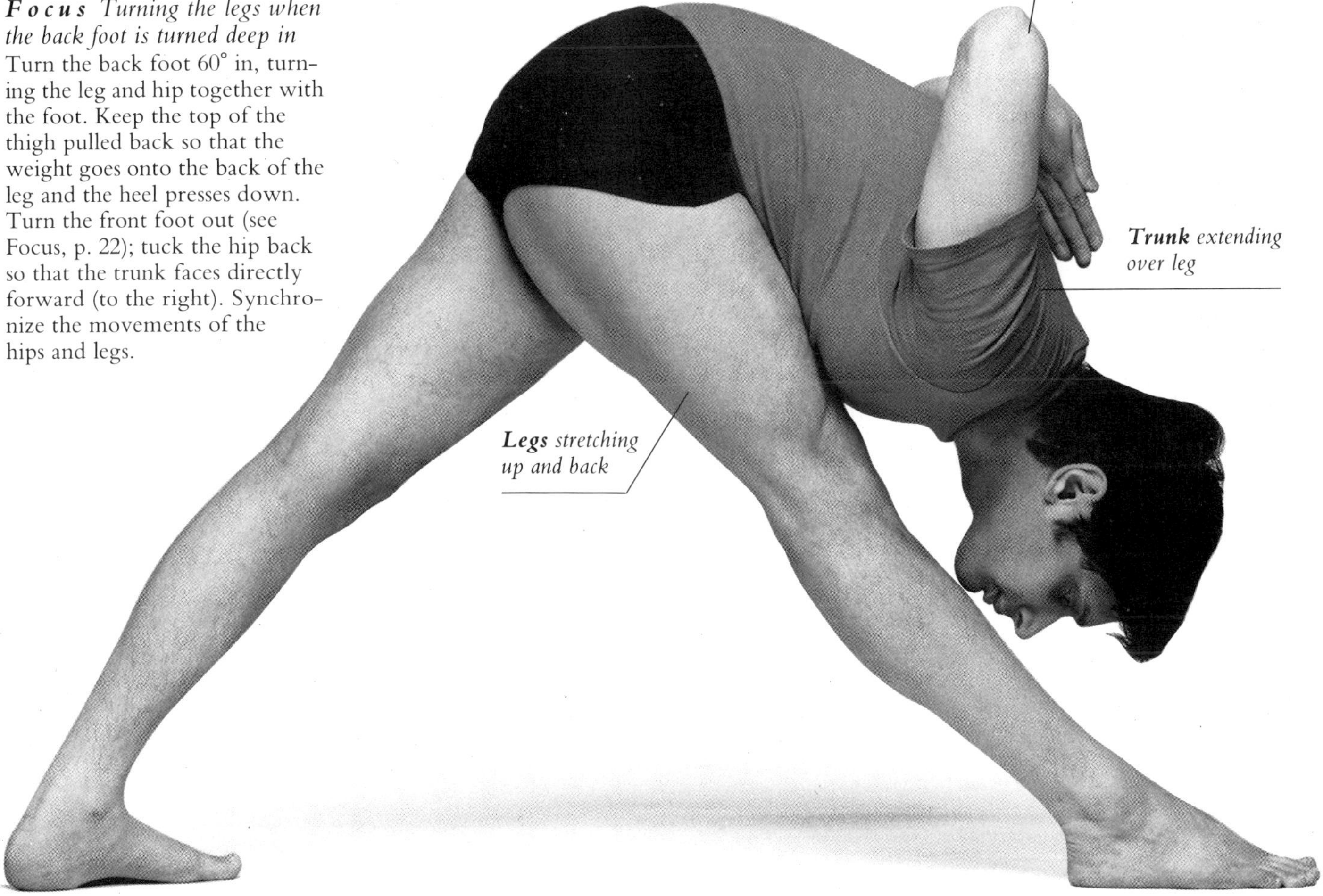

Elbows *lifting*
Trunk *extending over leg*
Legs *stretching up and back*

प्रसारित पादोत्तानासन १

Prasārita Pādottānāsana I

PRASĀRITA = spread out, expanded; *PĀDA* = foot, leg;
UTTĀN = extended, stretched

THIS IS a resting pose with the legs spread wide apart and stretching up.♦

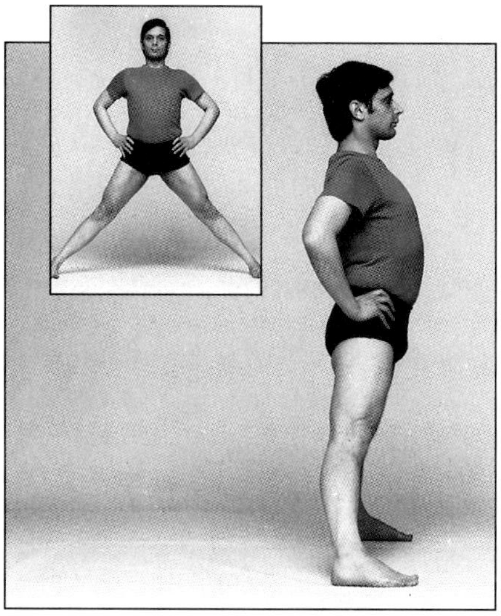

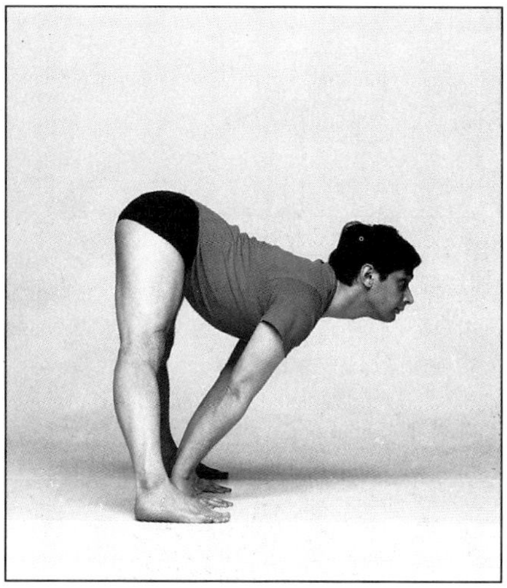

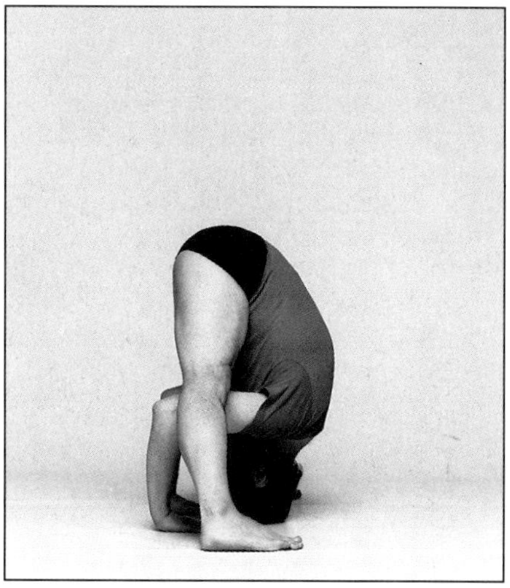

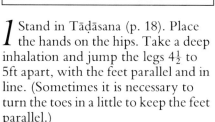

1 Stand in Tāḍāsana (p. 18). Place the hands on the hips. Take a deep inhalation and jump the legs $4\frac{1}{2}$ to 5ft apart, with the feet parallel and in line. (Sometimes it is necessary to turn the toes in a little to keep the feet parallel.)

Stretch the legs up and hit the inner ankles, shins, knees, and thighs outward (see Focus, opposite). Extend the trunk up from the base of the hips. Take two or three breaths. Lift the chest and take the shoulders back.

2 With an exhalation bend the trunk about halfway down, placing the palms on the floor between the legs, a shoulder's-width apart. Spread the buttock bones away from each other to "create space" in the sacroiliac joint and to prevent strain in the lumbar. Press the heels of the hands down and stretch the palms and fingers forward. Lock the elbows and stretch the arms from the wrists up.

Keep the tops of the thighs pulled back and extend the trunk from the buttock bones to the head. Take the hips, waist, and rib cage down and move the top of the chest forward to make the back concave. Lift the chin and look up. Stay for 20 to 30 seconds, breathing evenly.

3 Exhale, bend the elbows back in line with the shoulders. Take the trunk down, placing the crown of the head on the floor.

Keep the forearms vertical and the upper arms parallel to the ground. Relax the trunk and the head. Stay for 30 seconds, breathing evenly.

Inhale and come up; place the hands on the hips and straighten the trunk. If necessary, bring the feet in a little. Exhale, jump the legs together, and bring the arms down.

WAYS OF PRACTICING

In step 2, keep the hands underneath the shoulders, with the arms vertical.

In the final pose, place the head on a bolster or brick.

प्रसारित पादोत्तानासन १

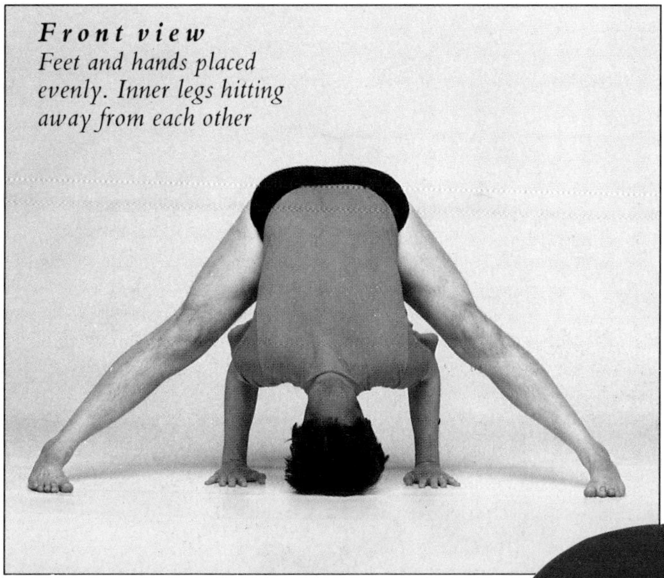

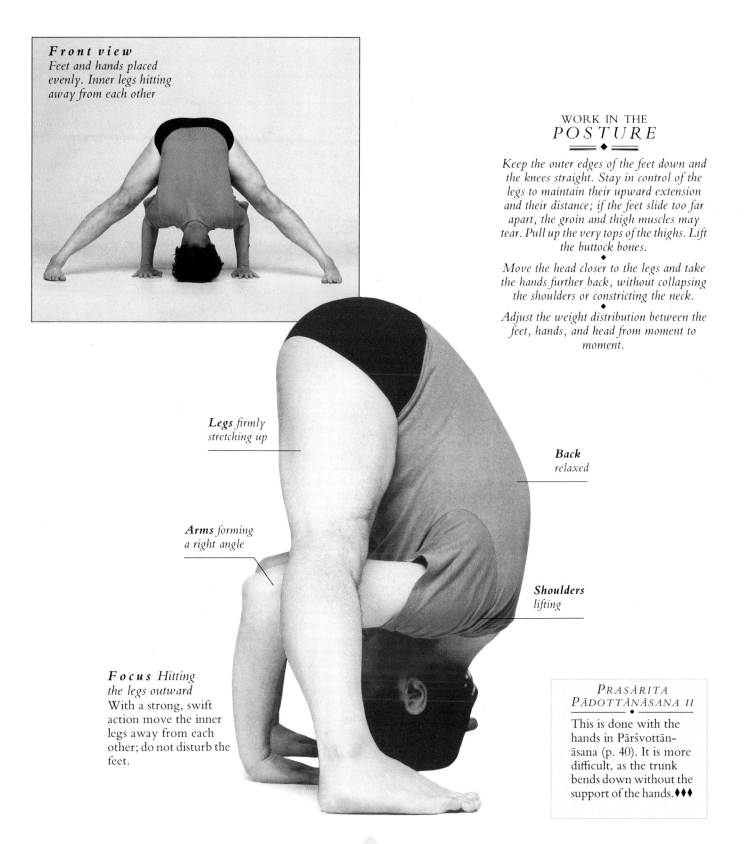

Front view
Feet and hands placed evenly. Inner legs hitting away from each other

WORK IN THE
POSTURE

Keep the outer edges of the feet down and the knees straight. Stay in control of the legs to maintain their upward extension and their distance; if the feet slide too far apart, the groin and thigh muscles may tear. Pull up the very tops of the thighs. Lift the buttock bones.

◆

Move the head closer to the legs and take the hands further back, without collapsing the shoulders or constricting the neck.

◆

Adjust the weight distribution between the feet, hands, and head from moment to moment.

Legs *firmly stretching up*

Back *relaxed*

Arms *forming a right angle*

Shoulders *lifting*

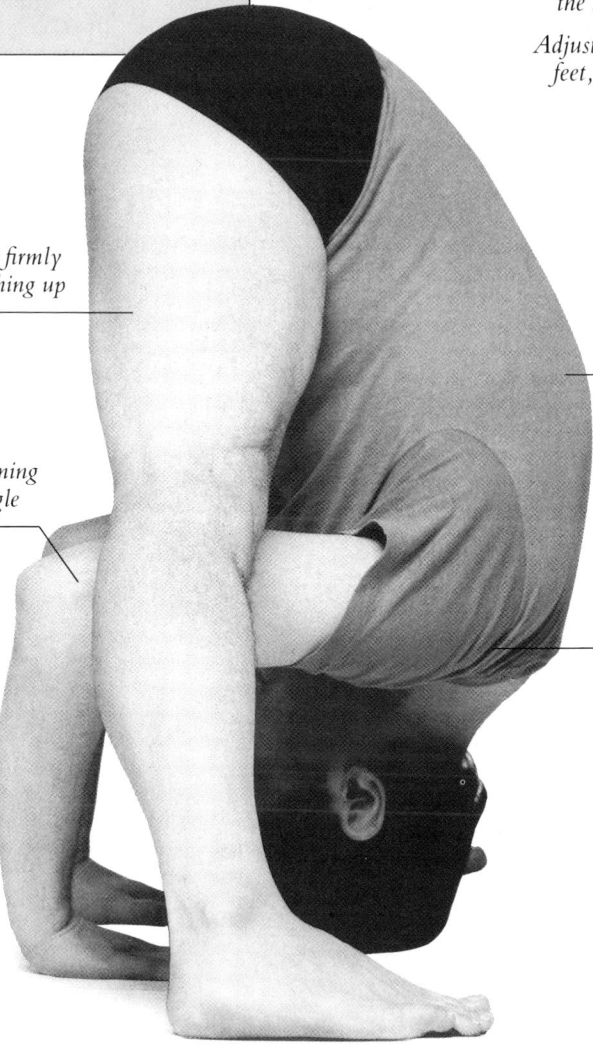

Focus *Hitting the legs outward*
With a strong, swift action move the inner legs away from each other; do not disturb the feet.

PRASĀRITA PĀDOTTĀNĀSANA II
◆
This is done with the hands in Pārśvottānāsana (p. 40). It is more difficult, as the trunk bends down without the support of the hands. ◆◆◆

उत्तानासन १

Uttānāsana I

UTTĀNA = extension

THIS IS a version of Uttānāsana done for relaxing purposes, in which the body elongates passively.♦

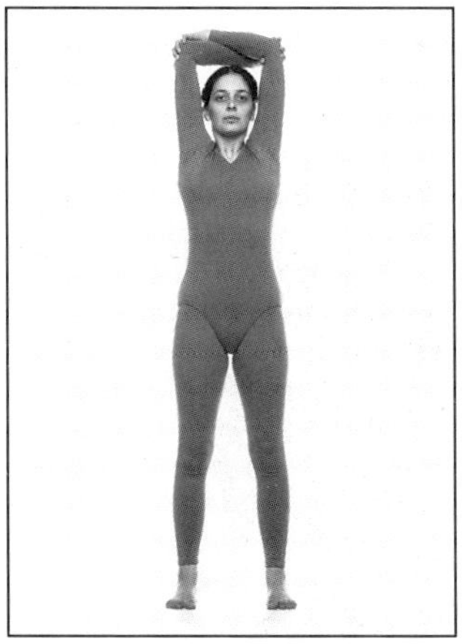

1 Stand with the feet about 1ft apart. Clasp the elbows, inhale, and stretch the arms over the head. Take the elbows back.

2 Exhale and take the trunk and arms down, keeping the legs firmly stretched up and vertical. Pull on the elbows and extend the whole body down. Relax the head and neck.

WAYS OF PRACTICING

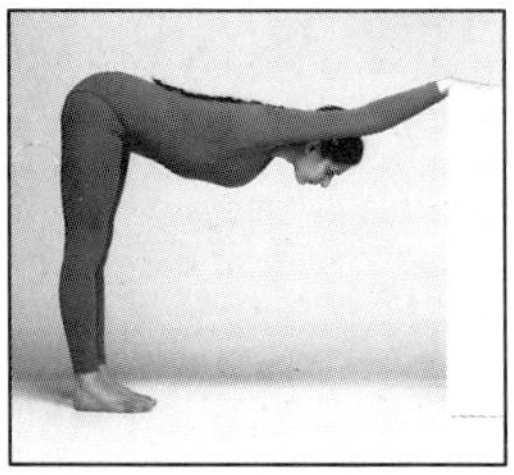

If you have a bad back or cannot bend, place the hands on a ledge, at hip level. Stretch forward.

Take the legs further apart.

For sciatica, take the heels out and the toes in.

WORK IN THE POSTURE

Separate the buttock bones.

Keep the abdomen relaxed and moving towards the chest. Bring the hips and lower abdomen toward the thighs.

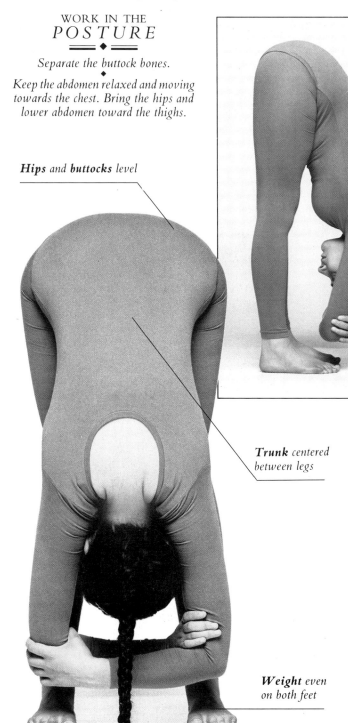

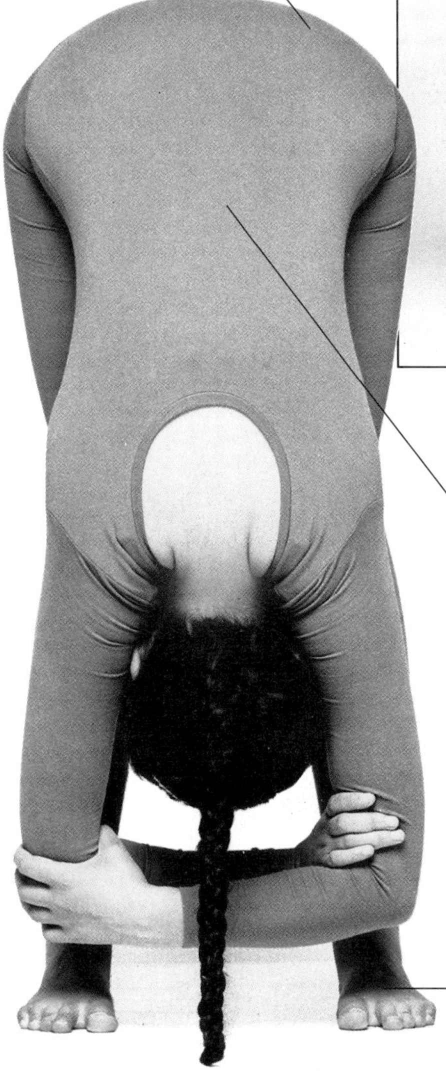

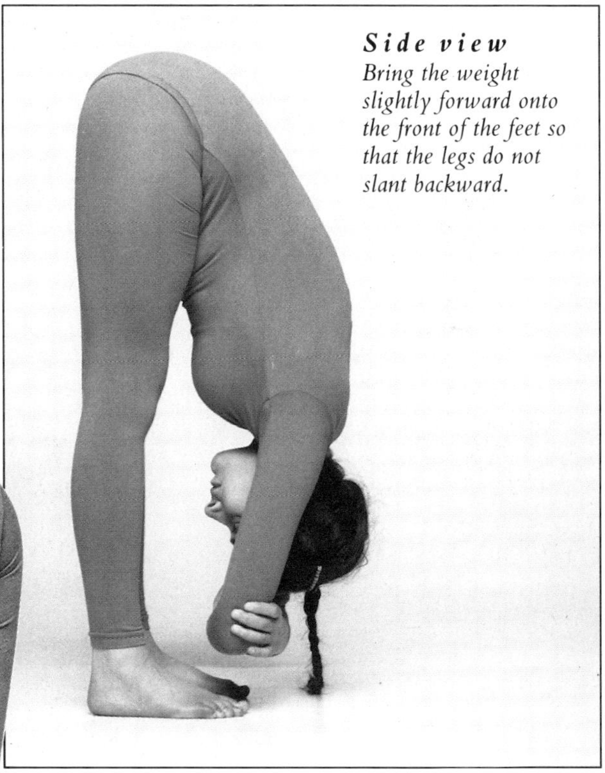

Side view
Bring the weight slightly forward onto the front of the feet so that the legs do not slant backward.

Focus *Straightening the knees*
Take the tops of the shin bones back and up. Stretch the knees up and tuck first the bottom corners of the kneecaps into the knee joints, and then the top corners. Move the bottom of the thigh bones in, then pull up the thigh muscles, and press them back to grip the bones. Open the backs of the knees horizontally from the center and vertically from the base. Do not jerk the knees but make the actions smooth and sensitive.

उत्तानासन २

Uttānāsana II

AN INTENSE upward stretch of the legs is matched by a strong downward extension of the trunk.♦♦

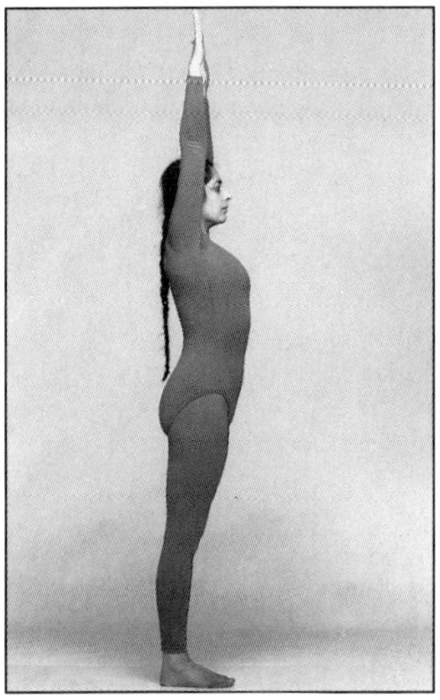

1 Stand in Tāḍāsana (p. 18). Inhale and stretch the arms up as in Ūrdhva Hastāsana (p. 19).

WAYS OF PRACTICING

If you are stiff, keep the feet 1ft apart.

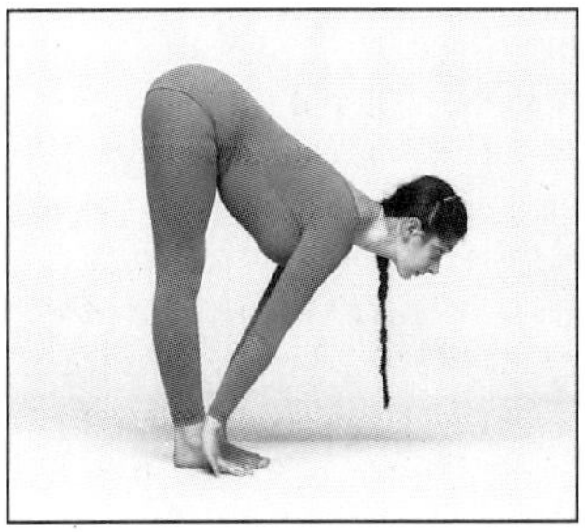

2 With an exhalation sweep the trunk and the arms down, placing the hands on the floor beside the feet or a little further back. Look up.

In going down, move the buttock bones outward and lift them away from the thighs.

3 Bring the hips, abdomen, and chest closer to the legs and place the head on the shins. Extend the trunk down. Relax the abdomen, the head, and the neck. Keep the knees straight and draw up the thigh muscles. Stay for 20 to 30 seconds, breathing evenly.

Inhale and come up, stretching the arms up. Exhale and take the arms down.

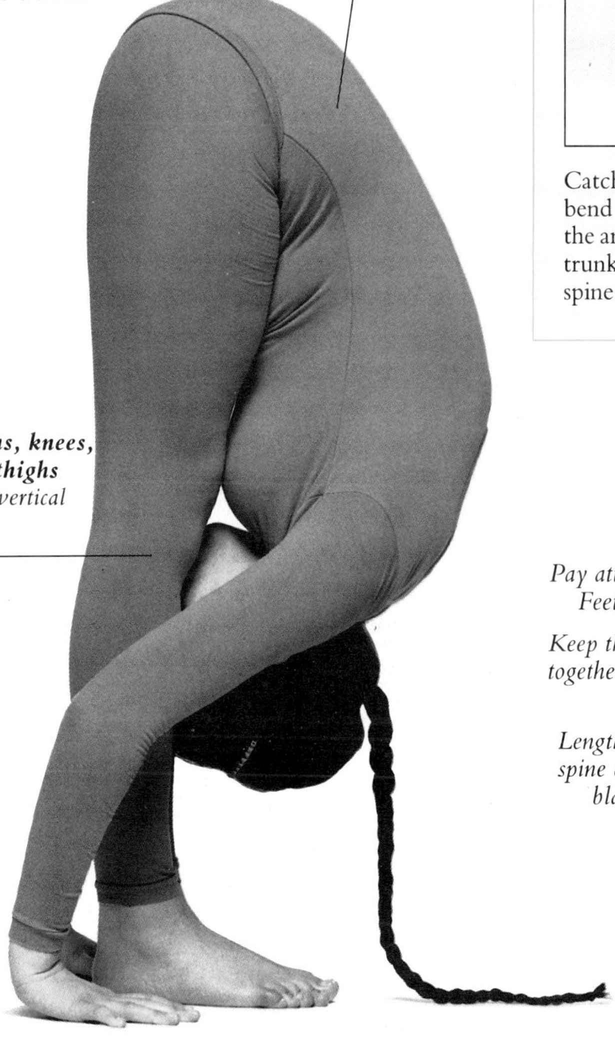

VARIATION

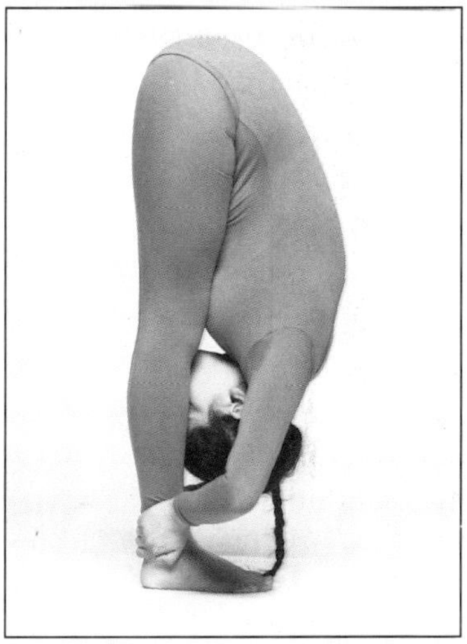

Catch the ankles from behind and bend the elbows outward. Pull on the ankles to stretch the sides of the trunk down and to release the spine.♦♦♦

WORK IN THE
POSTURE

Pay attention to the feet (see Tāḍāsana, Feet, p. 18). Keep the toes active.

Keep the inner ankles, knees, and thighs together. Stretch to the tops of the thighs. Roll the hip sockets in.

Lengthen the front of the body and the spine downward, keeping the shoulder blades pulled toward the waist.

गरुडासन

Garuḍāsana

GARUḌA = the eagle deity in Indian mythology

IN THIS balancing posture the arms and legs are intricately entwined.♦

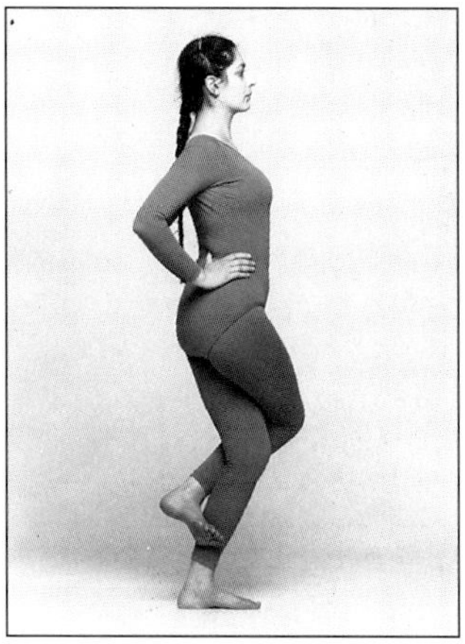

1 Stand in Tāḍāsana (p. 18). Keep the hands on the hips. ▷Bend the legs slightly. Raise the right leg and balance on the left. With an exhalation cross the right thigh and knee over the left, and take the right shin behind the left calf. Hook the toes of the right foot around the inside of the left shin.

2 Bend the elbows and cross them in front of the chest with the forearms stretching up and the thumbs facing the head. Cross the left elbow over the right, fitting it snugly into the notch of the elbow. Moving the right hand toward the head and the left away from it, cross the hands and place the fingers of the right hand on the left palm.

Raise the elbows to shoulder level. Stretch the hands and fingers up. Stay, breathing evenly, for 20 to 30 seconds.

Release the arms and legs and stand straight.◁ Repeat from ▷to◁, standing on the right leg.

Focus *Synchronizing arm and leg movements*
Gradually learn to swing the right leg into place in one movement and the arms together in another movement. Later synchronize the actions of the legs and arms.

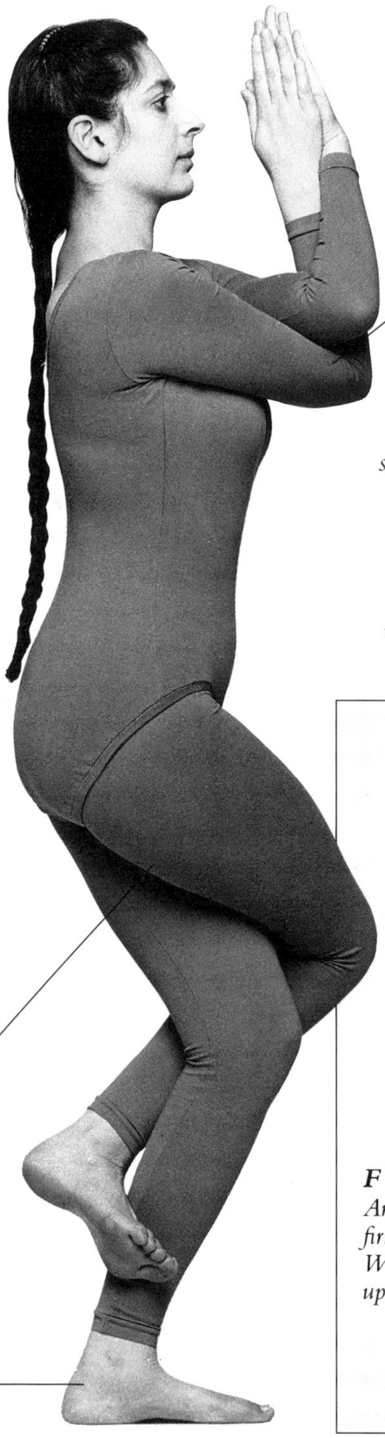

WORK IN THE
POSTURE

Concentrate on balance. Be steady on the left foot and keep the heel and big toe down.

♦

Do not let the knee turn outward.

♦

Learn to extend the trunk upward though the legs are bent.

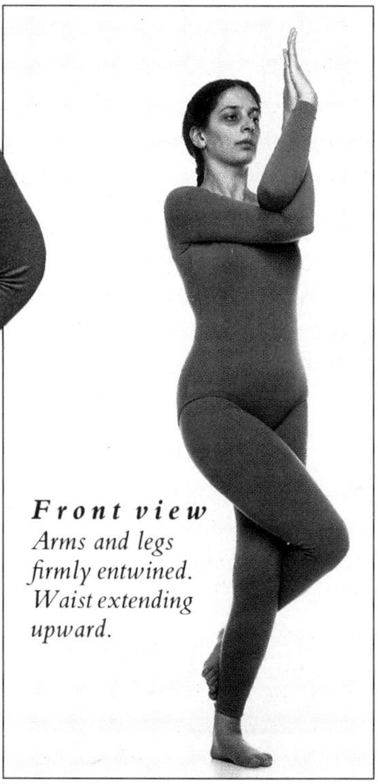

Front view
Arms and legs firmly entwined. Waist extending upward.

उत्कटासन

Utkaṭāsana

UTKAṬA = powerful, mighty

THE BENT legs and upstretched trunk and arms form a dynamic zigzag. The heels and arms extend in opposite directions while the hips move down as if to sit.♦

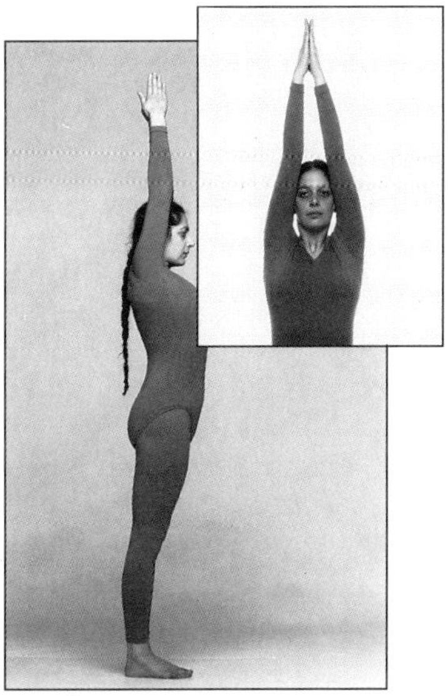

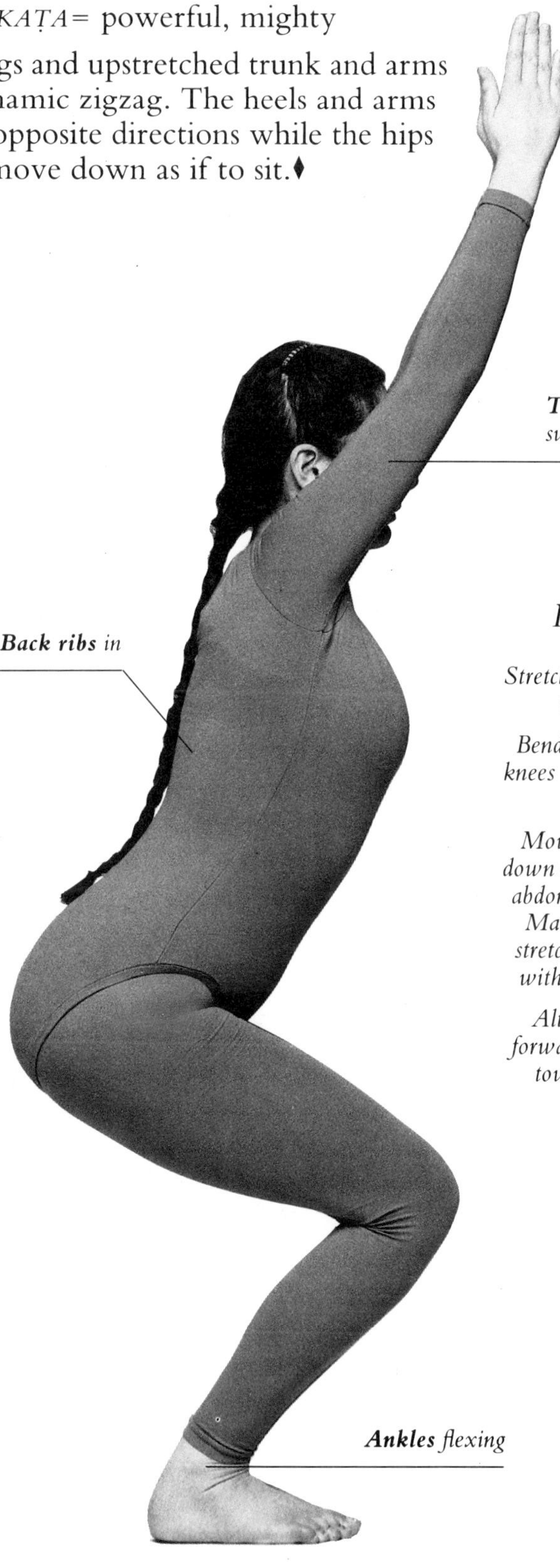

1 Stand in Tāḍāsana (p. 18). Inhale and stretch the arms forward and up. Join the palms (or keep the arms parallel).

2 Keeping the heels down and the arms and upper torso lifted, exhale and bend the legs by about 60°. Bend the ankles, knees, and hips.

Keep a firm grip on the back of the body. Stretch it up, moving the kidney area, back ribs, and shoulder blades deep in. Extend the abdomen, lift the rib cage and stretch the armpits. Pull the waist, the top of the trunk, and the arms back. Keep the elbows straight. Look ahead. Stay for 20 to 30 seconds, breathing evenly.

With an exhalation straighten the legs and bring the arms down.

WORK IN THE POSTURE

Stretch the Achilles tendons and the calf muscles up.

♦

Bend more in the ankles and knees to make the angles of the joints more acute.

♦

Move the tops of the thighs down more and lift the hips and abdomen away from the legs. Maintain a strong upward stretch of the trunk and arms without creating any strain.

♦

Although the trunk leans forward, keep pulling it back toward the vertical axis.

परीघासन

Parīghāsana

PARĪGHA = gate, crossbar

FROM A kneeling position the trunk extends to the side, creating a gate with a crossbar.♦

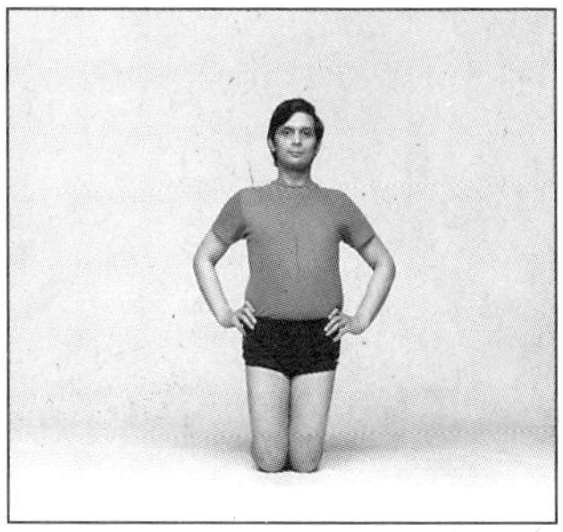

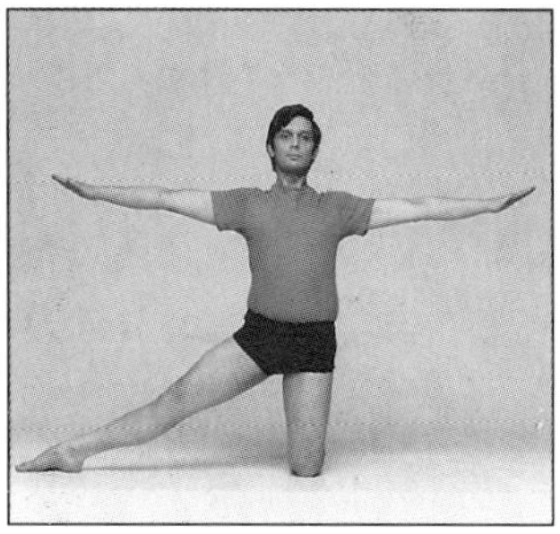

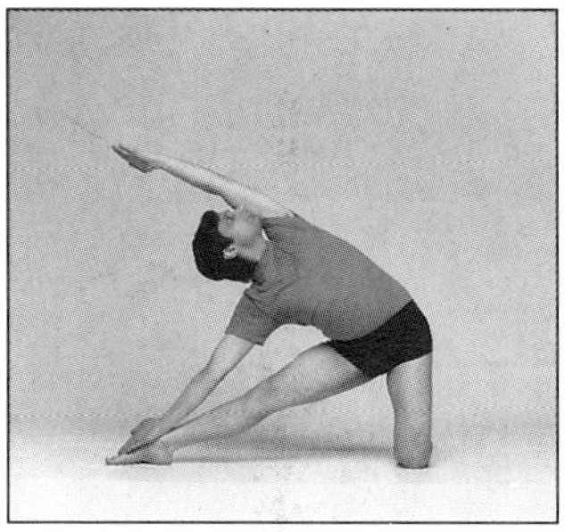

1 Kneel with the thighs perpendicular, knees and feet together and in line, hands on the hips.

Press the hips down and extend the trunk up. Open the chest and take the shoulders back. Bring the tops of the thighs and the hips slightly forward and move the coccyx in.

Take a few breaths. Pay attention to alignment.

2 ▷Exhale and stretch the right leg out to the right; simultaneously extend the arms to the sides. Straighten the right knee and turn the thigh outward in its socket; keep the knee facing the ceiling and the leg in line with the hip.

Extend the right heel along the floor; stretch the sole up, then put the foot down, in line with the leg.

3 With an exhalation bend the trunk sideways toward the right leg. Extend the right arm and rest the back of the hand on the shin; stretch the left arm over the ear. Revolve the front of the body up and the left side back, to keep the trunk facing forward.

4 As the trunk goes down, start turning the arms and palms. (Synchronize the movements of the trunk and the arms.) Extend the right arm further and rest the hand on the foot; at the same time extend the left arm down toward the right hand.

Turn the head and look up. Stay for 20 to 30 seconds, breathing evenly.

Inhale, come up, bring the right leg up to kneeling position, and stretch up. Line yourself up.◁

Repeat from ▷to◁ on the left.

WAYS OF PRACTICING

Keep the sole of the right foot raised on a pad.

WORK IN THE POSTURE

Tuck the top of the right thigh in toward the hip. Bend more in the hip joint and slide the trunk closer toward the leg.

♦

Keep the trunk extended and the arms straight. Make the right side of the back concave.

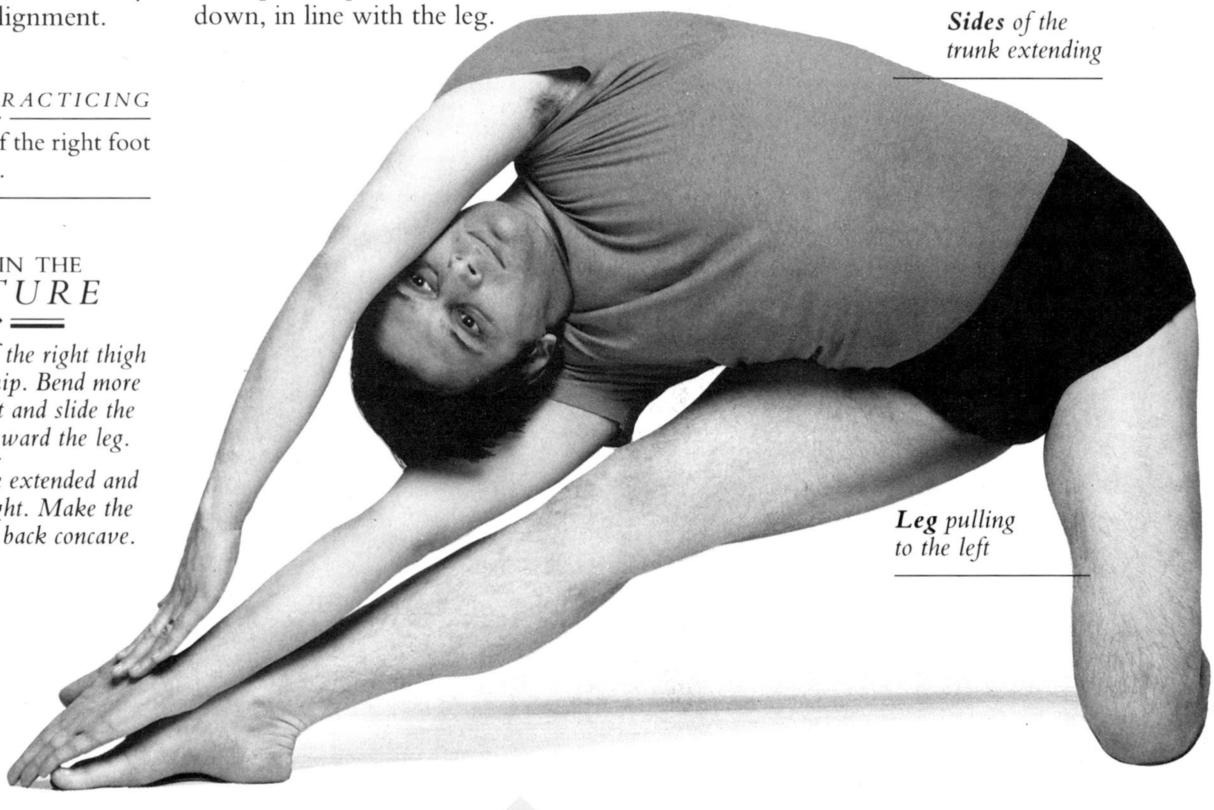
***Sides** of the trunk extending*
***Leg** pulling to the left*

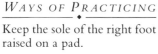

SITTING POSES

Extension brings space, space brings freedom, freedom brings precision. Precision is truth and truth is God.

B. K. S. IYENGAR

The sitting poses are calming. They remove fatigue, refresh the brain, and soothe the nerves. They regularize blood pressure and aid recovery from illness. They promote healthy sleep.

They fall into two categories: upright postures that involve flexing the legs into different positions, and forward bends where the trunk bends over the legs.

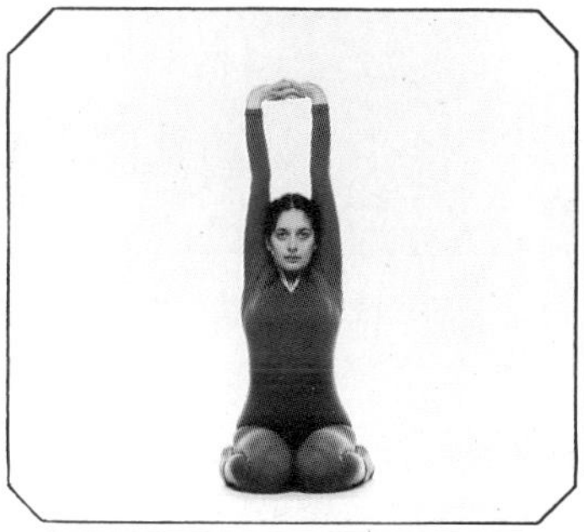

GUIDELINES FOR PRACTICE

It is best to sit on one or two folded blankets to give the lower back freedom to move.

The body should be lined up with the room. When the forward bends are done thoughtfully, with quiet breathing, they induce a calm, meditative frame of mind. They can also be done energetically, with vigorous breathing. This is refreshing, as tremendous freedom is created in the spine through stretching. Another way of working is to stretch up with a concave back. This strengthens the spine and helps the front of the body to extend.

When using a belt around the foot, the foot should press into it and the hands should pull on it, to bring the trunk forward.

The minimum length of time has been given for staying in the postures. This should be gradually increased as the muscles of the back are toned, as long as there is no strain anywhere.

Forward bends done with the forehead resting on a bolster or stool (see p. 64) are recuperative and may be held for several minutes at a time.

The forward bends are particularly suitable for practicing during menstruation.

Sometimes the bent knee may feel strained, particularly if it is weak or injured. In this case it is essential to support it and to work carefully (see pp. 50-51, 54-5). With correct practice it will gradually become stronger.

Twists may be done after forward bends if the back feels strained.

CAUTIONS: Do forward bends with concave movements if the lower back is weak and prone to backache or if suffering from depression.

During pregnancy take care to avoid strain: use a belt to catch the foot so that the lower back and the abdomen can lift.

वीरासन

Vīrāsana

VĪRA = a hero

THIS IS wonderful for refreshing and relaxing the legs when they are tired. It may be used for sitting in meditation.♦

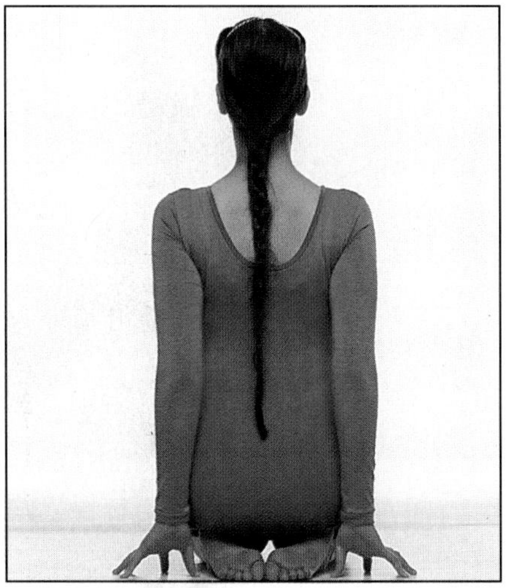

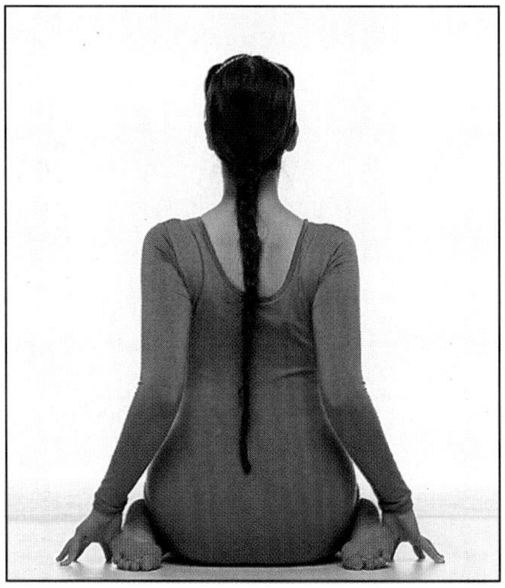

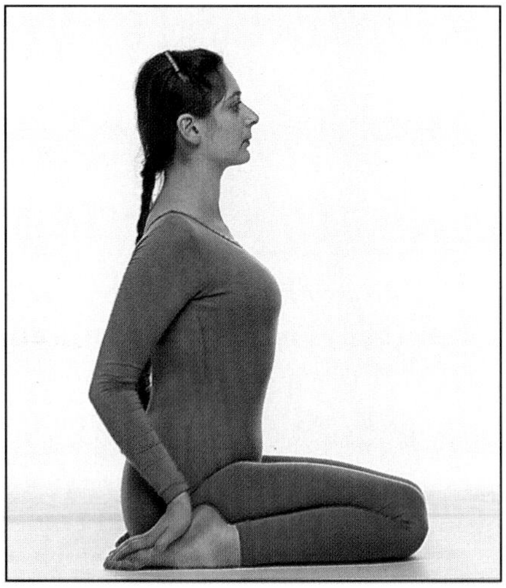

1 Sit upright on the heels, with the knees level and facing forward. Be on the centers of the feet.

WAYS OF PRACTICING

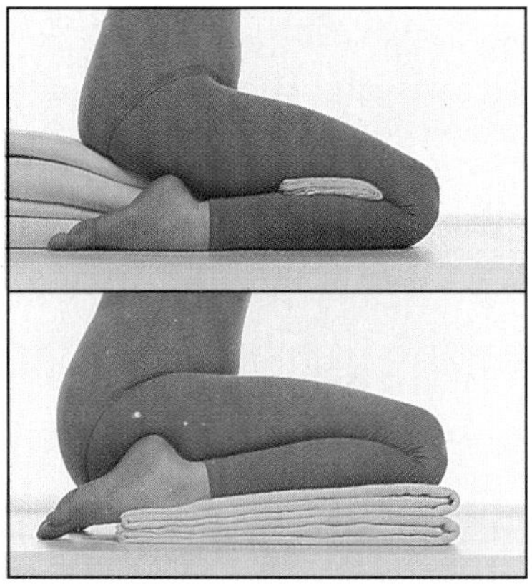

To prevent strain, sit on folded blankets to lift the lower back and to make the legs comfortable.

Place a thinly folded towel behind the knees.

For stiff feet and ankles, kneel with the shins on two or three blankets, with the feet hanging over the edge.

2 Take the feet a little apart and sit on the edges of the heels. Lift the buttocks for a moment and, with the fingers, ease the outer calf muscles to the sides and away from the knees. Then separate the feet still further and sit between them. Keep the knees together.

Alternative method
Kneel as in step 1 of Parīghāsana (p. 48). Spread the feet apart and sit between the legs.

3 Turn the arms out and place the hands on the feet, fingers on the toes. Revolve the thighs and knees outward so that the shins face the floor and the front thighs face the ceiling. Center the trunk and stretch both sides up evenly. Keep the head straight and draw the gaze inward. Once the legs are comfortable, stay for 5 to 10 minutes.

Release the legs.

वीरासन

WORK IN THE POSTURE

Raise the hips, keeping the buttock bones down; stretch the abdomen and the trunk up.

◆

Move the lumbar and the kidneys in without projecting the floating ribs forward.

◆

Lift the diaphragm. Keep the shoulders balanced over the hips and sit with the back erect.

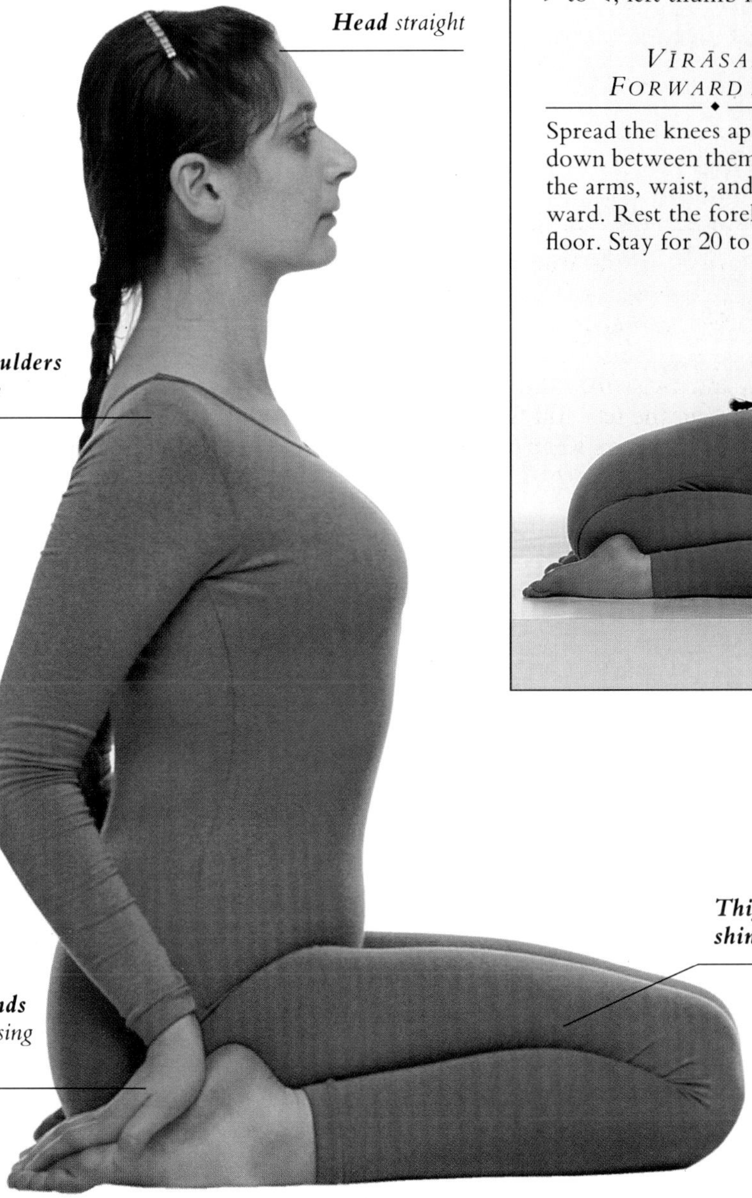

PARVATĀSANA

PARVATA = mountain

▷Interlock the fingers with the right thumb base over the left, base of the fingers in contact. Turn the palms out and stretch the arms forward and up. Lock the elbows. Open the armpits. Pull up the trunk with the arms. Take the arms further back. Stay for 15 to 20 seconds. Bring the arms down.◁ Repeat from ▷to◁, left thumb in front.♦

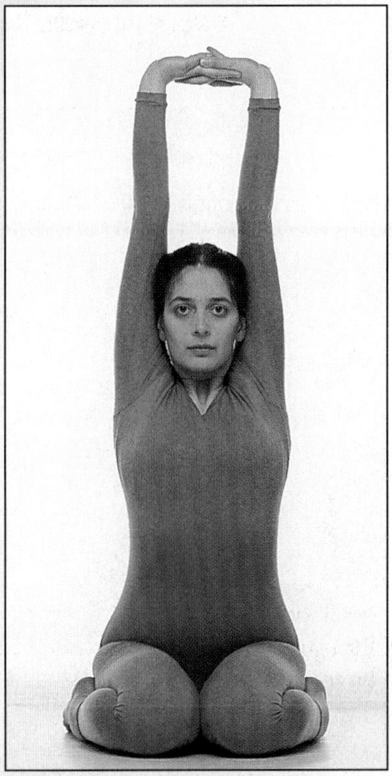

VĪRĀSANA FORWARD BEND

Spread the knees apart, bend down between them, and extend the arms, waist, and chest forward. Rest the forehead on the floor. Stay for 20 to 30 seconds.♦

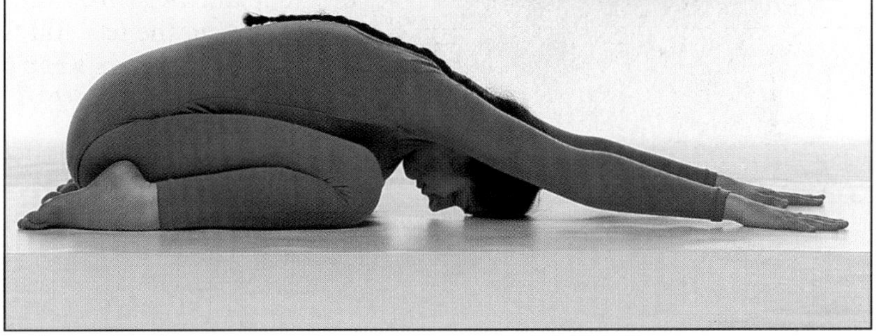

दंडासन

Daṇḍāsana

DAṆḌA= a stick or staff

THIS POSTURE is the basis of the sitting poses and twists. The trunk is erect and the legs are stretched straight.♦

Sit on the floor with the legs stretched out in front and the trunk upright. Join the inner knees and inner ankles. Place the palms on the floor beside the hips, fingers pointing forward. Stay for 15 to 20 seconds.

Legs and Feet

Extend the legs and heels forward, keeping them parallel and centered. Stretch the soles, the tops of the feet, and the toes up. Keep the feet parallel: move the inner edges of the feet away from the legs and draw the outer edges slightly back.

Straighten the knees by pressing the kneecaps into the knee joints and stretching the backs of the knees. Press the thighs, knees, and shins down. Tuck the tops of the thighs in toward the trunk.

Ways of Practicing

If the lower back sags, sit on two folded blankets.

Front view *Keep the chest lifted and broad*

Trunk and Arms

Pressing the hands into the floor, extend the sides and the back of the body up. Stretch the sacrum and lumbar. Lift the rib cage; press the shoulder blades into the back. Rotate the upper arms outward and lock the elbows.

Extend the front of the body from the pubis up. Keep the lower abdomen slightly pulled back, without tensing it. Lift the sternum, the top ribs and the collarbones. Move the shoulders back and down. Open the chest and breathe evenly.

Head

Do not let the head tilt. Keep it straight and look ahead.

Focus *Alignment*
(See also Tāḍāsana, p. 18). Keep both sides of the body parallel. Center the face and the trunk.

Reflection
Paying attention to detail brings precision in the postures. Precision leads to perfection and truth. Truth is divinity. Being observant trains the inner eye to see subtle movements within the body. As practice becomes more accurate, the body responds with pointers to further refinements. In this way practice is filled with the light of understanding, and clarity in Yoga is attained.

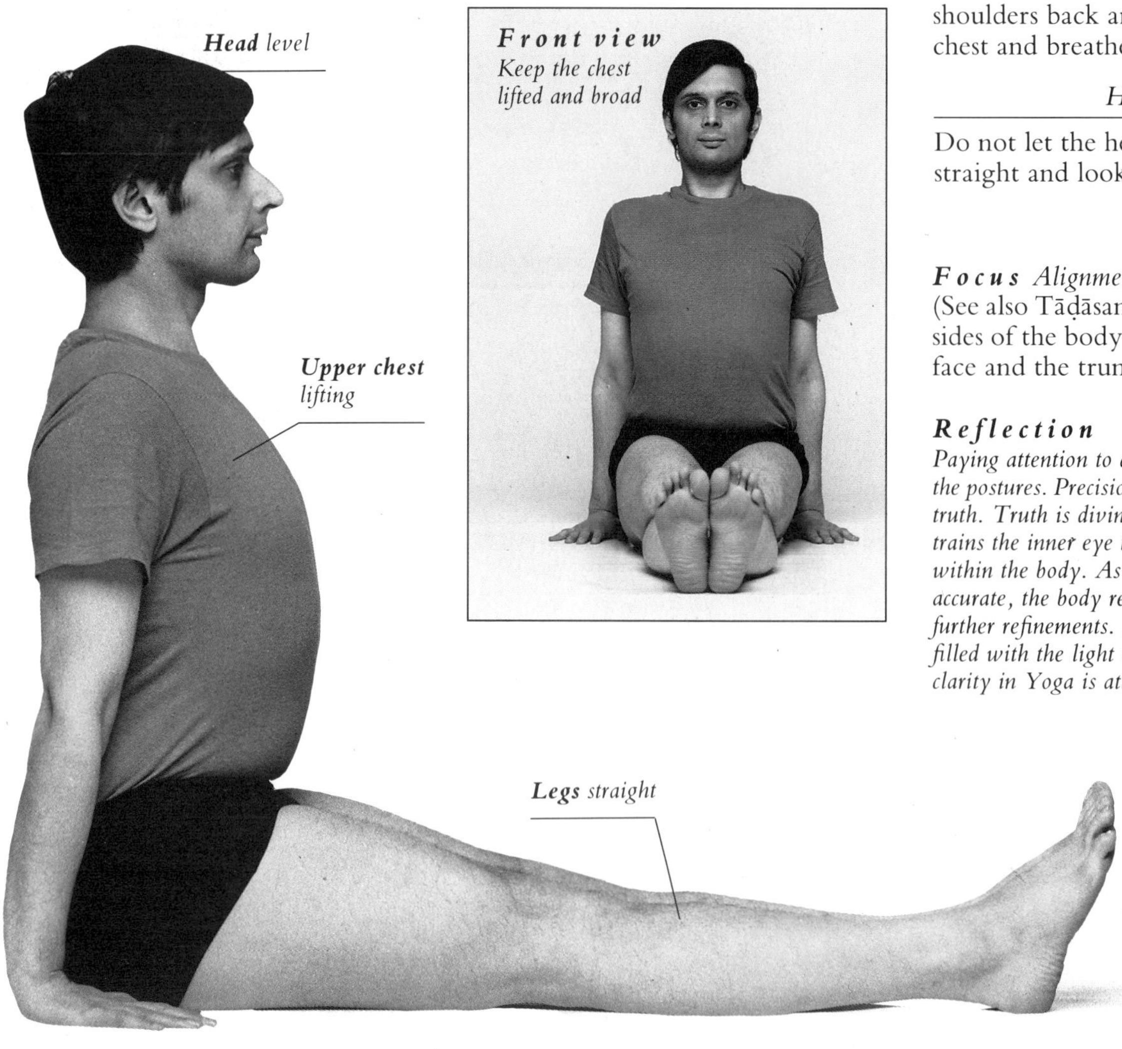

सुखासन

Sukhāsana

SUKHA = happy, easy, comfortable

THIS IS an easy posture, where the legs are crossed simply.♦

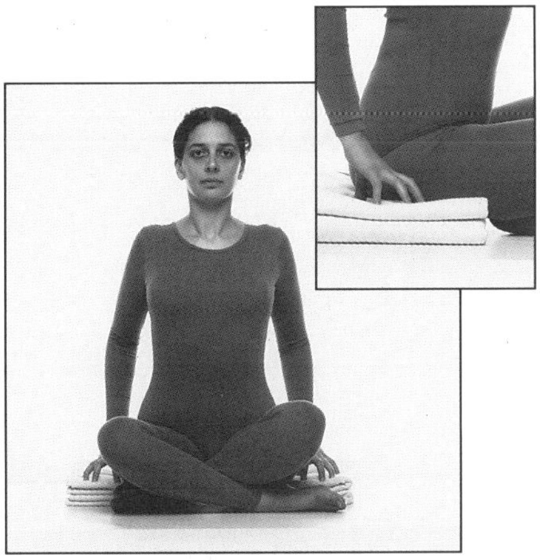

1 Sit in Daṇḍāsana (p. 52) ▷ Bend the legs and cross the right shin over the left. Draw the knees closer together. Place the hands beside the hips, cupping the fingers.

WAYS OF PRACTICING

Sit on two or three folded blankets.

Support the thighs on blankets.

If the back is weak, sit against a wall with a small cushion behind the waist or chest.

2 Keep the seat firm. Press the fingertips into the floor to lift the trunk up vertically. Rest the hands on the knees. (To sit straighter, stretch the arms over the head. Maintaining the upward lift, bring the arms down.)

Breathe evenly. Stay for 20 to 30 seconds, keeping the head straight, the eyes relaxed. ◁

Repeat from ▷ to ◁, crossing the left shin over the right.

PARVATĀSANA

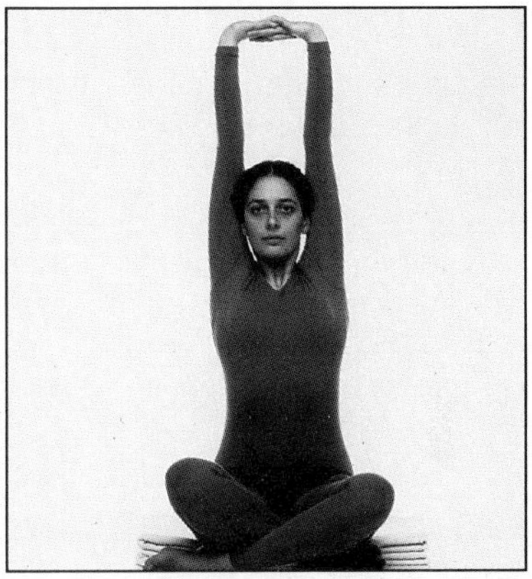

Do Parvatāsana as in Vīrāsana (p. 51). Repeat on the other side.♦

SUKHĀSANA FORWARD BEND

Bend over the legs, stretching the arms forward, head on the floor.♦

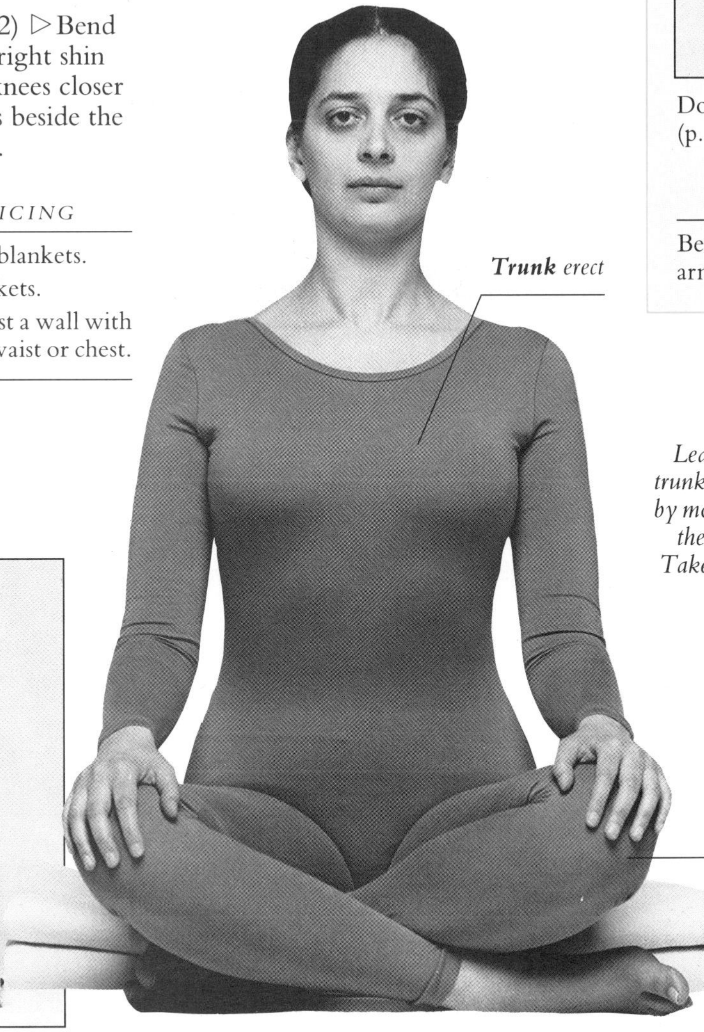

WORK IN THE POSTURE

Learn to sit straight. Stretch the lower trunk up without tensing it. Open the chest by moving the dorsal spine in and widening the front ribs away from the sternum. Take the shoulders back. Drop the upper arms down.

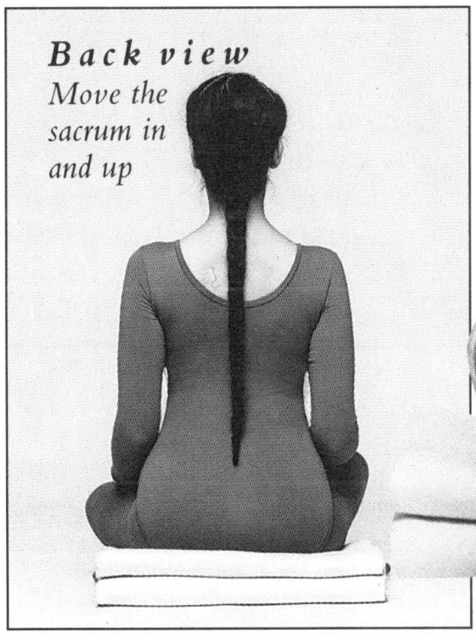

पद्मासन

Padmāsana

PADMA = a lotus, symbol of creation

THE TRUNK rises from the compact support of the crossed legs. This is one of the principal postures used in meditation.♦♦

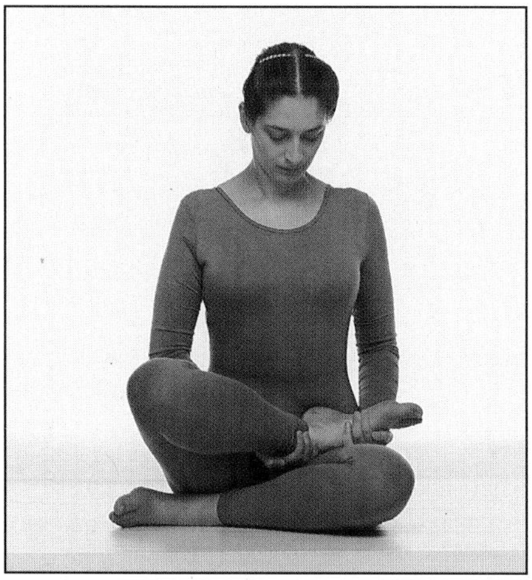

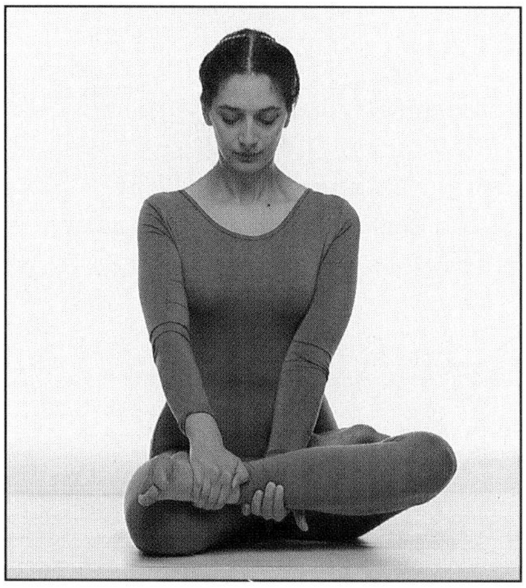

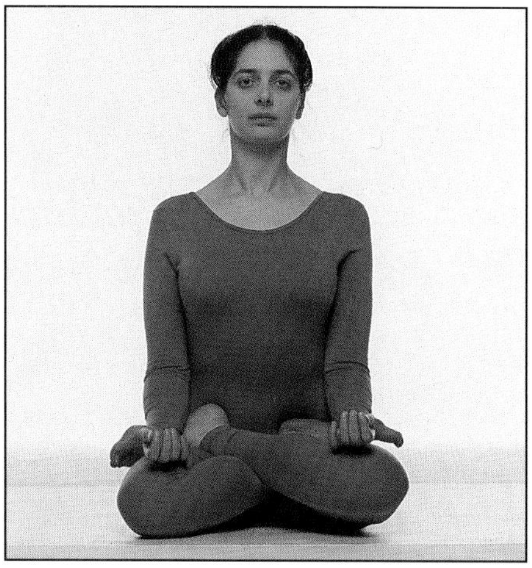

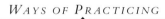

1 Sit in Sukhāsana (p. 53). ▷Hold the right foot. Place it on top of the left thigh with the outer edge of the foot pressed into the groin. Roll the right hip in; bring the knee in to face almost forward.

2 Bring the left foot forward, in front of the right shin; then lift it over into the right groin.

WAYS OF PRACTICING

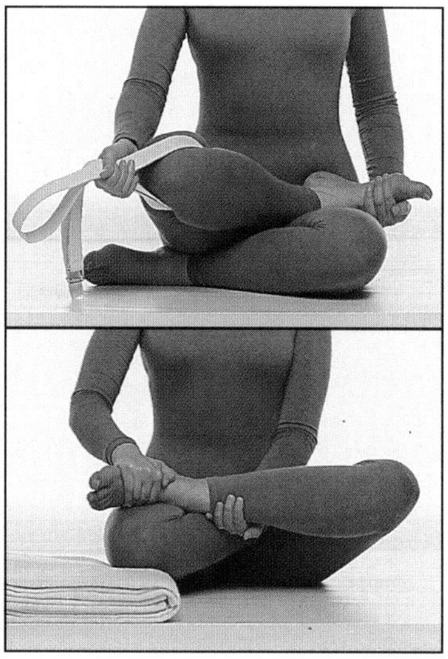

For knee problems, open the back of the knee by pulling on a belt. Place a thin pad into the back of the knee joint.

Sit on folded blankets to raise the lumbar.

If the right knee does not reach the floor, support it on a blanket. Then take the left foot up.

3 Move the feet further up into the groin and bring the knees closer together.

Sit straight, extending the trunk up. Open the chest and take the shoulders back. Make the posture stable. Rest the hands on the thighs, palms facing up.

Stay for 20 to 30 seconds, breathing evenly. Do not strain the knees. Once they are strong, stay for 5 to 10 minutes or longer.

With an exhalation release the legs.◁ Repeat from ▷to◁ on the left.

Focus *Bending the legs in Padmāsana* Before the foot is in place, bend the leg carefully. With the fingers, press in the skin and flesh of the back of the knee. This creates space in the knee joint and helps it to bend without strain. Then draw the thigh and calf together. When the foot is in place, ease the skin and flesh of the inner calf and thigh up, using the fingers.

पद्मासन

WORK IN THE POSTURE

◆

Squeeze the thighs toward each other.

◆

Maintain the lift of the body. Pull up the coccyx and the buttock muscles.

◆

Move the shoulder blades in. Lift the diaphragm. Sit steadily, keeping the face relaxed.

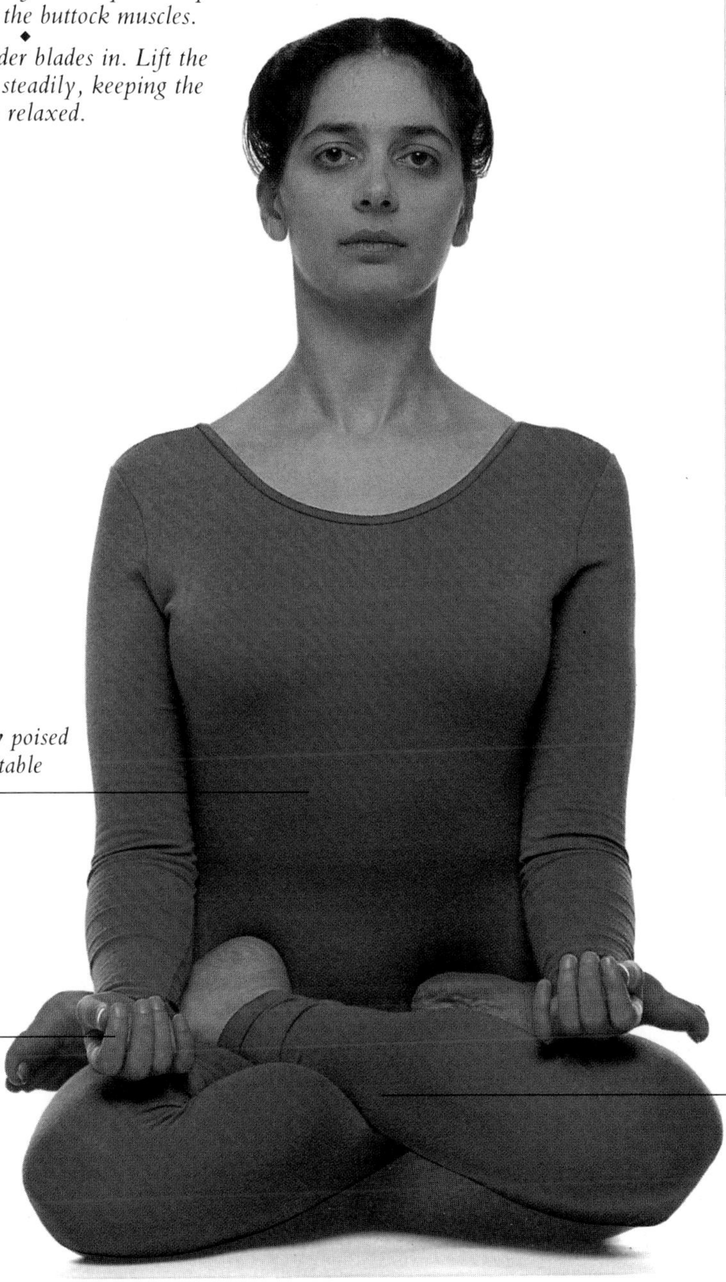

***Body** poised and stable*

***Palms** relaxed*

***Shins** crossed*

BADDHA PADMĀSANA

◆

BADDHA = bound

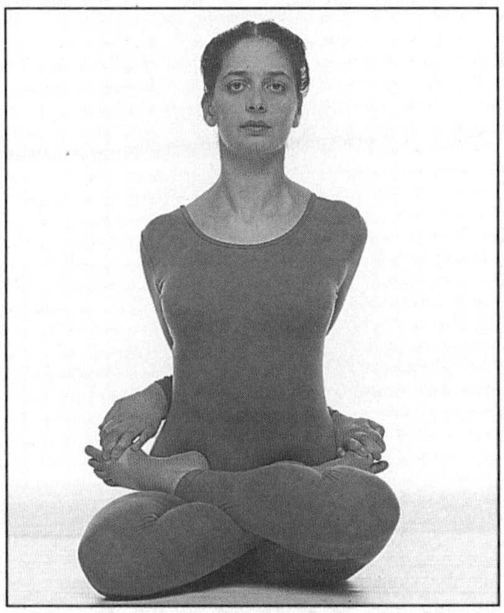

Here the feet are caught from behind.

▷In Padmāsana, swing the arms back and hold the left foot from behind with the left hand, and the right foot with the right hand. (Catch the top foot first.)

Grip the toes firmly and catch further. Draw the elbows closer together, pull the shoulders back and make them level. Pull the trunk back to make it upright. Stay for 20 to 30 seconds.◁ Repeat from ▷ to◁ , changing the legs and the arms. ♦♦♦

PARVATĀSANA

◆

Do Parvatāsana as in Vīrāsana (p. 51). Repeat on the other side.♦♦

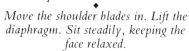

गोमुखासन

Gomukhāsana

GO = cow; *MUKHA* = face, aspect

THE CLOSELY crossed thighs and the hands clasped behind the back give this posture an asymmetrical balance.♦♦

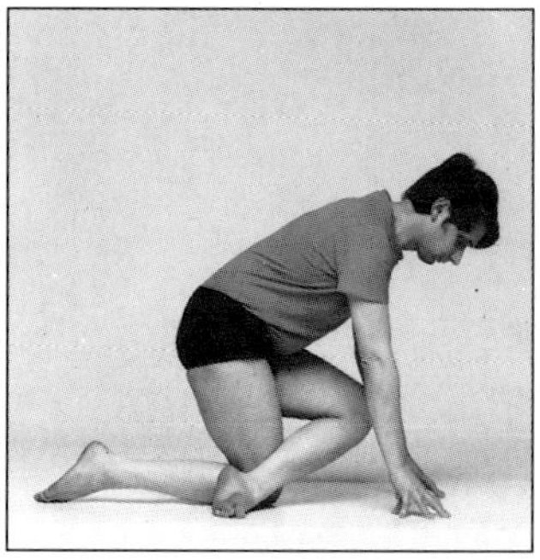

1 Sit in Daṇḍāsana (p. 52). ▷ Bend the right leg and pass the foot under the left thigh toward the buttock; turn the foot to face back. Bend forward, place the fingertips on the floor and raise the hips; bend the left leg over the right, placing the foot beside the right thigh.

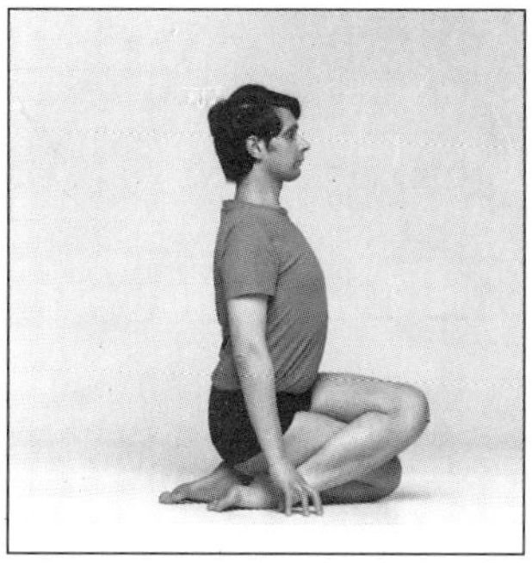

2 Cross the thighs well, rolling the left thigh from the outside in. Draw the left foot further back, as close as possible to the right foot. Be on the tops of the feet with the toes pointing back. Sit on the heels. Take the hands back and place them beside the feet.

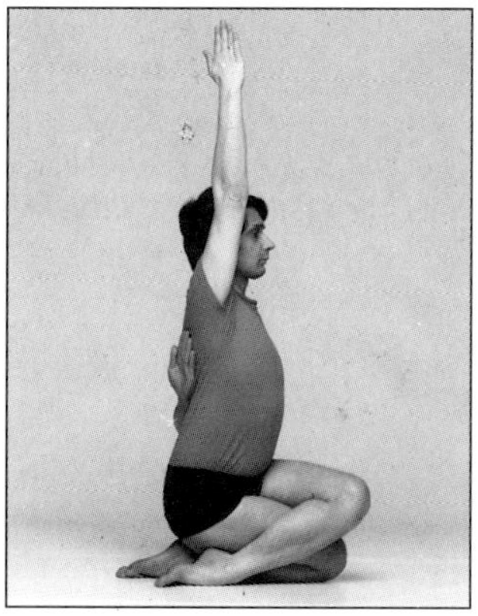

3 Keep the trunk facing forward and extend it up. Bend the left elbow behind the back and take the back of the hand high up the spine. Stretch the right arm up. (Taking the right arm back and the left arm up gives a different balance.)

4 Bend the right elbow back, stretch the hand down, and clasp the left hand or wrist with the palms facing. Stay, breathing evenly, for 15 to 20 seconds. Keep the head straight and look ahead. Release the arms and legs. ◁ Repeat from ▷ to ◁.

WAYS OF PRACTICING

Use a belt to catch the hands.

If it is difficult to sit, place a blanket on the heels, or one blanket on the heels and another under them.

WORK IN THE *POSTURE*

Learn to sit without leaning to one side. Keep the trunk balanced and centered.

♦

Open the right armpit and roll the left shoulder back. Press the shoulder blades in.

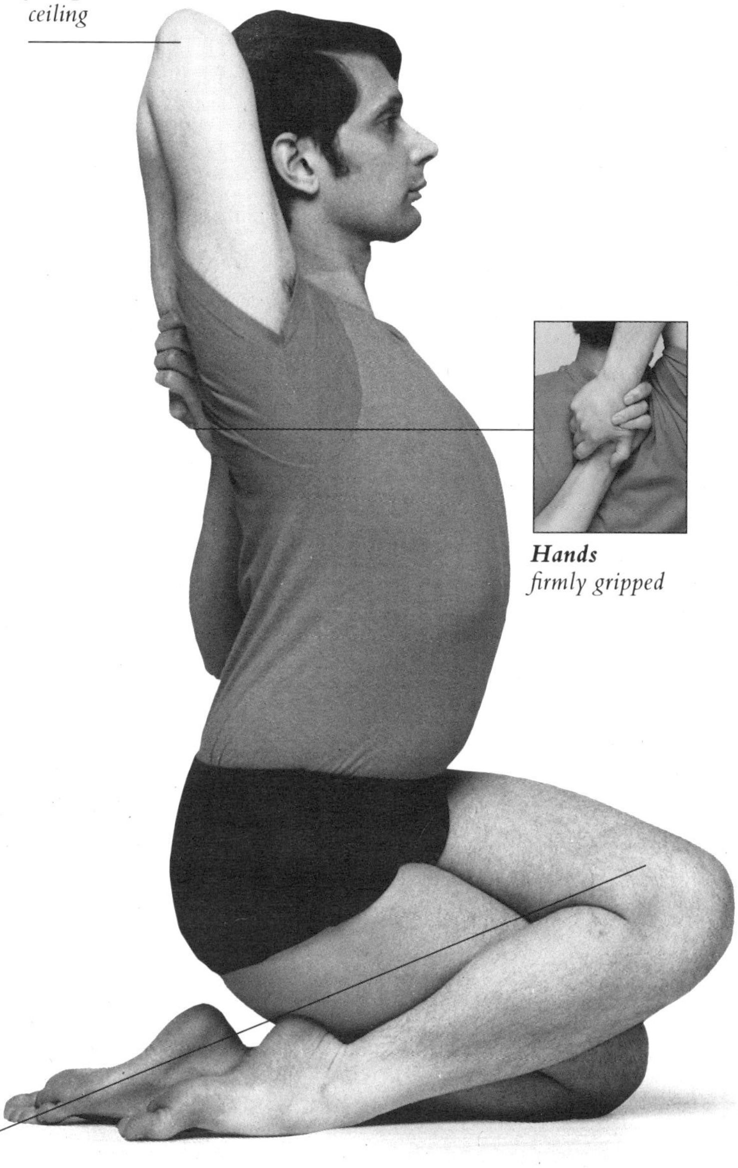

बद्ध कोणासन

Baḍdha Koṇāsana

BADDHA = bound; *KONA* = angle

THIS IS the "cobbler" pose. It strengthens the bladder and is invaluable for menstrual problems and in pregnancy.♦

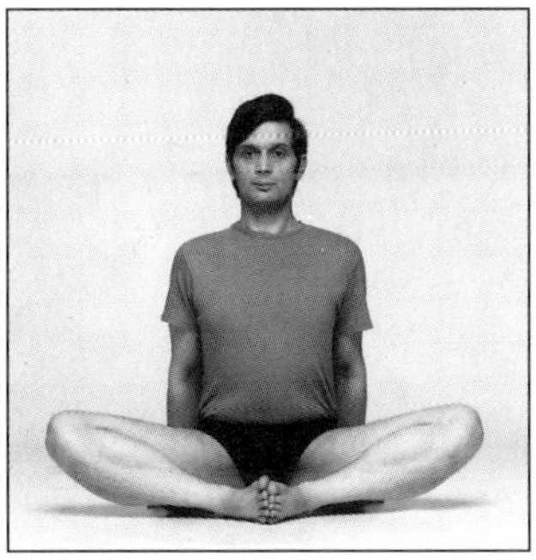

1 Sit in Daṇḍāsana (p. 52). Bend the knees to the sides and draw the heels in towards the pubis. Join the soles of the feet.

Hold the ankles and bring the feet close to the perineum. With the fingers, open the inner calf and thigh muscles upward. Keep the heels, toes, and inner and outer edges of the feet in line. Press the feet lightly together. Make both arches a similar shape.

Open the thighs outward and keep the knees level. Raise the hips. For a moment place the fingertips behind the hips and stretch the back of the body upward.

2 Clasp the fingers around the toes and pull up the abdomen, waist, and chest. Open the groin, bring the sacrum forward, and take the knees down to the ground.

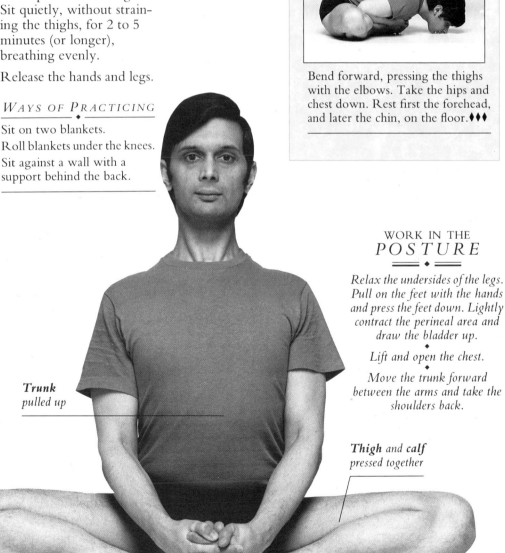

Keep the head straight. Sit quietly, without straining the thighs, for 2 to 5 minutes (or longer), breathing evenly.

Release the hands and legs.

Ways of Practicing

Sit on two blankets.

Roll blankets under the knees.

Sit against a wall with a support behind the back.

Baddha Koṇāsana Forward Bend

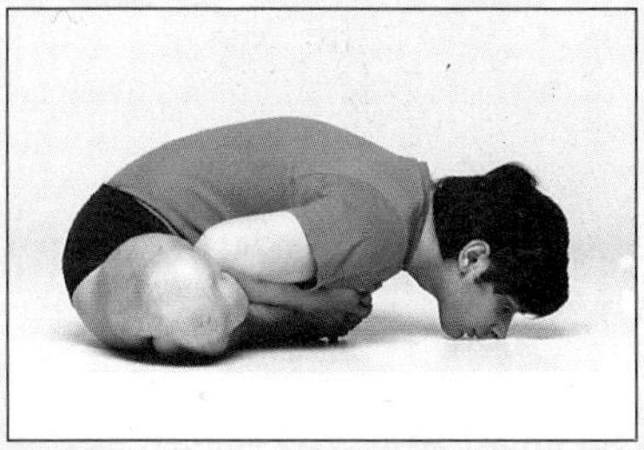

Bend forward, pressing the thighs with the elbows. Take the hips and chest down. Rest first the forehead, and later the chin, on the floor.♦♦♦

Trunk *pulled up*
Thigh *and* **calf** *pressed together*
Hands *clasping feet*

WORK IN THE POSTURE

Relax the undersides of the legs. Pull on the feet with the hands and press the feet down. Lightly contract the perineal area and draw the bladder up.

Lift and open the chest.

Move the trunk forward between the arms and take the shoulders back.

नावासन

Paripūrṇa Nāvāsana

PARIPŪRṆA = full, complete; *NAU* = boat

IN THIS posture the body is like a boat, with the arms as oars.

Sit in Daṇḍāsana (p. 52). With an exhalation raise the legs to 60° and lower the trunk by 30°; simultaneously raise the arms to shoulder level and stretch them toward the legs. Keep the palms facing each other.

Balance on the front of the buttock bones. Elongate the trunk toward the head and the legs toward the feet. Keep the knees and elbows locked. Lift the chest and look toward the feet. Do not tense the abdomen.

Stay for 20 to 30 seconds, breathing evenly.

Come down.

ARDHA NĀVĀSANA

ARDHA = half;
NAU = boat

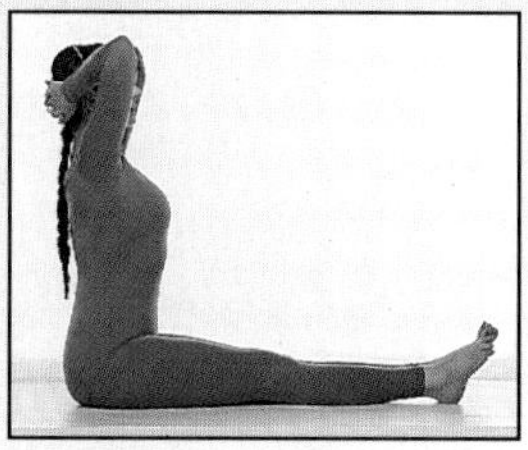

1 Sit in Daṇḍāsana (p. 52). Clasp the hands behind the head; bring the elbows slightly in so that the arms form a semicircle.

2 Exhale, lean back, lower the trunk, and raise the legs to 30°. Balance, with the legs and trunk extended above the ground. Extend the front of the body but do not tense the abdomen. Stay for 15 to 20 seconds, looking toward the feet. Release the hands and come down.

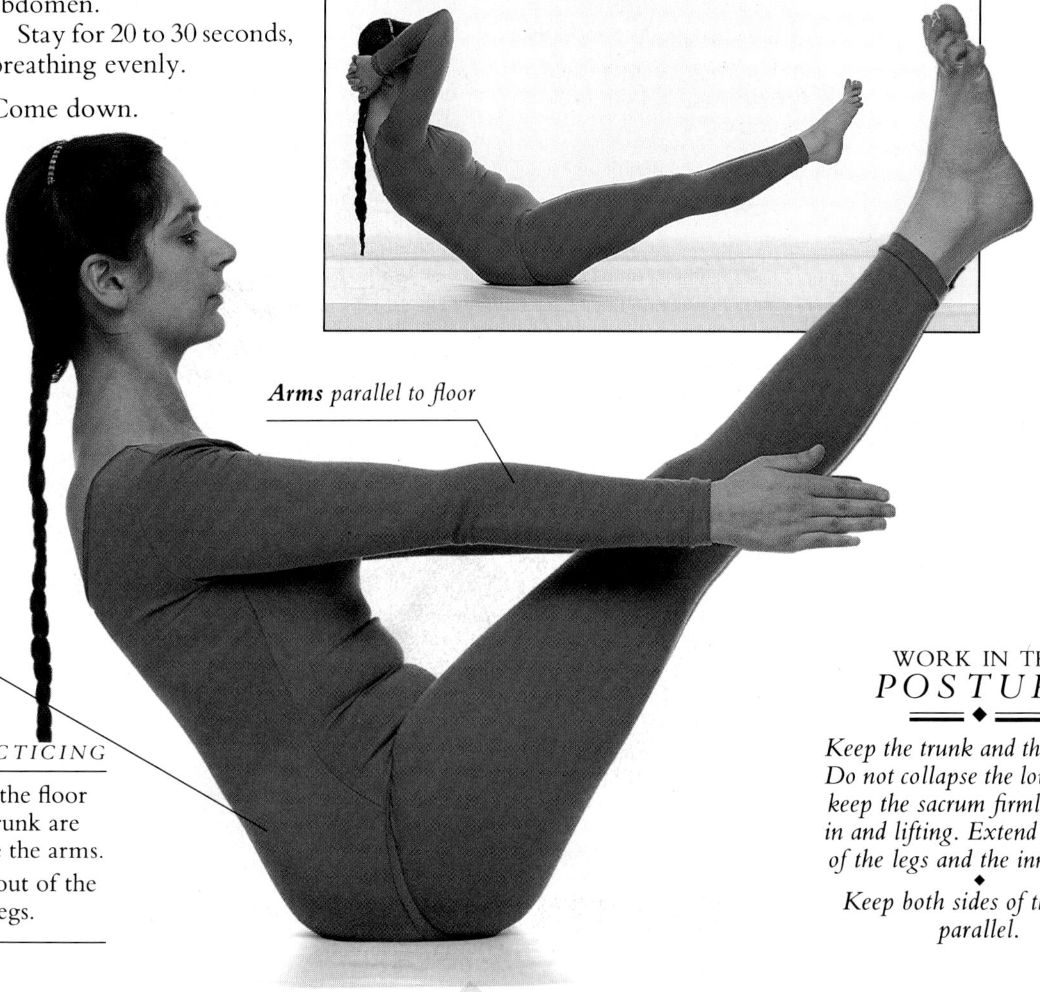

WAYS OF PRACTICING

Keep the hands on the floor until the legs and trunk are balanced; then raise the arms.

Go into and come out of the posture with bent legs.

WORK IN THE POSTURE

Keep the trunk and the legs up. Do not collapse the lower back: keep the sacrum firmly pressed in and lifting. Extend the backs of the legs and the inner heels.

Keep both sides of the body parallel.

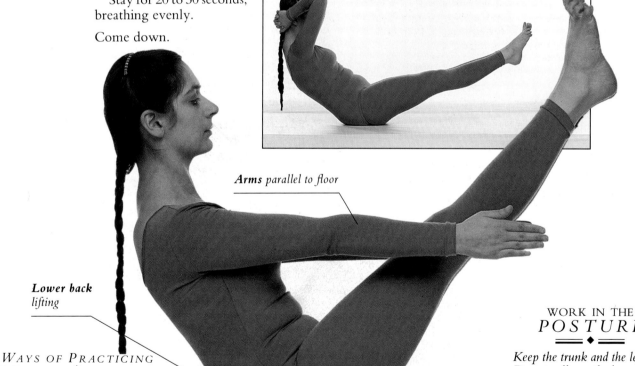

जानु शीर्षासन

Jānu Śīrṣāsana

JĀNU = knee; *ŚĪRṢA* = head

WITH ONE leg bent to the side, the trunk stretches forward.♦

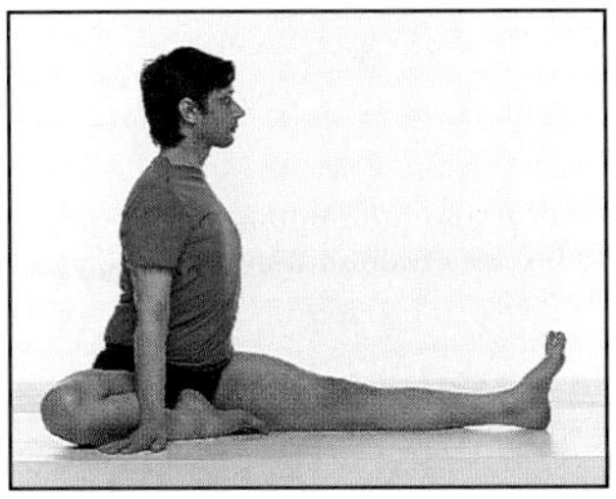

1 Sit in Daṇḍāsana (p. 52). ▷ Without disturbing the left leg, bend the right knee to the side and take it back as far as possible. Press the heel into its own thigh and let the toes touch the left inner thigh.

Bring the right hip slightly forward and turn the pubis, lower abdomen, and chest to the left, so that the sternum faces the center of the left leg. Tuck the bottom of the left hip slightly back.

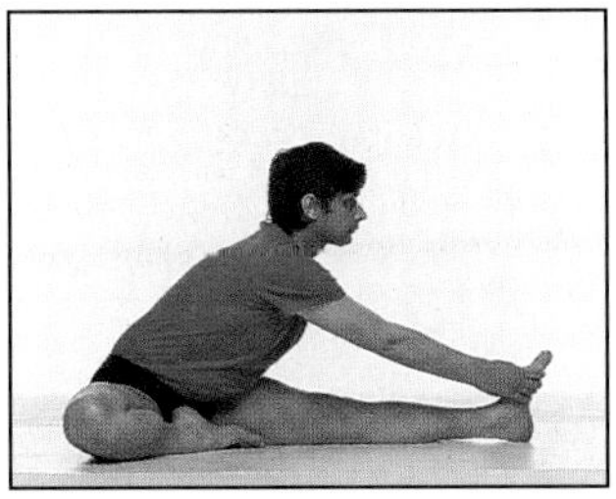

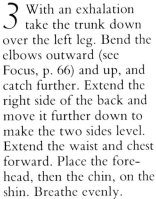

2 With an exhalation bend the hips and trunk down, stretch the arms forward, and hold the left foot.

Inhale, pull on the foot to bring the trunk forward and up. Make the back concave and take the kidneys in. Keep both sides of the body parallel. Take the shoulders back and look up.

3 With an exhalation take the trunk down over the left leg. Bend the elbows outward (see Focus, p. 66) and up, and catch further. Extend the right side of the back and move it further down to make the two sides level. Extend the waist and chest forward. Place the forehead, then the chin, on the shin. Breathe evenly.

Stay for 15 to 20 seconds and gradually longer, relaxing the trunk, the neck, and the head.

Inhale, come up. Straighten the right leg. Line up the trunk with the legs. ◁ Repeat from ▷ to ◁ on the left.

WAYS OF PRACTICING

Sit on folded blankets. Rest the forehead (see p. 64).

Support the bent knee or use a pad or belt behind it.

***Focus** Catching the foot*

The following methods are in order of difficulty, starting with the easiest.

Catch with a belt.
Hold the toes.
Clasp the hands.
Invert the hands behind the foot and catch the wrist.

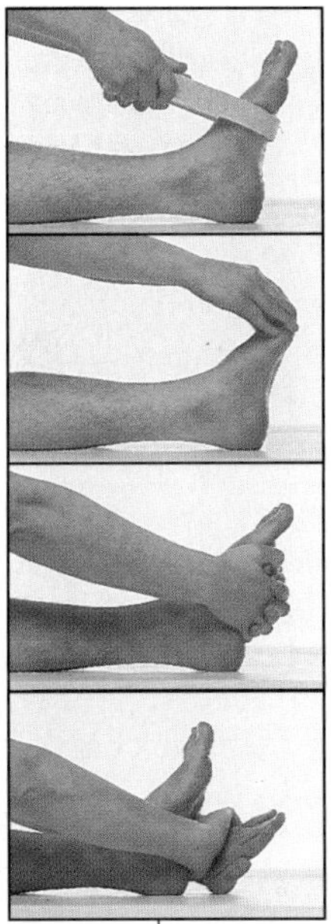

WORK IN THE POSTURE

Keep the left leg straight. Go on revolving the abdomen to the left. Extend the front of the body as well as the back. Keep the back soft. Every now and then, go down further on an exhalation.

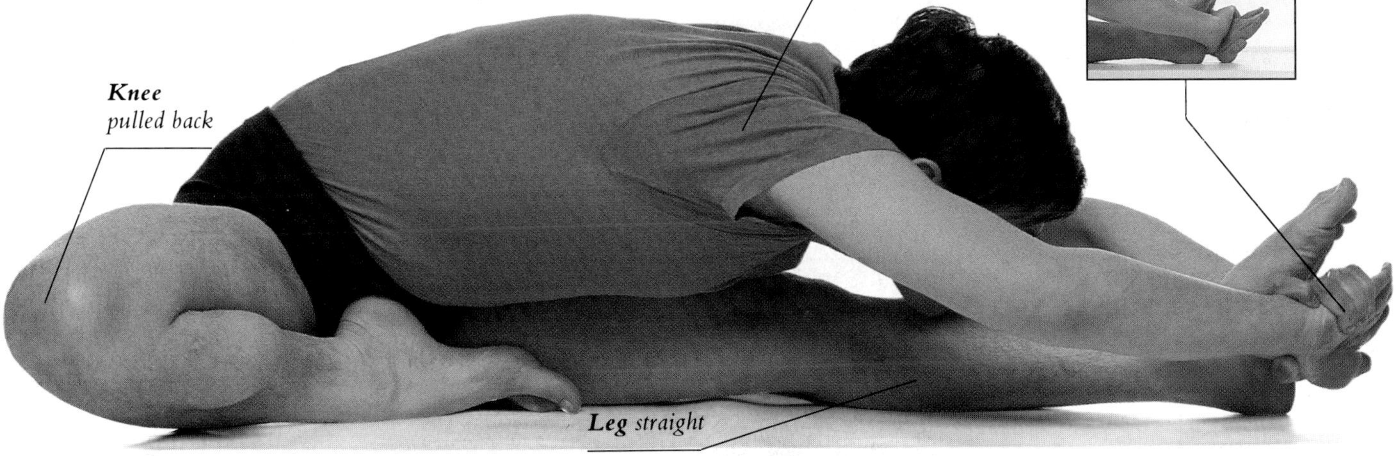

अर्ध बद्ध पद्म पश्चिमोत्तानासन

Ardha Baddha Padma Paścimottānāsana

ARDHA = half; *BADDHA* = bound; *PADMA* = lotus; *PAŚCIMOTTĀNA* = posterior stretch

THE HEEL presses into the abdomen, which extends over it.♦♦

1 Sit in Daṇḍāsana (p. 52). ▷Keep the left leg firm. Bend the right leg and bring the outer edge of the foot into the left side of the groin. Draw the calf and thigh together and bring the right knee in toward the center. Cup the fingers beside the hips and stretch up.

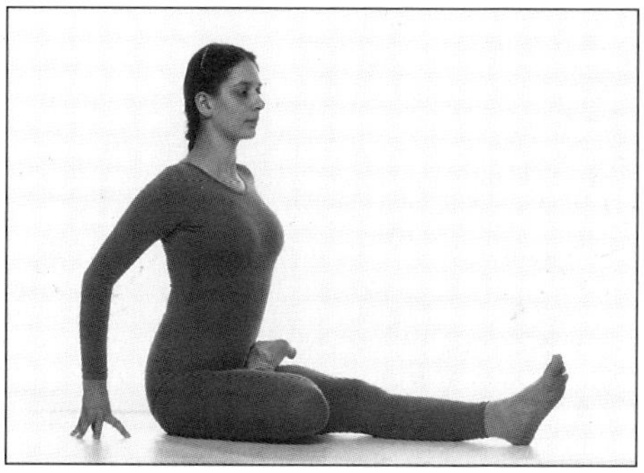

2 Lean forward, stretch the arms and hold the left foot.

Inhale, stretch the trunk up, and look up. Make the back concave.

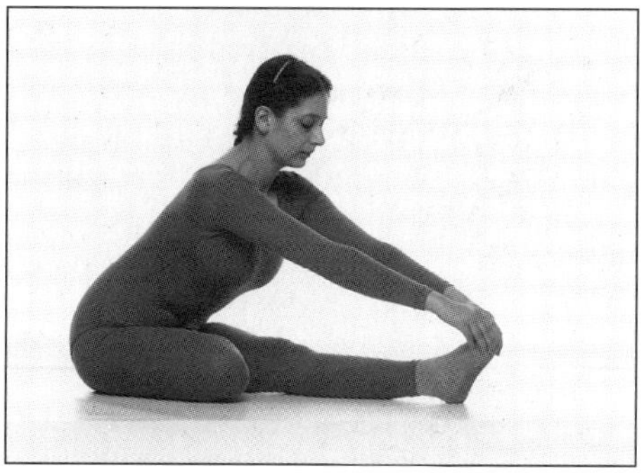

WAYS OF PRACTICING

See methods in Ways of Practicing, p. 59.

3 Exhale and bend down, extending the trunk along the left leg. Take the hips down. Rest the forehead, and then the chin, on the shin. Do not strain the back.

Stay, breathing evenly, for 20 to 30 seconds, keeping the head relaxed. (Come out of the posture if there is strain in the bent knee.)

Inhale, come up. Release the right leg.◁ Repeat from ▷to◁ on the left.

FULL POSTURE

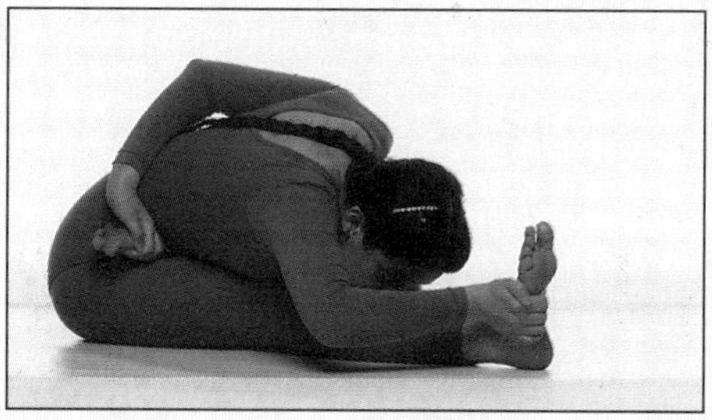

From Step 1 swing the right arm back to hold the right foot. Turn the trunk forward, then continue the pose. (If necessary, use a belt around the foot.)♦♦

WORK IN THE POSTURE

Keep the left leg straight. Press the right knee down and keep it facing forward. Press the right heel into the abdomen in a massaging action and move the abdomen over the heel.

Stretch the arms and trunk forward and relax the back and the neck.

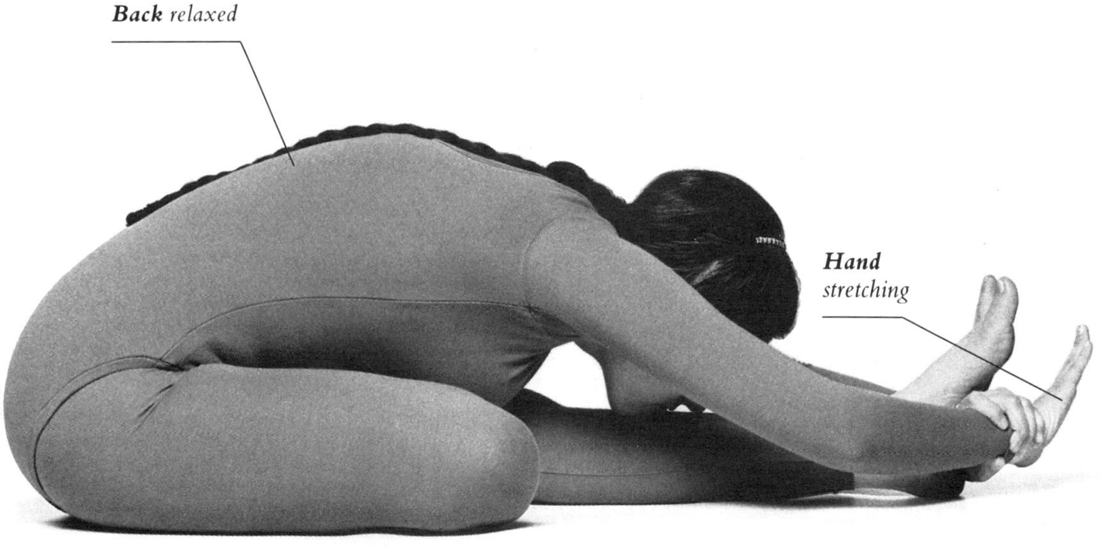

त्रिअंग् मुखैकपाद पश्चिमोत्तानासन

Triaṅg Mukhaikapāda Paścimottānāsana

TRI = three; *AṄGA* = limb; *MUKHA* = face; *EKA PĀDA* = one foot or leg; *PAŚCIMOTTĀNA* = posterior extension

HERE THE trunk extends freely; the problem is to keep the hips balanced.♦

1 Sit in Daṇḍāsana (p. 52). ▷Do not disturb the left leg. Bend the right leg back as in Vīrāsana (p. 50), with the inner heel close to the thigh. Keep the knees together. Open the right calf muscle out and turn the thigh outward. Extend the left leg forward. Press the outer edge of the right buttock bone down.

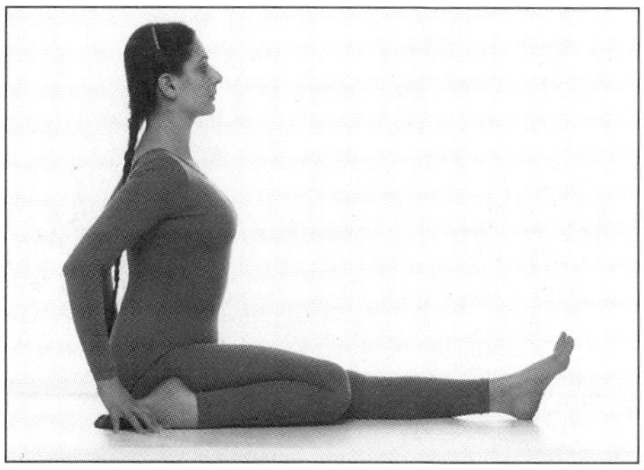

2 Stretch the arms and hold the left foot. Inhale and stretch up, making the back concave and lifting the front of the body from the pubis. Raise the head and look up.

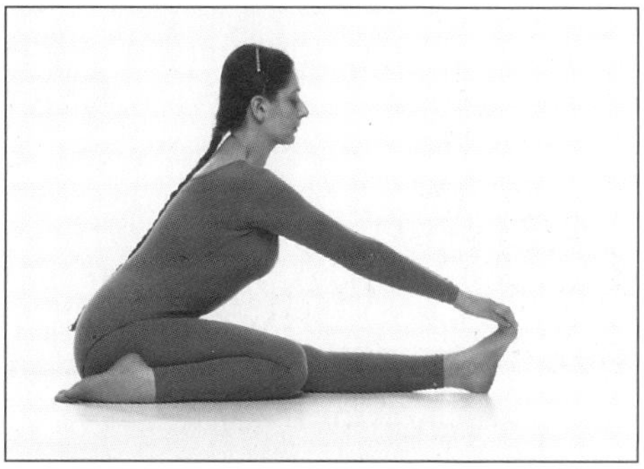

3 Exhale and move the hips and the trunk down toward the left leg. Make the seat light and extend the skin and flesh of the buttocks from the backs of the thighs toward the lumbar. Catch further (see Focus, p. 59) and continue to extend.

Place the head on the shin. Stay for 20 to 30 seconds, breathing evenly.

Inhale, come up. Bring the right leg forward.◁ Repeat from ▷to◁ on the left.

WAYS OF PRACTICING

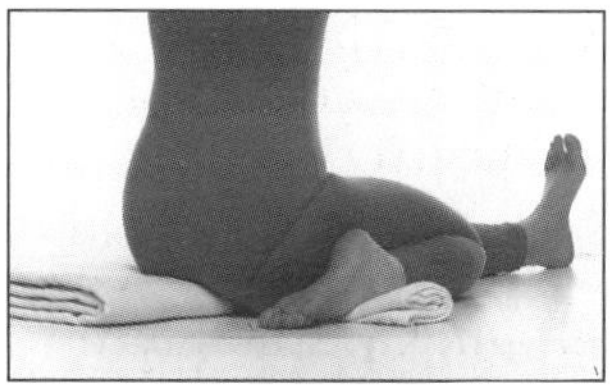

If the right hip lifts off the ground, place a folded blanket under the left buttock or under both buttocks.

Place a rolled blanket under the front of the ankle, if the foot is not flexible.

WORK IN THE POSTURE

Relax the head and neck.

♦

Be on the center of the top of the right foot and press the knee down. Do not let the body weight roll onto the left leg. Keep the chest centered over it. Bring the hips closer to the thighs.

***Whole body** extending from right foot to left*

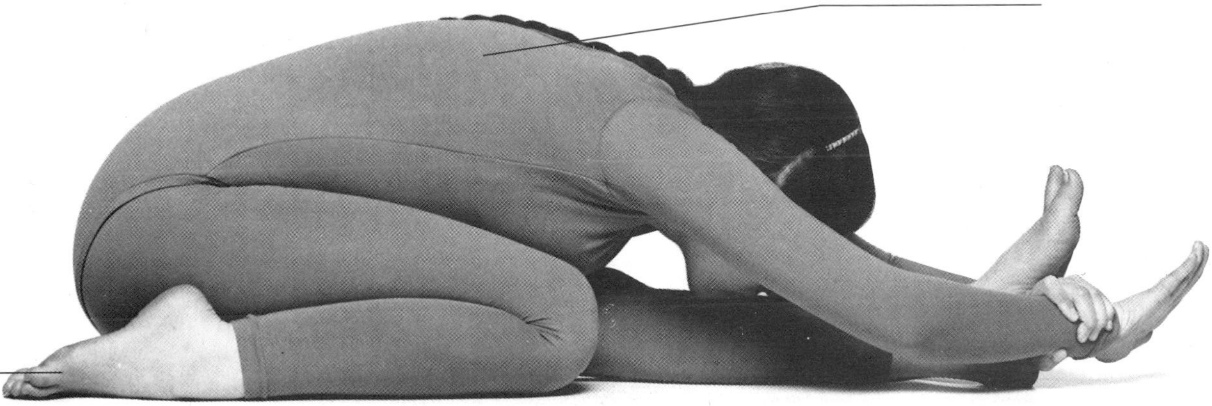

***Toes** stretching back*

क्रौंचासन

Krauñcāsana

KRAUÑCA = a heron

THE TRUNK and raised leg meet in an upward stretch; the bent leg grips the ground.♦♦♦ *Avoid this posture during menstruation.*

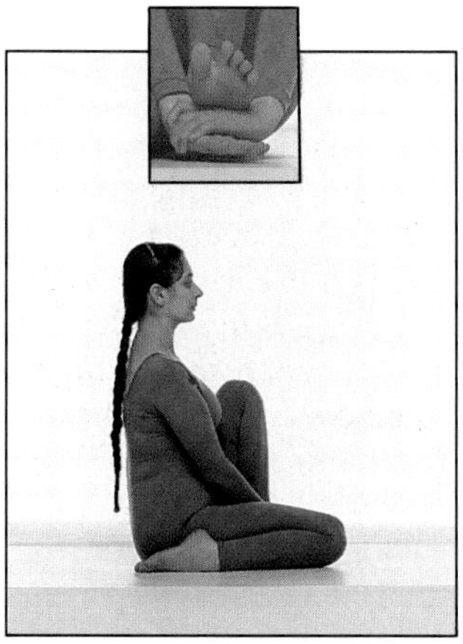

1 Sit in Daṇḍāsana (p. 52). ▷Bend the right leg back as in Vīrāsana (p. 50). Bend the left knee up, bring the foot in, and hold it or clasp the hands underneath.

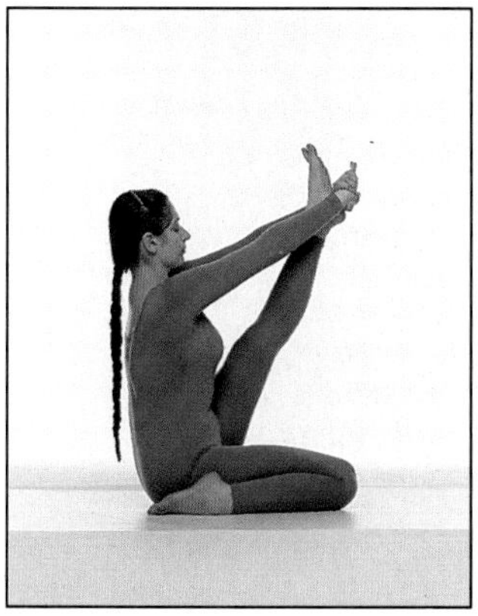

2 Raise the left leg and straighten it upward, extending the back of the leg toward the heel. Keep the center of the thigh, knee, and big toe facing directly forward.

Straighten the arms; with an inhalation lean back and stretch the trunk from the buttock bones up. Lift the abdomen and chest. Move the sacrum, lumbar, kidneys, and back ribs forward and up. Keep the sternum facing the middle of the left shin. Take the head back and look up. Take one or two breaths.

● *If you cannot straighten the leg, or if the hamstrings are strained, do not proceed to the final pose.*

3 Exhale, bend the elbows outward, and bring the left leg toward the trunk and the hips and trunk toward the leg. Extend the trunk along the leg and rest the head on the shin.

Stay for 15 to 20 seconds.

Inhale, lean back again as in step 2, then release the arms and legs.◁ Repeat from ▷to◁ on the other side.

WAYS OF PRACTICING

Learn to catch the foot in stages (see Focus, p. 59).

Use a belt to catch the foot.

WORK IN THE POSTURE

Press the toes of the right foot down. Go on stretching the left leg, locking the knee, and extending the hamstrings.

Move the trunk closer to the leg. Do not collapse the back.

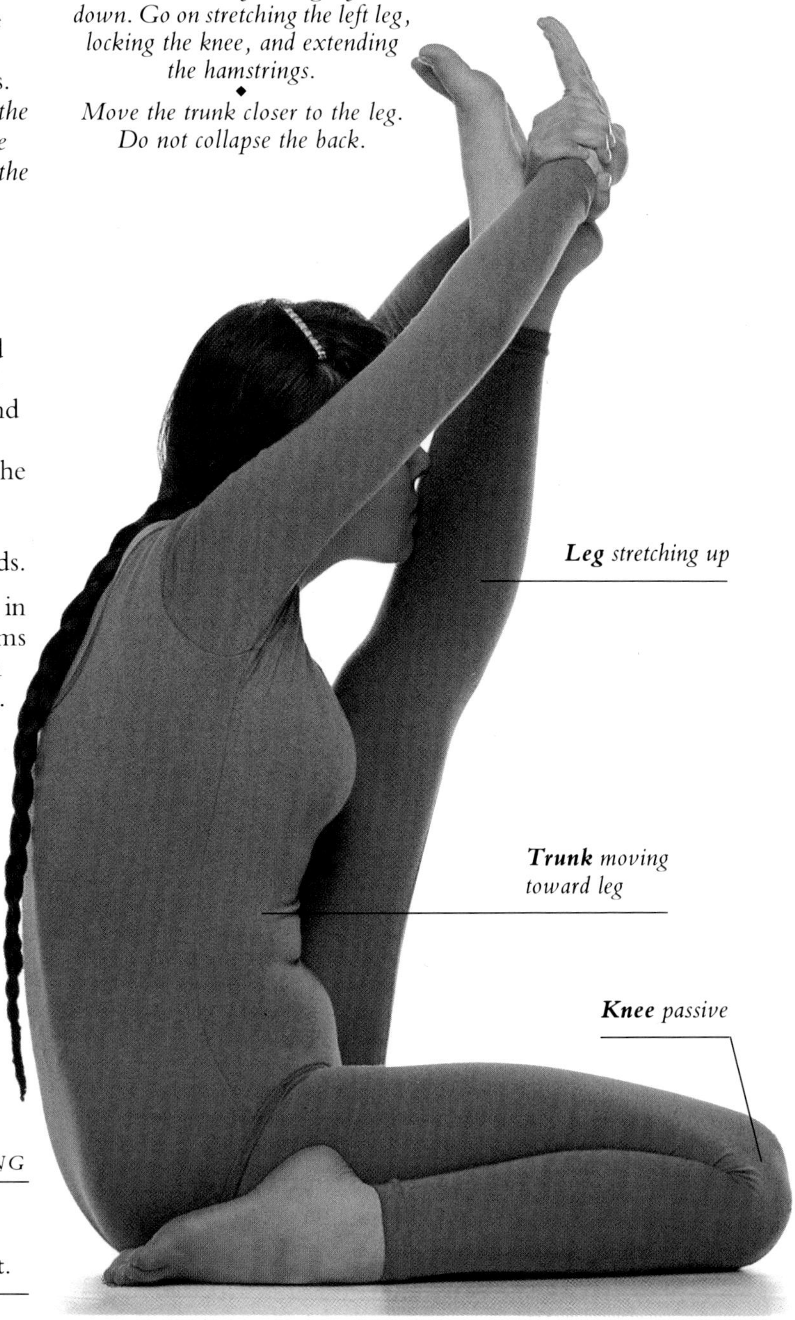

मरीच्यासन १

Marīcyāsana I

MARĪCI = the name of a sage in Indian mythology

THIS IS a complex pose where the body first twists to the side and then bends forward.♦♦

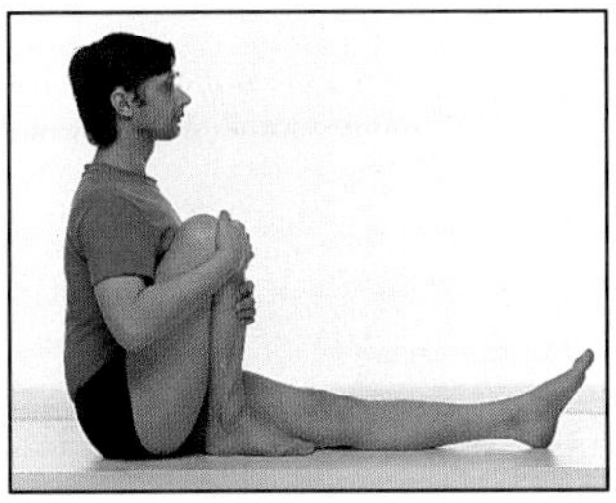

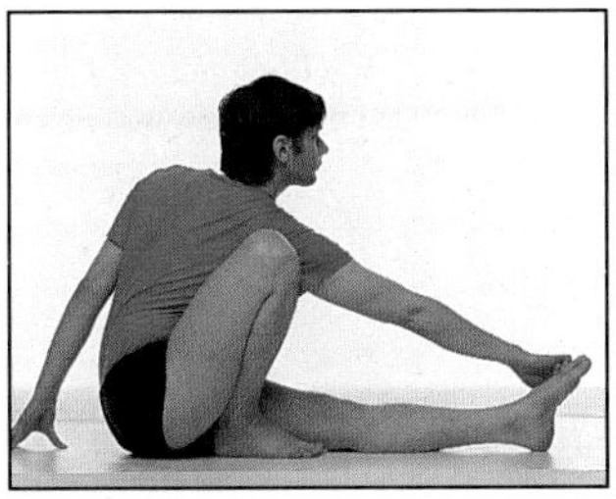

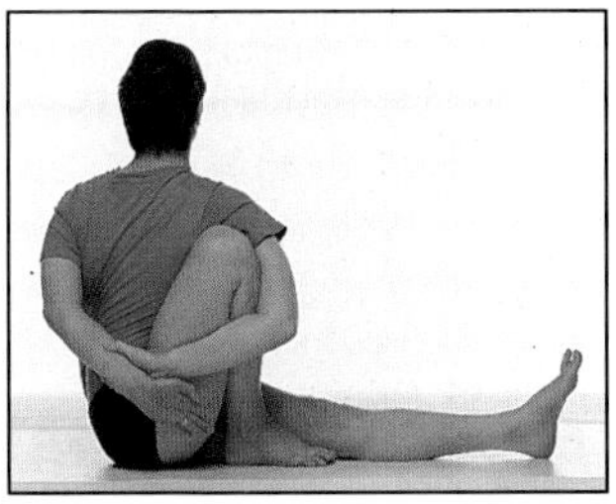

1 Sit in Daṇḍāsana (p. 52). ▷Keep the left leg firm. Bend the right leg up with the knee facing the ceiling; draw the heel close to its own thigh and to the left inner thigh.

Focus *Entwining the arms*
After catching the hands, take the shoulders back, draw the upper arms down, and pull the elbows closer together. Catch further and pull the hands away from the trunk.

2 Turn to the left, take the left arm back, and place the fingertips on the floor. Extend the right arm toward the left foot, bringing the armpit to the inside of the right knee. (For a moment hold the foot to bring the side of the body toward the bent leg; then release the hand.)

WAYS OF PRACTICING

Use a belt to catch the foot.

3 Revolve the right arm inward to the maximum, palm facing back. Then take the arm around the bent leg. Bend the left arm back and clasp the right hand or wrist (or vice versa). Lift the chest and turn further to the left, without dropping the bent leg to the side.

4 Exhale, turn to the front, and bend down over the left leg. Swing the left side down more to make it level with the right. Elongate the trunk toward the foot, pulling the left shoulder back and lifting the elbows. Rest the head on the shin. Stay for 20 to 30 seconds, breathing normally.◁

Inhale, come up. Repeat from ▷to◁ on the right.

WORK IN THE
POSTURE

Relax into the posture. Keep the abdomen passive.

Do not constrict the floating ribs; move them forward. Keep the right and left sides of the chest parallel, with the sternum over the center of the left leg.

Keep the bent knee upright and increase the grip of the hands.

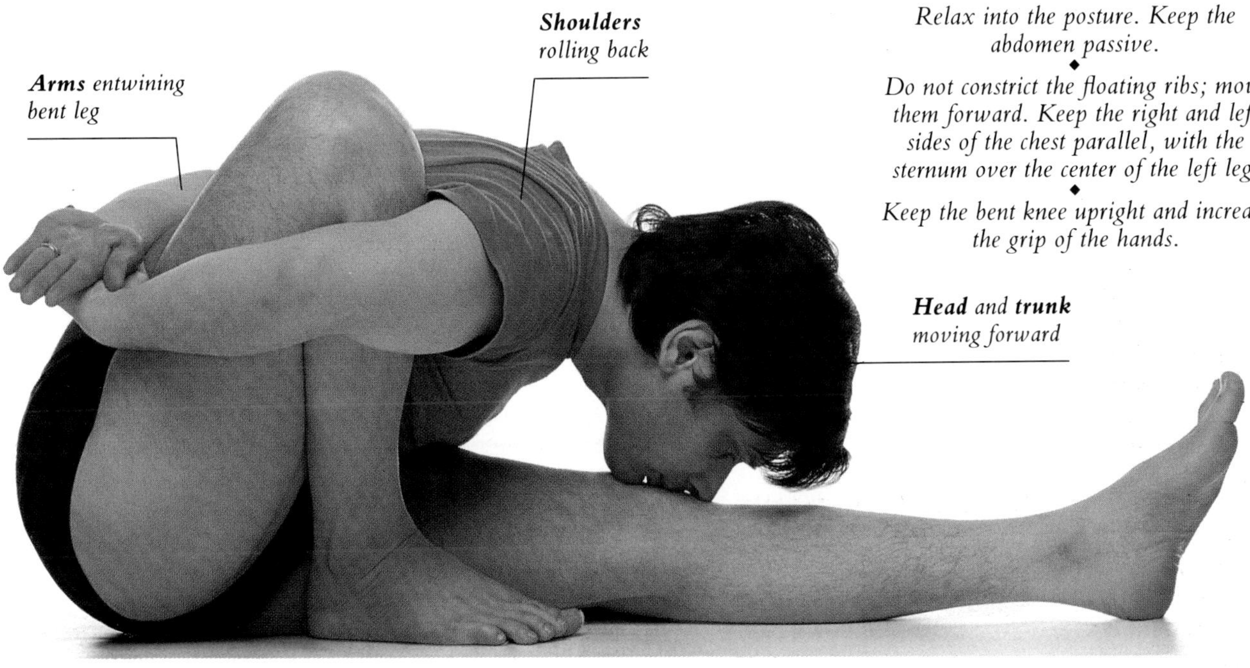
Shoulders *rolling back*
Arms *entwining bent leg*
Head *and* **trunk** *moving forward*

पश्चिमोत्तानासन

Paścimottānāsana

PAŚCIMA = back; *UTTĀNA* = extension

IN THIS extreme extension of the back of the body the ego becomes subdued and the mind quiet.♦♦

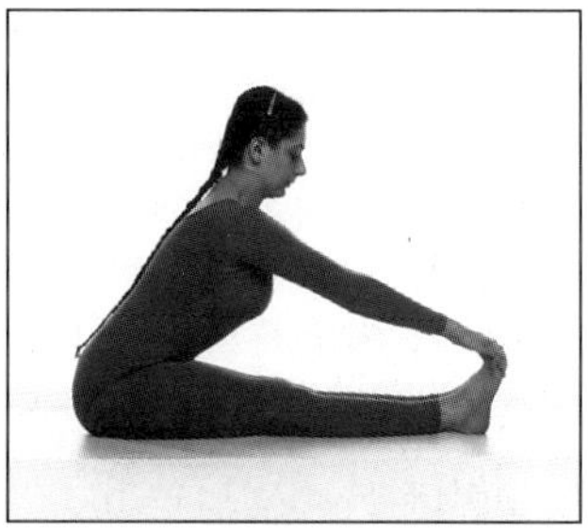

1 Sit in Daṇḍāsana (p. 52). With an exhalation lean forward, extend the arms, and hold the feet. Inhale, pull on the feet, and extend the trunk up from the pubis. Stretch both sides of the trunk and open the chest. Make the back concave. Look up.

Focus *Stretching the feet*
Keep the feet and ankles together. Lengthen the Achilles tendons. Pressing the heels lightly, stretch the soles and toes up. Stretch the tops of the feet away from the legs so that the ankles are not rigid. Project the heels and balls of the feet forward, while drawing the arches back.

2 Exhale, bend the elbows outward, and take the trunk toward the legs. Move the pubis back to bring the hips closer to the thighs. Open the buttock bones away from each other.

Extend the front, sides, and back of the body simultaneously toward the feet. Move the navel and the side ribs forward. Catch further (see Focus, p. 59).

Rest the head on the shin. Stay, breathing evenly, for 30 to 60 seconds (or longer). Keep the back and the head relaxed.

Inhale, come up.

WAYS OF PRACTICING

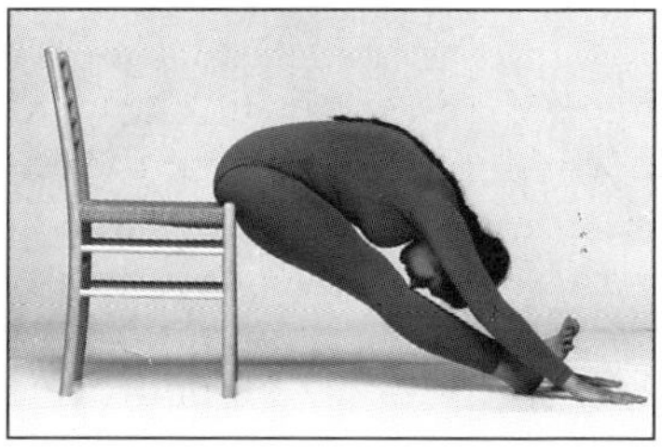

Place a chair against a wall. Sit on the edge and bend down over the legs. Keep the hands on the floor.

RESTFUL VARIATION

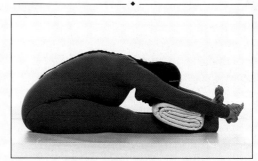

Rest the forehead on a folded blanket (or bolster) placed on the shins or on a stool. Stay for 2 to 3 minutes. Do not strain the back. (All the forward bends may be done in this way.)♦

WORK IN THE POSTURE

Maintain the extension of the legs and trunk without becoming tense.

♦

Do not let the legs roll outward; pull up the outer thigh muscles and keep the knees pressed down. Stretch the trunk forward and rest the front of the body on the legs.

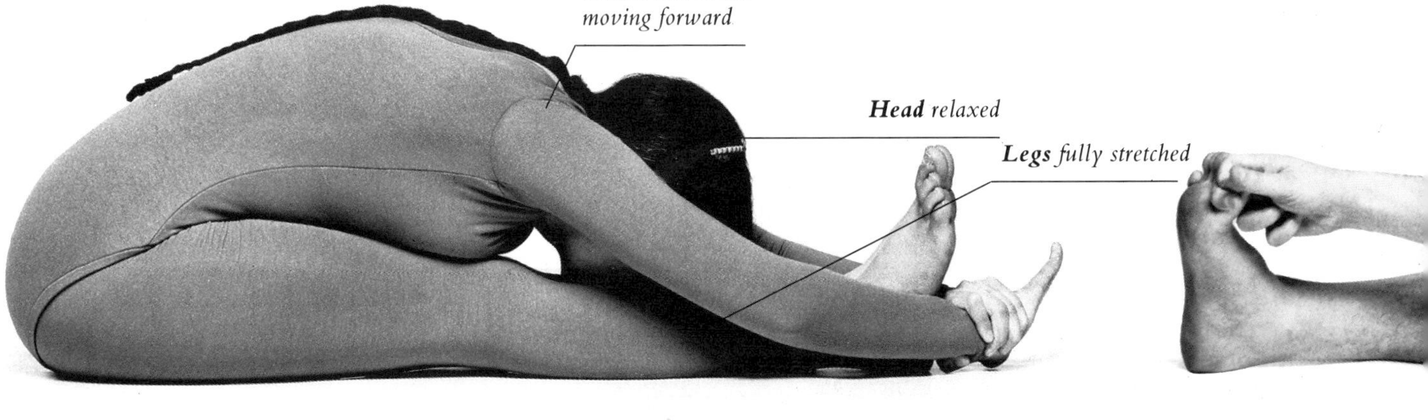

उपविष्ट कोणासन

Upaviṣṭa Koṇāsana

UPAVIṢṬA = seated; KOṆA = angle

HERE THE legs are spread wide apart. Sitting upright in this posture is beneficial for gynecological problems and can be practiced during menstruation and pregnancy *as long as there is no strain.*♦♦♦

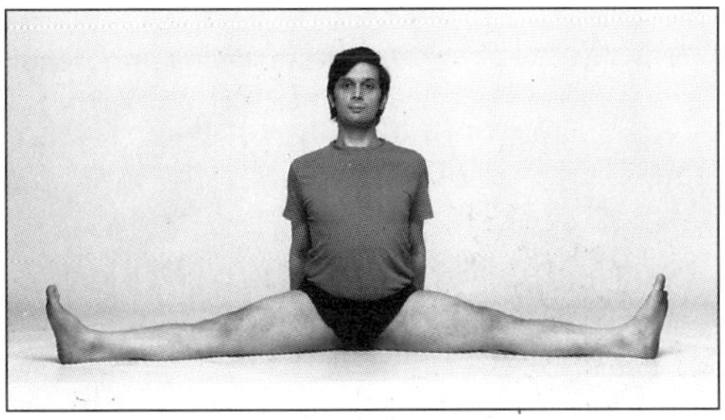

1 Sit in Daṇḍāsana (p. 52). Spread both legs simultaneously wide apart. Keep the knees and toes facing up, and the knees straight.

Press the fingertips into the floor beside the hips and draw the trunk up. Check that the legs are equidistant from the trunk. Extend the inner legs and the inner edges of the feet forward and draw the outer legs slightly back. Stretch the feet up.

WORK IN THE
POSTURE

Control the separation of the legs: as they stretch away from each other, do not let them roll outward. Keep the knees pressed down.

♦

Every so often exhale and move the trunk further down, taking the chest and chin forward.

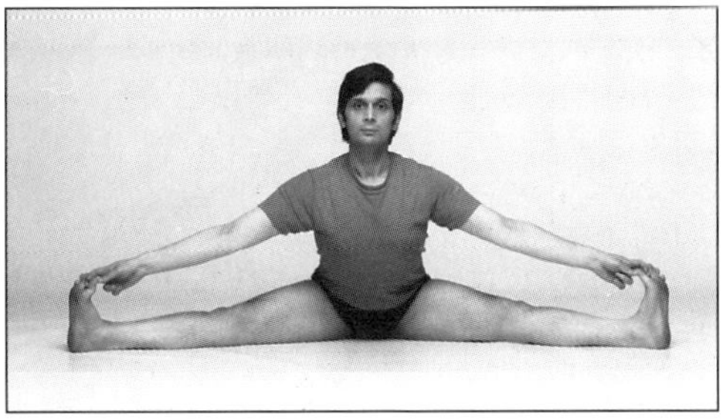

2 Lean forward and extend the arms toward the feet. Make a ring around the big toes with the thumbs, index, and middle fingers. Straighten the arms; pull the hips and trunk forward and up. Make the back concave (see Focus, below right). Raise the head and look up. Stay for two or three breaths. ● *If the hamstrings pull, do not continue to the next step.*

3 Exhale and bend the trunk toward the floor, pulling on the big toes, and at the same time resisting the pull.

Move the waist and chest forward, then take the shoulders and upper chest down. Rest the head on the floor.

Stay for 20 to 30 seconds, breathing evenly.

Inhale, come up. Bring the legs together.

WAYS OF PRACTICING

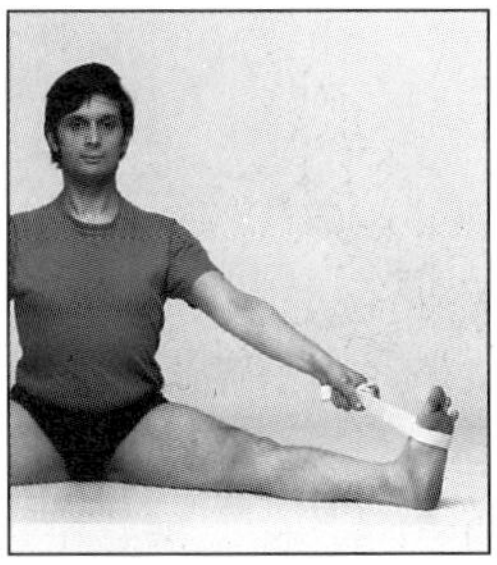

Use a belt around each foot. Sit on two folded blankets against a wall.

Focus *Making the back concave*

Raise the coccyx. Move the sacrum, lumbar, kidneys, and dorsal spine in, then extend the front as well as the back of the body up. Extend the cervical vertebrae and take the head back.

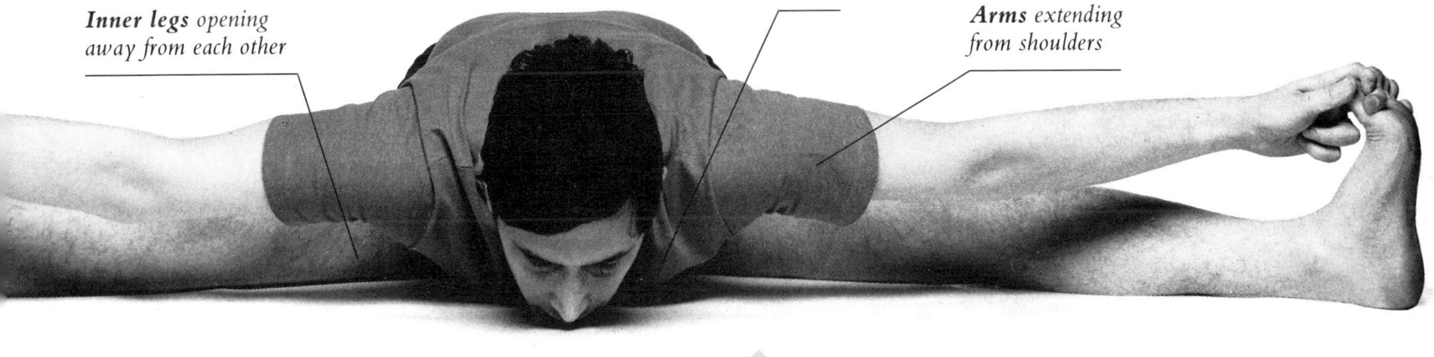

पार्श्व उपविष्ट कोणासन

Pārśva Upaviṣṭa Koṇāsana

PĀRŚVA = sideways; *UPAVIṢṬA* = seated; *KOṆA* = angle

THIS COMBINES a wide spread of the legs with a lateral extension of the trunk.♦♦♦

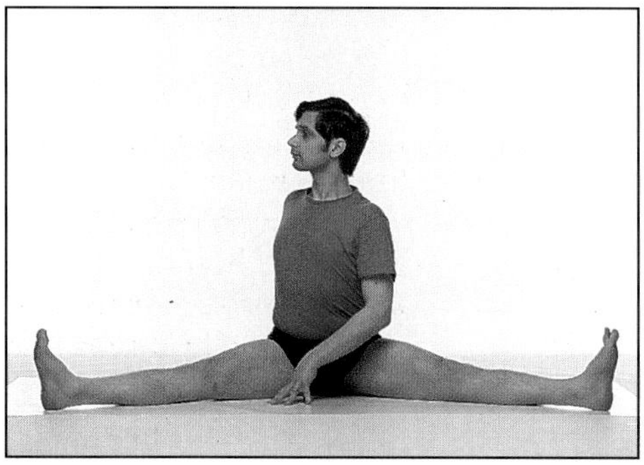

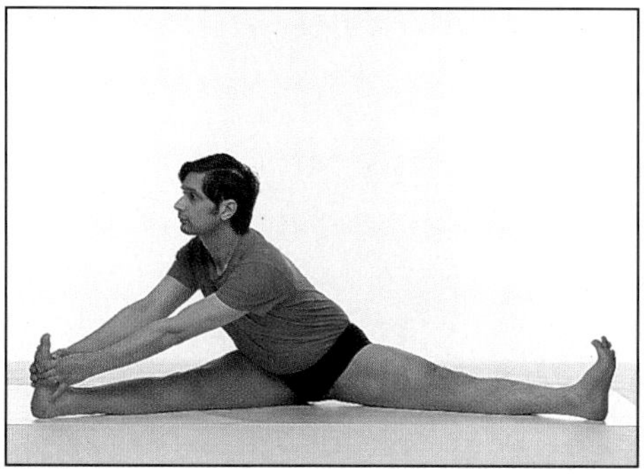

1 Sit in Upaviṣṭa Koṇāsana, step 1 (p. 65). ▷Keeping the left leg firm, turn the hips, waist, and chest to the right. At the same time place the fingertips of the right hand behind the right hip and the left hand by the inside of the right thigh. Bring the left hip further around and tuck the right hip slightly back so that you are facing the middle of the right leg. Keep both sides of the body parallel.

WAYS OF PRACTICING

See Ways of Practicing and Focus, p. 59.

2 Keeping both thighs down, lean over the right leg; extend the arms and catch the foot. Move the hips forward and stretch up. Make the back concave (see Focus, p. 65) and look up.

3 Exhale, bend the elbows outward, and take the trunk down over the leg. Rest the head on the shin.

Stay for 20 to 30 seconds, breathing evenly, keeping the head relaxed.

Inhale, come up. Turn to the center.◁ Repeat from ▷to◁ on the other side. Bring the legs together.

PARIVṚTTA UPAVIṢṬA KOṆĀSANA

PARIVṚTTA = revolved

Study the text and illustrations opposite for Parivṛtta Jānu Śīrṣāsana. Do the pose with the legs in Upaviṣṭa Koṇāsana.♦♦♦

Focus *Bending the elbows out*

After catching the foot, pull the elbows strongly out to the sides and up. Stretch the sides of the trunk and take the shoulders and shoulder blades down. Keep the shoulders away from the neck. Stretch the armpits forward.

WORK IN THE POSTURE

Press the left thigh down.

Turn the hips more. Revolve the abdomen to the right. Extend the trunk further along the leg and catch the hands further.

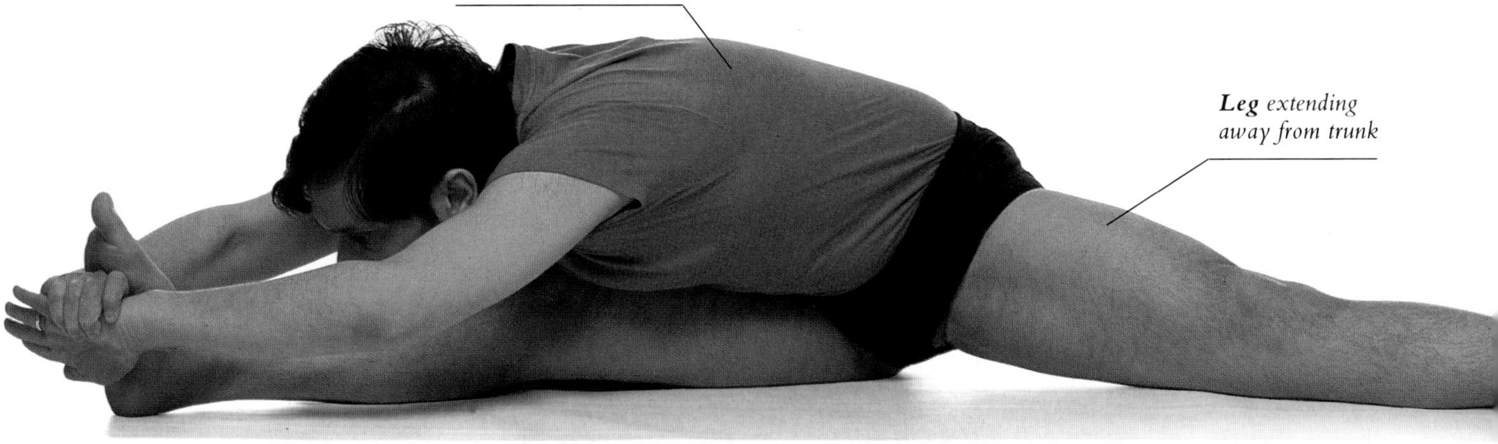
Trunk extending away from left leg
Leg extending away from trunk

परिवृत्त जानुशीर्षासन

Parivṛtta Jānu Śīrṣāsana

PARIVṚTTA = revolving; JĀNU = knee; ŚĪRṢA = head

WITH THE help of the arms the trunk revolves to face upward.♦♦♦

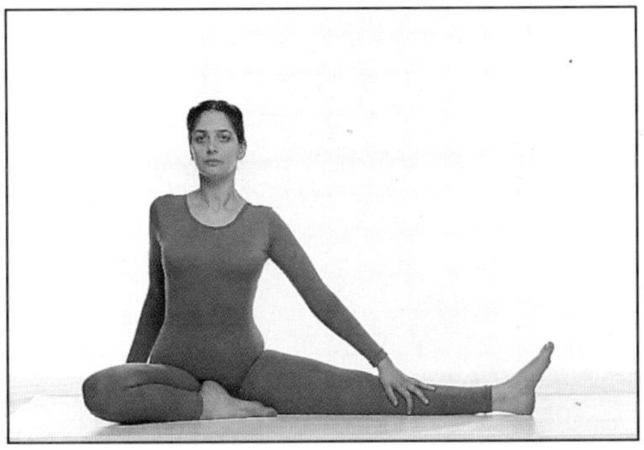

1 Sit in Daṇḍāsana (p. 52). ▷Bend the right knee as in Jānu Śīrṣāsana (p. 59); take it back as far as it will go, without disturbing the left leg. Turn to the right, with the hips and sides of the body almost in line with the left leg. Place the right hand behind the right hip and the left hand in front of the left thigh or on the leg. Stretch up.

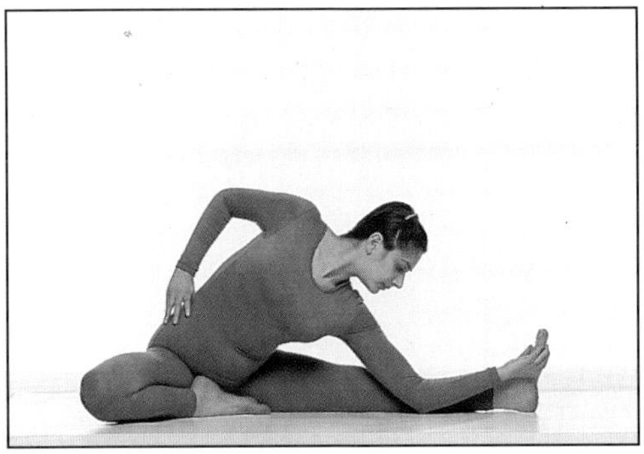

2 Pull the top of the left thigh slightly back. Exhale; bend the trunk sideways and extend it over the leg; at the same time turn it up, bringing the left side forward and turning the right side back.

As the trunk goes down, extend the left arm toward the foot; turn the hand up and hold the foot with the thumb on top and the fingers on the sole. Bend the elbow and place it on the floor in front of the left leg; use it as a lever to bring the left side of the body over the thigh.

3 Extend the right arm over the ear toward the left foot; hold the outer edge of the foot, with the thumb on top.

Turn the hips, waist, chest, and shoulders by pulling on the foot from both sides and pressing the right elbow back. Turn between the arms and look up. Stay for 20 to 30 seconds, maintaining the turn of the trunk.

Release the hands and turn to the front. Straighten the right leg. ◁

Repeat from ▷ to ◁ on the left.

WAYS OF PRACTICING

Put a belt around the foot; hold each end in one hand and pull on it.

WORK IN THE POSTURE

Turn more and more. Be strong in the elbows. Press the bent leg back. Lengthen the front of the body.

♦

Make two or three short repeated efforts when turning the trunk.

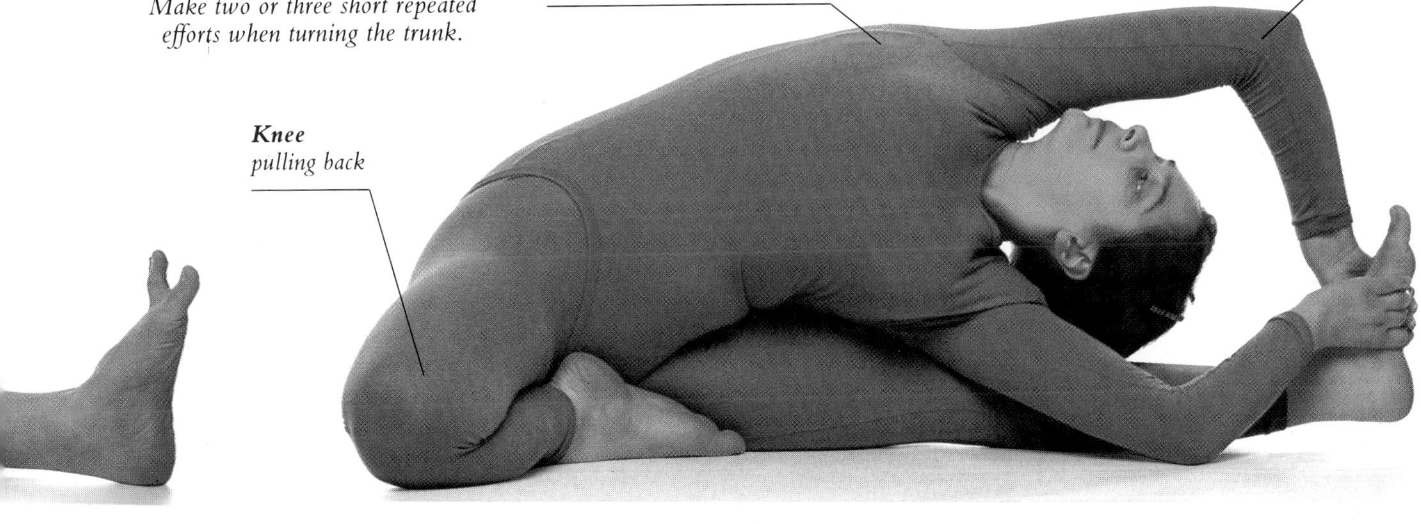

कूर्मासन

Kūrmāsana

KŪRMA = tortoise

THE BODY is enclosed by the arms and legs and the mind draws inward.♦♦♦♦

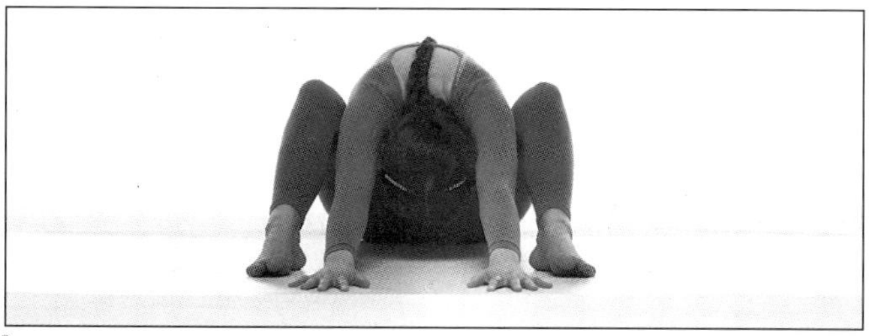

1 Sit in Daṇḍāsana (p. 52). Spread the legs about $1\frac{1}{2}$ft apart and bend them slightly. Exhale; bend the trunk down and extend it toward the feet. Stretch the arms forward and take the head down.

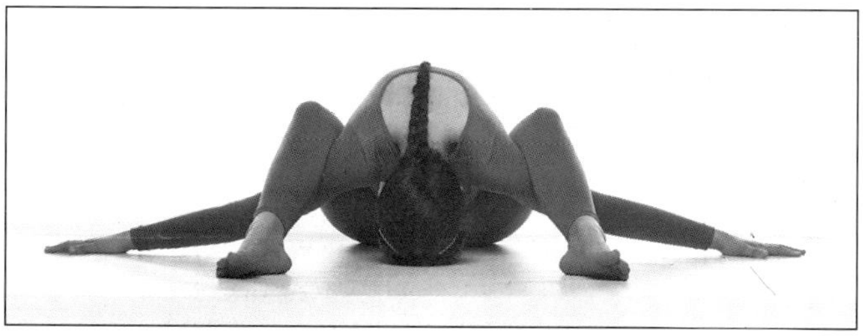

2 Bend the elbows; move the arms one at a time under the bent legs to the sides, palms down. Bring the backs of the knees over the shoulders and press the shoulders down.

3 Slide the heels forward and stretch the legs. Straighten the elbows and extend the arms and hands to the sides.

Rest the forehead, then the chin, on the floor and stay for 20 to 30 seconds, breathing evenly.

Inhale, bend the knees, release the arms, and come up, or continue to the next variation.

VARIATION

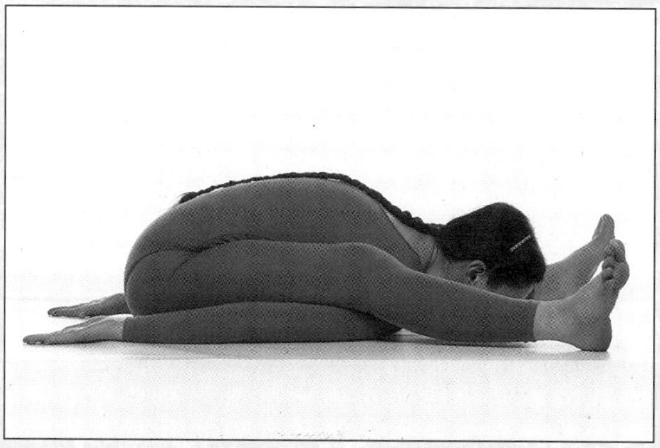

Turn the arms in, with the palms facing up, and stretch them back almost in line with the legs.
Extend the legs forward.

Take the head down. Move the chin forward and stay for a further 20 to 30 seconds.♦♦♦♦

WORK IN THE POSTURE

Settle and relax into the posture; let go mentally.

Roll the thighs and knees in. Move the trunk forward and take the chest down. Do not strain the back or the legs.

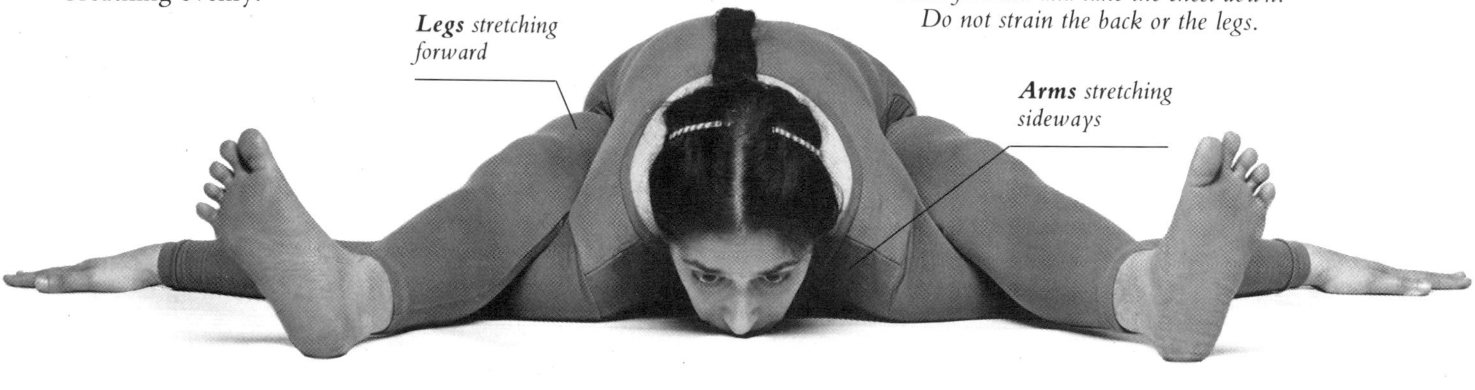
Legs stretching forward
Arms stretching sideways

TWISTS

Never perform the āsanas mechanically, for then the body stagnates.
B. K. S. IYENGAR

The twists are very effective in relieving backaches, headaches, and stiffness in the neck and shoulders. As the trunk turns, the kidneys and abdominal organs are activated and exercised. This improves the digestion and removes sluggishness. The spine becomes flexible and the hips move more easily.

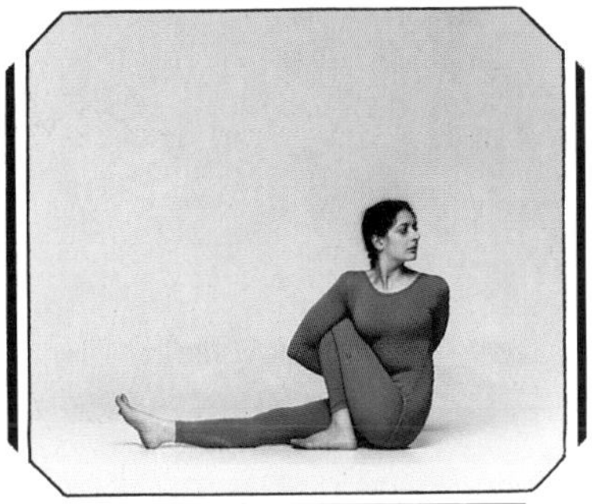

GUIDELINES FOR PRACTICE

The body should be lined up with the walls of the room. For maximum freedom of movement in the lower trunk, it is best to sit on one or two folded blankets.

In the final stage of the twists the abdomen may become compressed or the back rounded, and it is difficult to lift up. It is therefore helpful to remain working in the intermediate stage, with the elbow bent against the knee or the hands pressed into the ground. In this way the trunk can turn and extend well. Pressing the fingers of the back hand against a wall or ledge also helps the trunk to turn.

Twists may be done after forward bends or by themselves. After backbends, or to relieve a backache, they should be done gently at first.

The head can be turned in either direction.

CAUTIONS: Do not do twists after recent operations, or if suffering from hernia, stomach, or abdominal problems.

Do not practice twists during pregnancy, except for Bharadvājāsana (on a chair, p. 71), which should be done gently.

मरीच्यासन

Marīcyāsana (standing)

MARĪCI = name of a sage

THIS STANDING twist is very useful for relieving backaches.♦

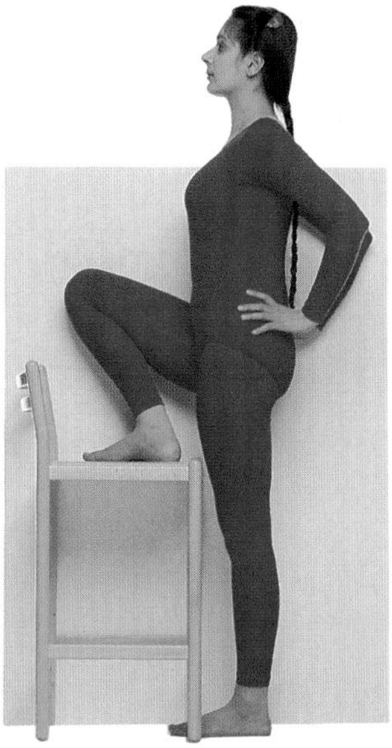

1 Place a tall chair or stool against a wall or piece of furniture with a ledge (as shown). ▷ Stand in Tāḍāsana (p. 18), facing the chair, with the right side against the wall. Keep the left leg perpendicular and draw the trunk up. Raise the right foot and place it on the chair directly ahead, with the toes facing forward and the knee in line with the foot. Keep the thigh against the wall.

2 Turn to the right and face the ledge. Raise the arms and hold the ledge. Grip well with the left hand to turn the left side of the trunk to the right; press the right hand to turn the right side back. Turn to the maximum. Turn the head further and look over the right shoulder. Stay, breathing evenly, for 20 to 30 seconds.

Exhale and turn to the front. Lower the arms and the right leg. ◁ Repeat from ▷ to ◁ on the left side.

WAYS OF PRACTICING

It is easier to lift and turn if the ledge has corners.

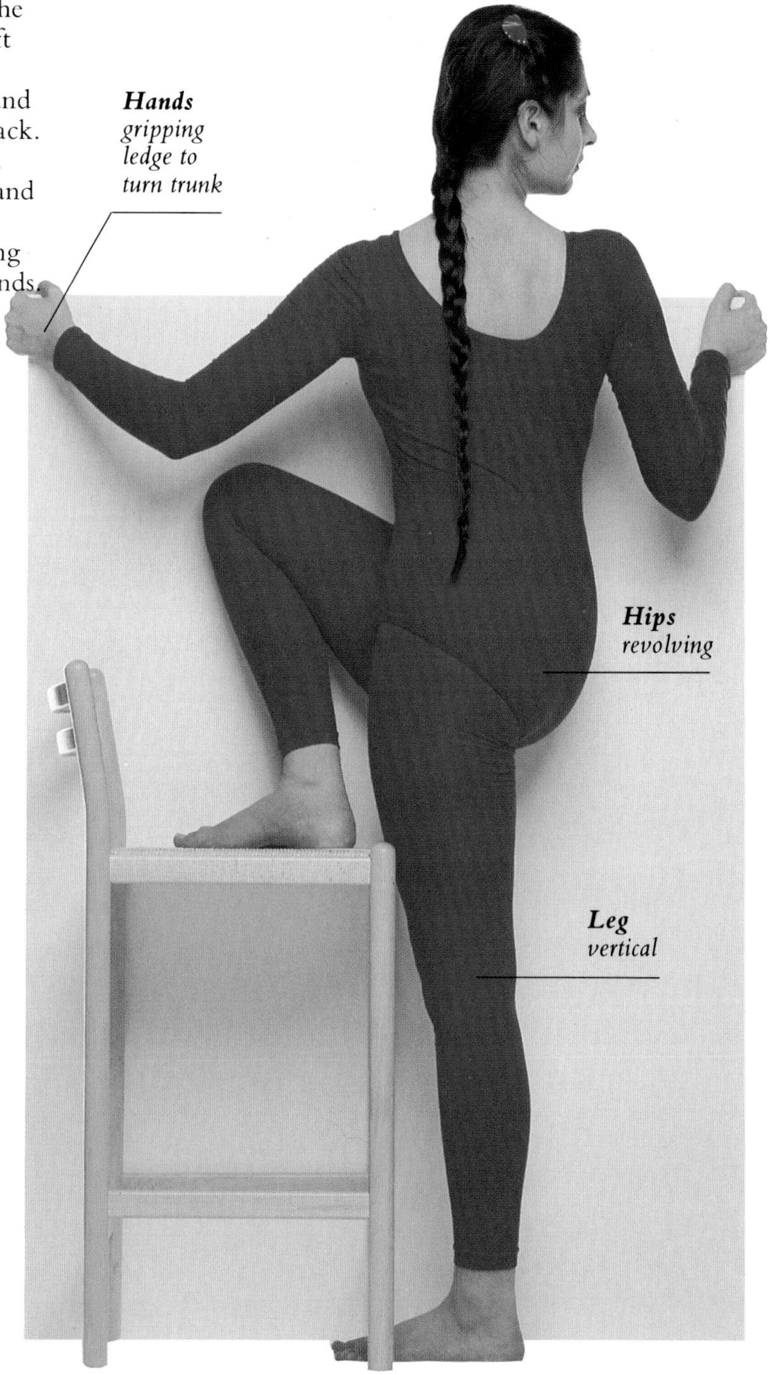

WORK IN THE POSTURE

Pull the left thigh back.

Keep the trunk upright. Every two or three breaths, turn more, on an exhalation. Alternately lift the trunk and turn it.

भारद्वाजासन

Bharadvājāsana (on chair)

BHARADVĀJA = name of a sage

THIS SIMPLE twist is invaluable for bad backs.♦

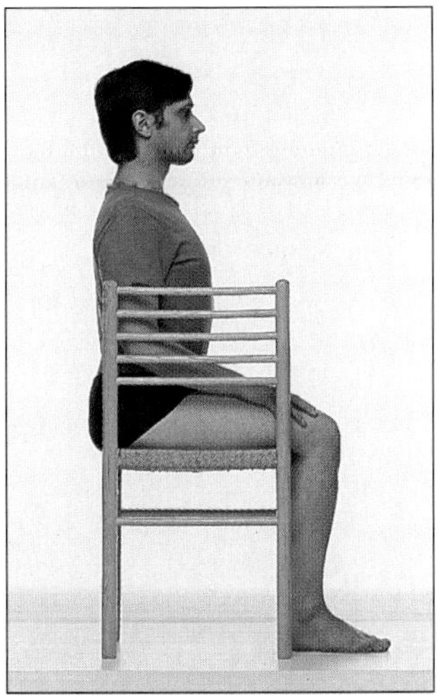

1 ▷ Sit sideways on a chair, with the right hip against the back of the chair. Sit on the whole seat. Stretch the trunk up and take the shoulders back. Line up the trunk with the legs. Keep the knees and feet together.

2 Exhale and turn toward the back of the chair, synchronizing the movements of the right and left sides. Move the back ribs in. Do not disturb the position of the legs.

Place the hands on the back of the chair. Pull with the left hand to bring the left side toward the back of the chair and push with the right hand to turn the right side away from it. Turn to the maximum, keeping the trunk upright.

Turn the head and look over the right shoulder. Stay for 20 to 30 seconds, breathing evenly.

Exhale, turn to the front. ◁ Repeat from ▷ to ◁ on the left.

Afterward, sit on the front of the chair. Spread the legs and bend down, relaxing the back and the head.

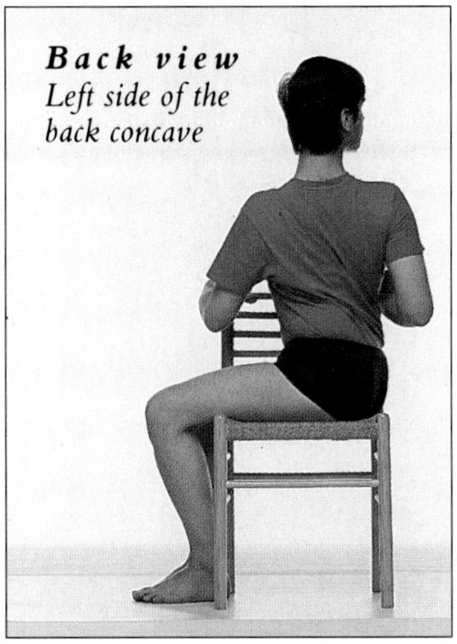

Back view
Left side of the back concave

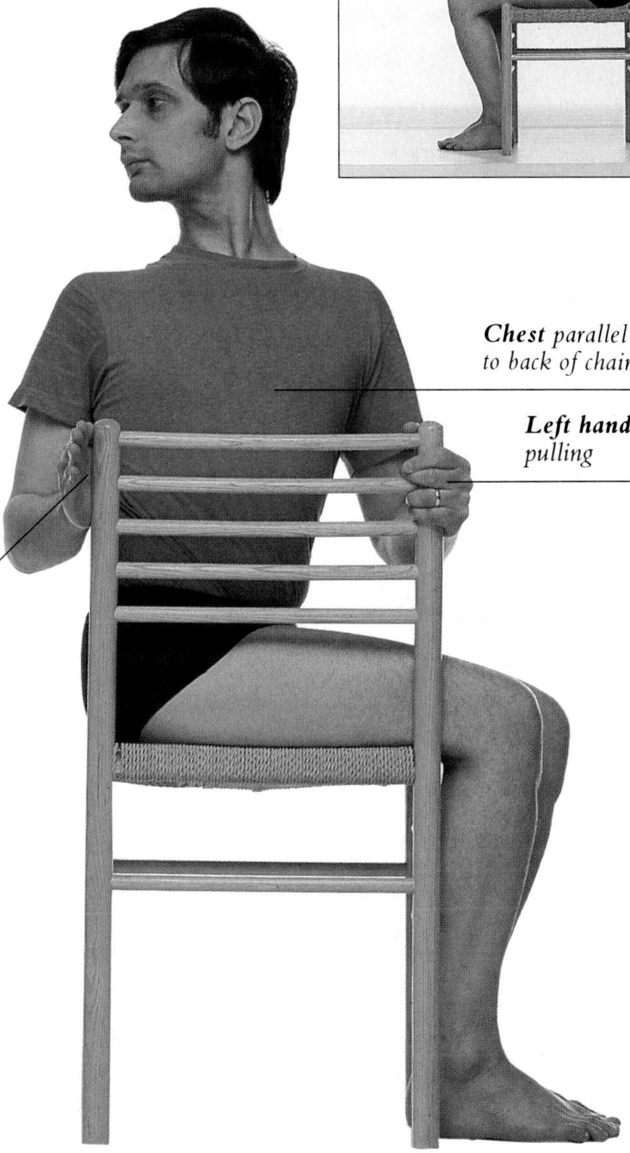

WORK IN THE
POSTURE

Turn the hips as much as possible, then the waist, chest, and shoulders. Move the left kidney in.

♦

Lift the rib cage and take the shoulders back.

♦

Squeeze the abdomen to the right.

भारद्वाजासन १

Bharadvājāsana I

BHARADVĀJA = name of a sage

HERE THE trunk turns in a spiraling movement from the hips.♦

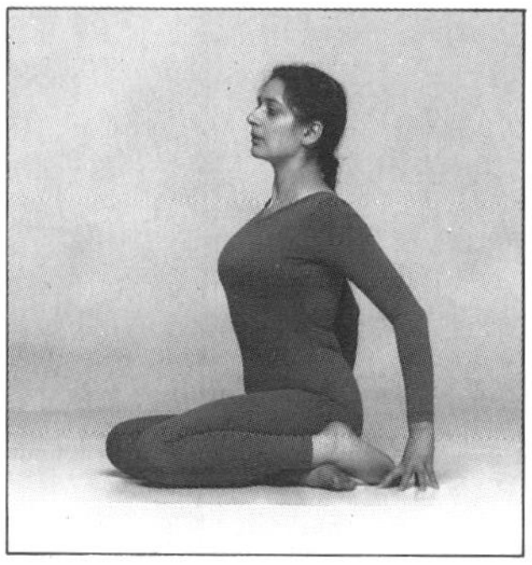

1 Sit in Daṇḍāsana (p. 52). ▷ Bend the legs back and place them beside the left hip. Keep the knees facing forward. Tuck the right foot under the left foot. Place the hands beside the hips, with the fingertips on the floor.

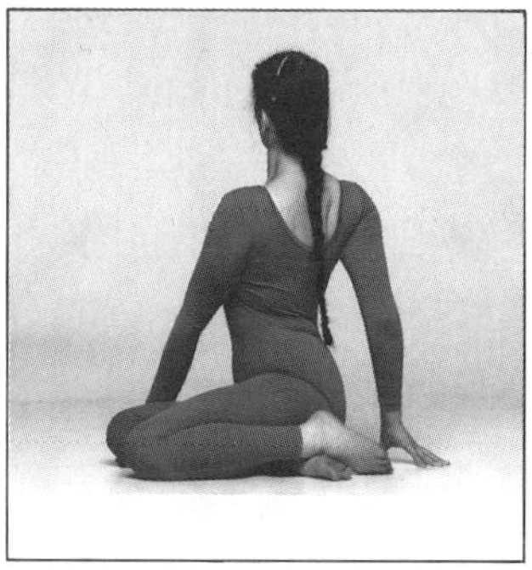

2 Turn to the right; place the left fingertips beside the right thigh and the right fingertips behind the right hip. Do not raise the left hip or thigh. Extend the spine and the trunk vertically up.

Stay for 20 to 30 seconds or continue to the final pose.

3 Turn the left arm out and place the palm under the right outer thigh, fingers pointing in. Swing the right arm back and, from behind, hold the left upper arm just above the elbow. Pull the right elbow and shoulder back, press the back of the body forward and swing the trunk further around.

Turn the head and look over the left shoulder. Stay for 20 to 30 seconds, breathing normally.

Release the hands and turn to the front; straighten the legs. ◁ Repeat from ▷ to ◁ on the left.

WAYS OF PRACTICING

Sit on two folded blankets.

Sit sideways near a wall, low ledge or baseboard.

Grip as in Marīcyāsana (standing) on p. 70, and turn.

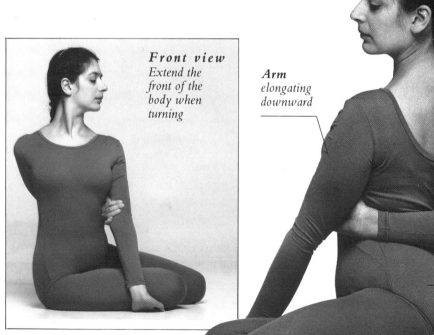

Front view *Extend the front of the body when turning*

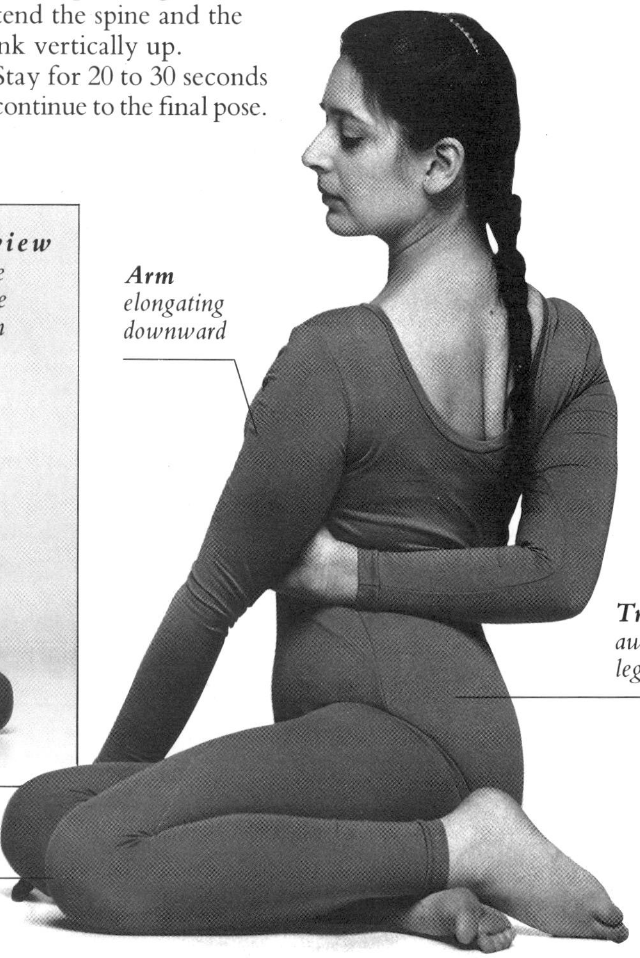

Arm *elongating downward*

Trunk *turning away from legs*

Legs *close together*

WORK IN THE POSTURE

Keep the legs firm.

Revolve from the hips. Move the lumbar and dorsal spine in. Be strong in the left side of the back.

Lift the upper chest, roll the shoulders back, and take the shoulder blades deep in.

मरीच्यासन ३

Marīcyāsana III

MARĪCI = name of a sage

ARMS ENTWINING the trunk and bent leg, the body turns.♦♦

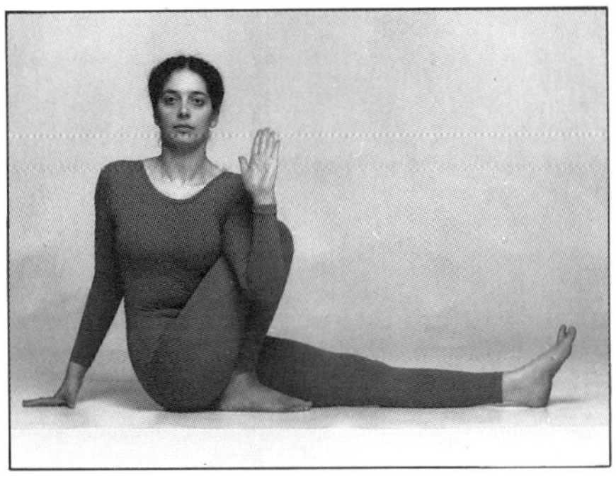

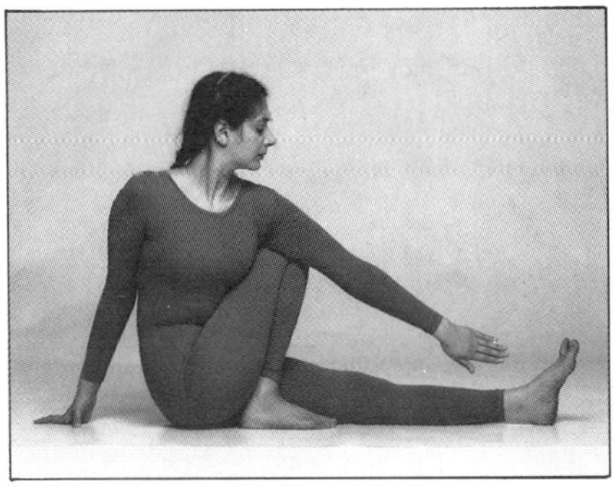

1 Sit in Daṇḍāsana (p. 52). ▷Bend the right knee up; bring the foot close to the perineum. Hold the knee to pull the trunk up. Keep the left leg firm.

Turn to the right. Bend the left elbow in front of the right knee, forearm vertical. Take the right arm back. Press the left arm and right knee against each other to bring the left side of the trunk forward. Press the right fingertips down on the floor to turn the right side back.

Stay for 20 to 30 seconds, breathing evenly, or continue to the final pose.

2 Move the trunk closer to the right leg and place the back of the left armpit over the right knee. Turn the hips more. Move the left hip toward the bent leg and the right hip away from it. Stretch the left arm down and turn it in, with the palm facing back.

3 Bend the left arm back around the right shin. Take the right arm behind the back; bend the elbow and clasp the left hand. Make the entwined side of the back concave.

Grip the hands well to increase the turn of the trunk. (Moving the hands away from the back intensifies the posture.)

Turn the head to gaze over the right shoulder. Stay for 20 to 30 seconds, breathing normally.

Release the hands and turn to the front. Straighten the right leg.◁ Repeat from ▷to◁ on the left.

Focus *Taking the arm around the legs* Stretch the arm from the shoulder and revolve it to keep the outer upper arm in contact with the outer bent leg. Move the upper arm further down. Then bend the elbow to take the arm around the leg. Do not leave space between the armpit and knee.

WORK IN THE POSTURE

Press the left side of the sacrum in.

♦

Extend the front of the body from the pubis to the neck. Lift the diaphragm and the sternum. Take the shoulders back and the shoulder blades in. Clasp further – the wrist if possible.

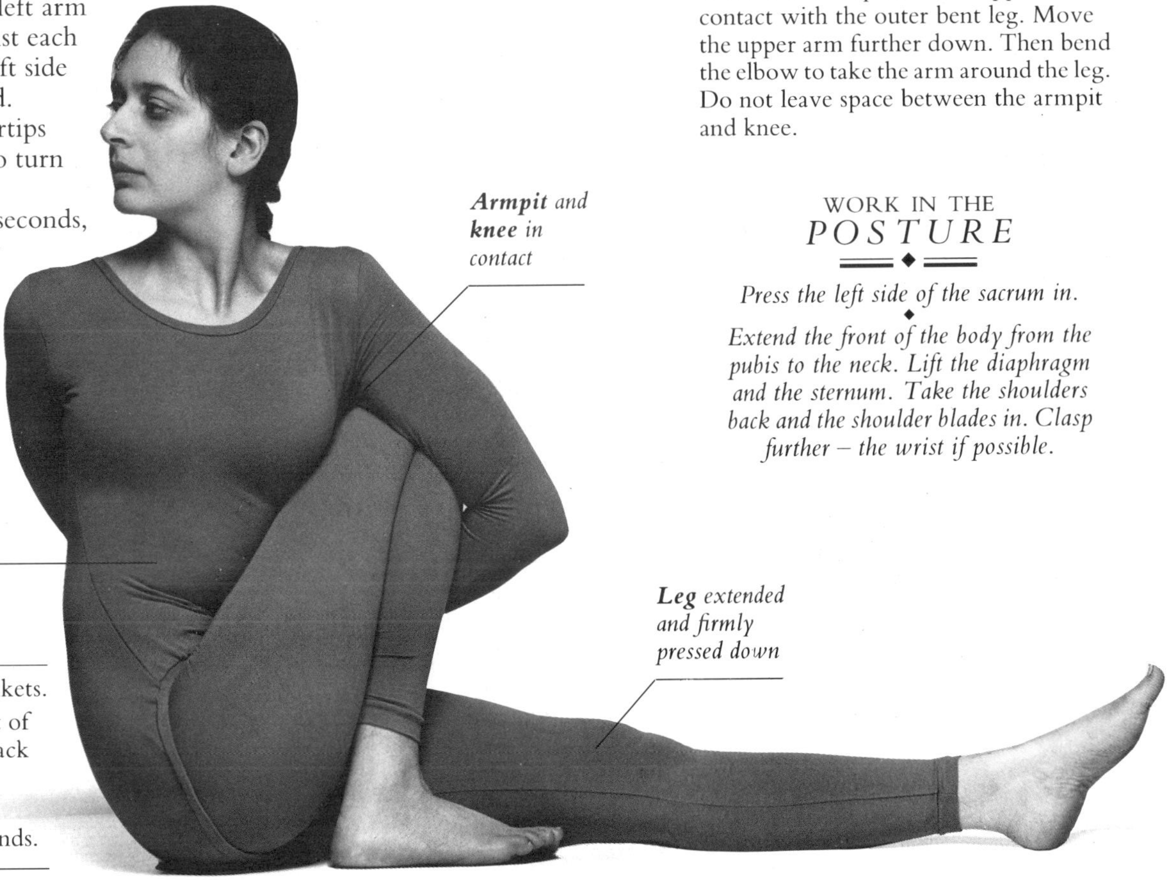
Armpit *and* **knee** *in contact*
Abdomen *revolving*
Leg *extended and firmly pressed down*

WAYS OF PRACTICING

Sit on two folded blankets.

To achieve a good lift of the trunk, place the back hand on a brick or baseboard.

Use a belt to catch hands.

अर्ध मत्स्येन्द्रासन १

Ardha Matsyendrāsana I

ARDHA = half; *MATSYENDRA* = Lord of the fishes, first teacher of Yoga to mankind

THIS IS a complicated twist, combining a strong turn with balance.♦♦

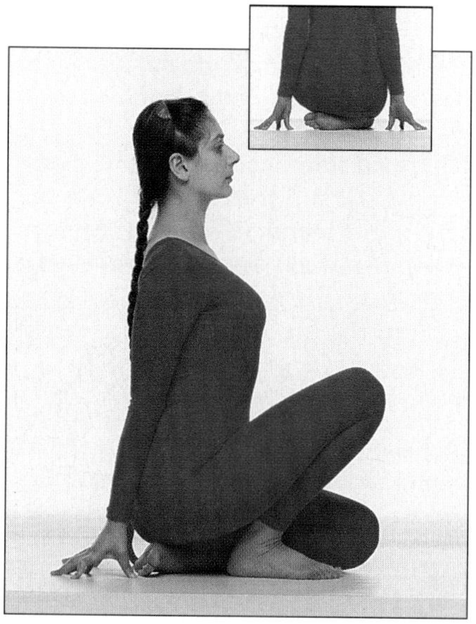

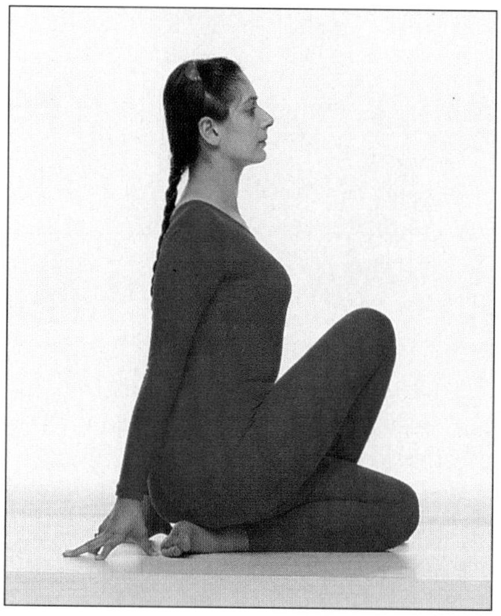

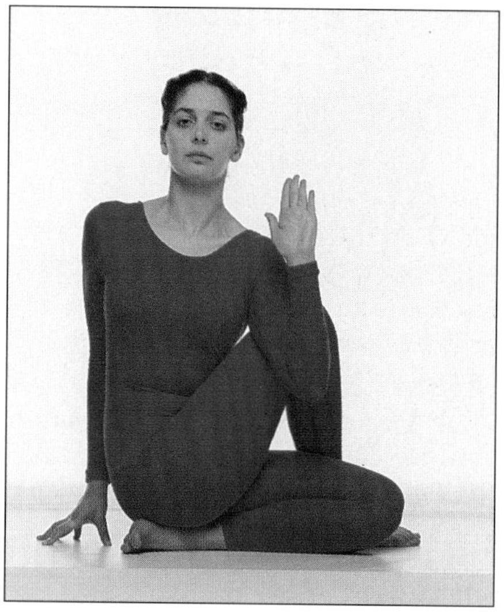

1 Sit in Daṇḍāsana (p. 52). ▷Bend the left leg in. Turn the foot at right angles to the shin with the inner heel under the left buttock, the toes under the right buttock, and the foot horizontal. Curl the outer edge of the foot back so that the edge, not the top, of the foot is on the floor. Keep the inner and outer edges parallel. Keep the left knee facing directly ahead. Bend the right knee up.

2 Take the right leg over the left, with the knee facing the ceiling. Place the foot by the left outer thigh, facing diagonally away from it. Keep the right thigh, knee, shin, and foot in line; do not let the leg drop to the side. Press the fingertips into the floor and draw the trunk up.

WAYS OF PRACTICING

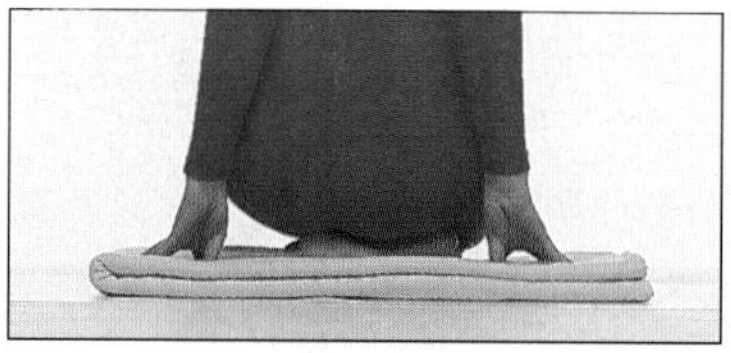

Place a folded blanket under the left foot and another, if necessary, between the heel and buttocks.

Put the left hand on a brick or low ledge to improve the lift and turn of the trunk.

Turn toward a wall and press the hands against it.

Use a belt to catch the hands.

3 Move the back ribs in. Exhale and turn to the right. Bend the left elbow, with the forearm vertical, in front of the right thigh and take the right arm back, cupping the hand on the floor. Press the bent arm against the right leg to bring the left side of the back forward and to move the left kidney in. Press the right hand into the floor to turn the front of the body to the right. Raise the diaphragm and turn the abdomen.

Stay for 20 to 30 seconds, breathing evenly, or continue to the final pose.

अर्ध मत्स्येन्द्रासन १

4 Exhale, bring the back of the left armpit over the right knee; bend the arm around the right leg as in the previous posture. Take the right arm behind the back and clasp the left hand or wrist. Take the dorsal spine and the shoulder blades deep in, and turn the chest more.

Turn the head and look over the left shoulder. Stay for 20 to 30 seconds.

Release the hands and turn to the front. Bring the legs forward. ◁

Repeat from ▷ to ◁ on the other side.

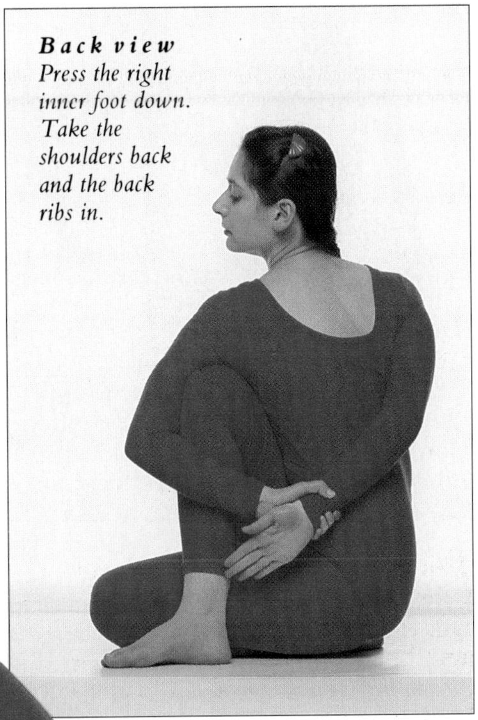

Back view
Press the right inner foot down. Take the shoulders back and the back ribs in.

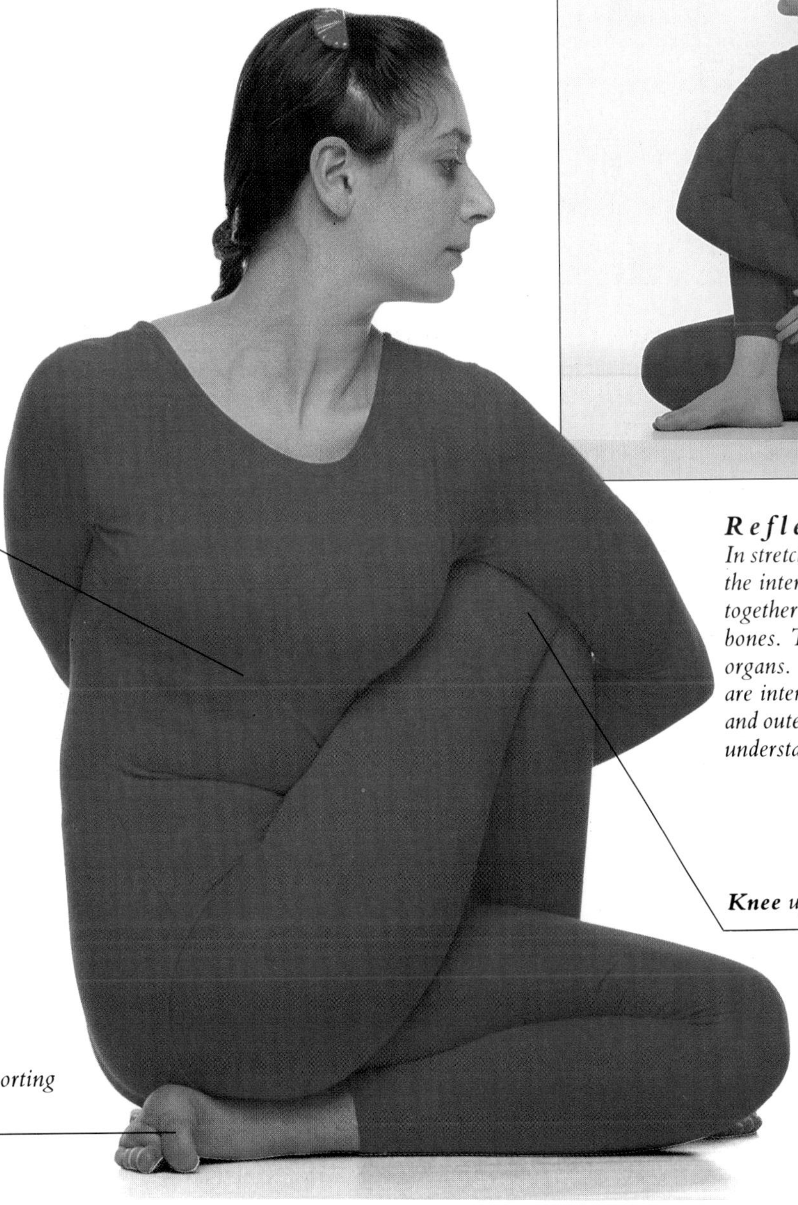

Reflection
In stretching or turning the trunk, the internal organs should move together with the skin, flesh, and bones. This stimulates the inner organs. The effects of the āsanas are intensified. When the inner and outer body work in harmony, understanding of Yoga deepens.

WORK IN THE
POSTURE

Keep both feet active; do not slide off the left foot.

Take the trunk closer to the legs. Leave no space between the armpit and knee.

Draw the elbows closer together and away from the trunk. Grip the hands strongly to increase the turn of the trunk.

पाशासन

Pāśāsana

PĀŚA = noose

THE ARMS form a noose around the legs and trunk.♦♦

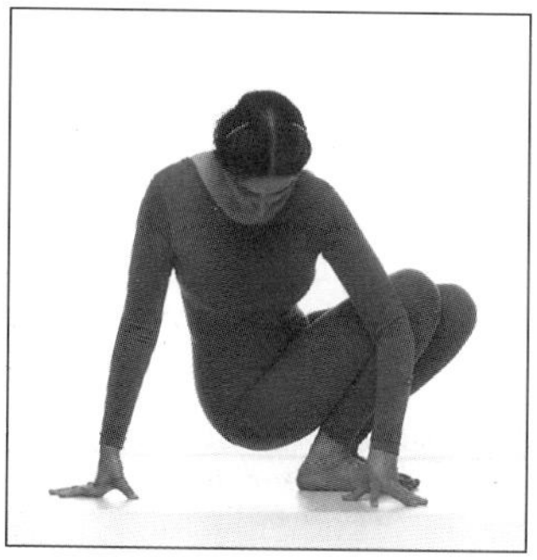

1 Squat with the heels down and feet together. ▷Exhale, turn to the right. Put the right hand on the floor beside the right hip and the left arm in front of the right thigh. Cup the hands on the floor.

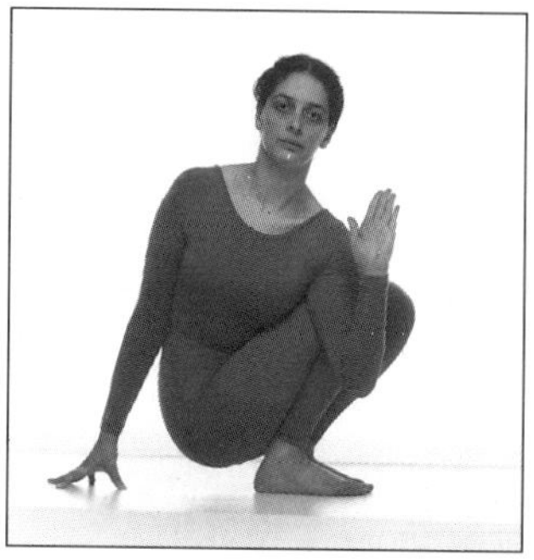

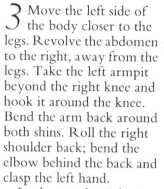

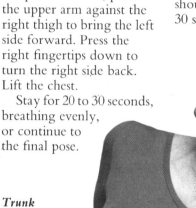

2 Bend the left arm up, palm forward; press the upper arm against the right thigh to bring the left side forward. Press the right fingertips down to turn the right side back. Lift the chest.

Stay for 20 to 30 seconds, breathing evenly, or continue to the final pose.

3 Move the left side of the body closer to the legs. Revolve the abdomen to the right, away from the legs. Take the left armpit beyond the right knee and hook it around the knee. Bend the arm back around both shins. Roll the right shoulder back; bend the elbow behind the back and clasp the left hand.

Look over the right shoulder and stay for 20 to 30 seconds.

Inhale, release the hands and turn to the front.◁ Repeat from ▷to◁ on the left.

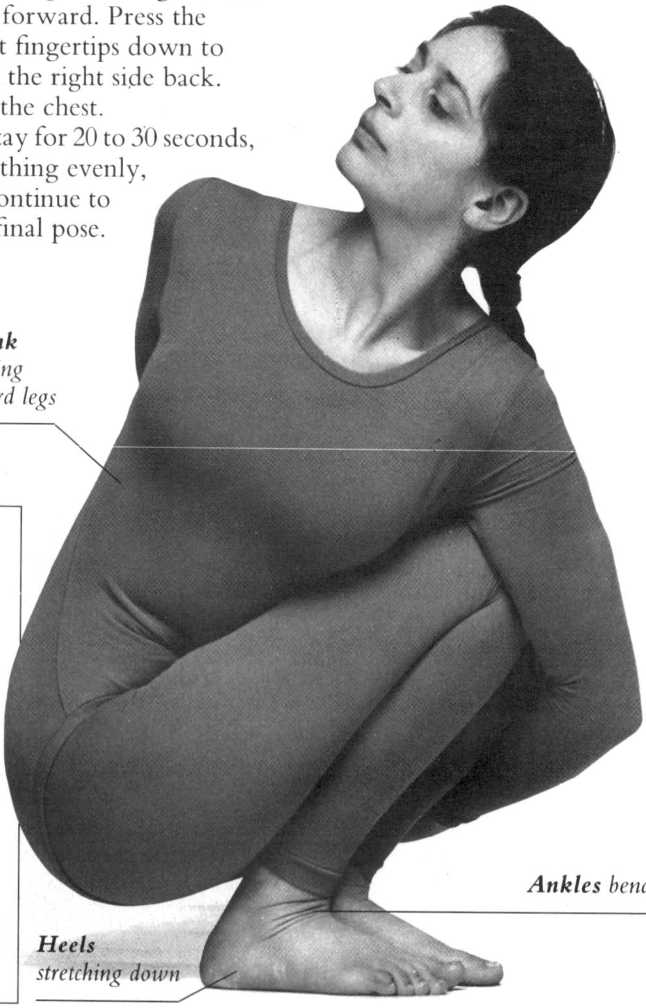

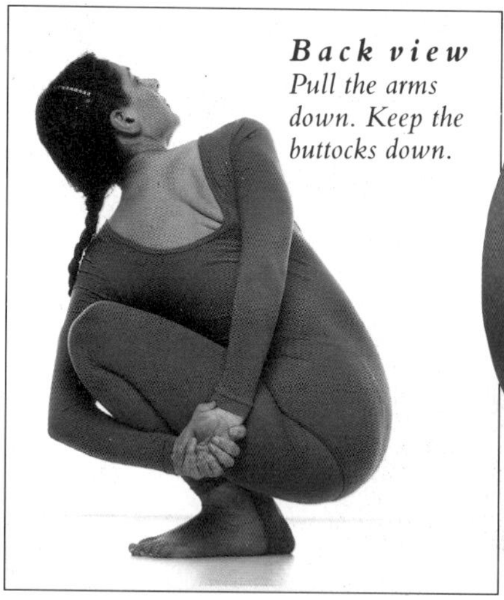

Back view *Pull the arms down. Keep the buttocks down.*

WAYS OF PRACTICING

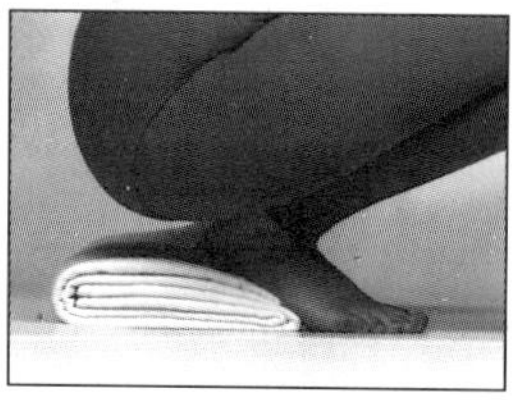

Place the heels on a rolled blanket.

Put the right hand on a brick.

Use a belt to catch the hands.

Press the hands on a wall or against a ledge to turn more.

WORK IN THE POSTURE

Keep the feet and knees together and compress the thighs.

♦

Make the back concave and stretch the front of the body up. Lift the diaphragm.

♦

Clasp the hands further to turn more.

भारद्वाजासन २

Bharadvājāsana II

BHARADVĀJA = name of a sage

THE LEGS are anchored, allowing the hips and trunk to turn strongly. ♦♦

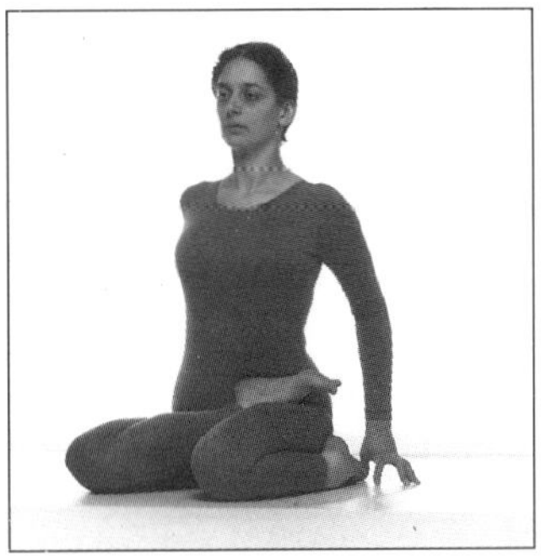

1 Sit in Daṇḍāsana (p. 52). ▷ Bend the left leg back with the foot beside the left hip; open the calf muscle out. Keep the heel and toes in line.

Bend the right leg in and place the foot on top of the left thigh. Bring the knee in to face forward. Open the right side of the groin and take the knee down. With the hands beside the hips, lift the trunk.

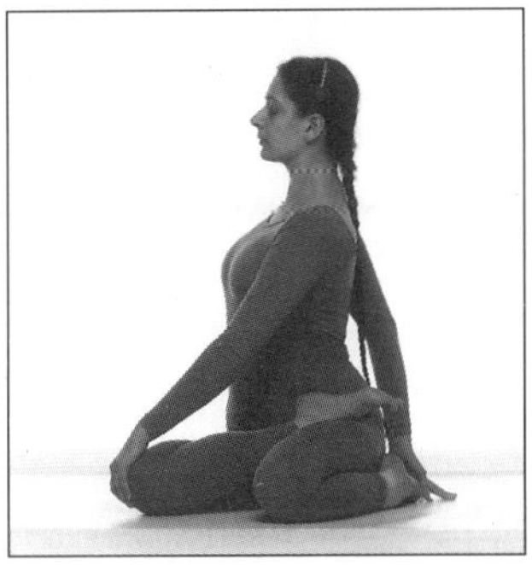

2 Exhale and turn to the right. Place the left hand on the right knee and take the right arm back. Pressing equally with both hands, turn the trunk between the arms, keeping it upright.

Stay for 20 to 30 seconds, breathing evenly, or continue to the final pose.

3 Straighten the left arm, turn the wrist out, and place the hand under the right thigh, with the fingers pointing in and the palm down. Bend the right arm behind the back and hold the right foot. Pull on the foot to turn the right side back; at the same time bring the left side forward.

Stay for 20 to 30 seconds, breathing evenly.

Inhale, release the arms, and turn to the front. Release the legs. ◁

Repeat from ▷ to ◁ on the left.

WORK IN THE POSTURE

Increase the turn of the trunk.

Extend the trunk up. Make the back concave and move the left kidney in.

Open the chest. Take the abdomen to the right.

WAYS OF PRACTICING

Sit on two folded blankets.

If the right knee does not go down to the floor, support it with a rolled blanket.

Put a belt around the right foot in order to catch it.

Keep the right hand on a brick (in step 2) to lift and turn more easily.

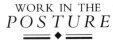

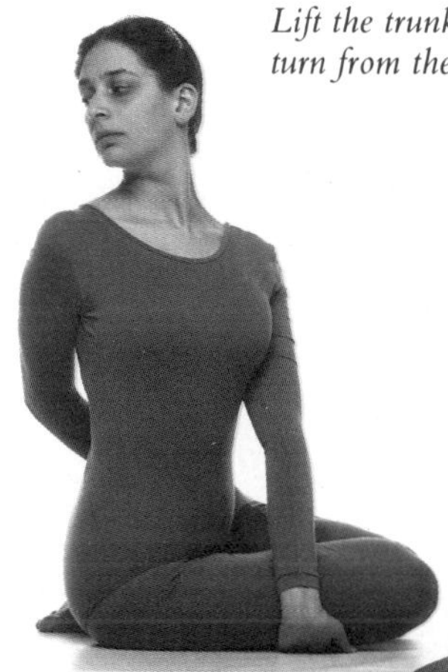

Front view
Lift the trunk and turn from the hips.

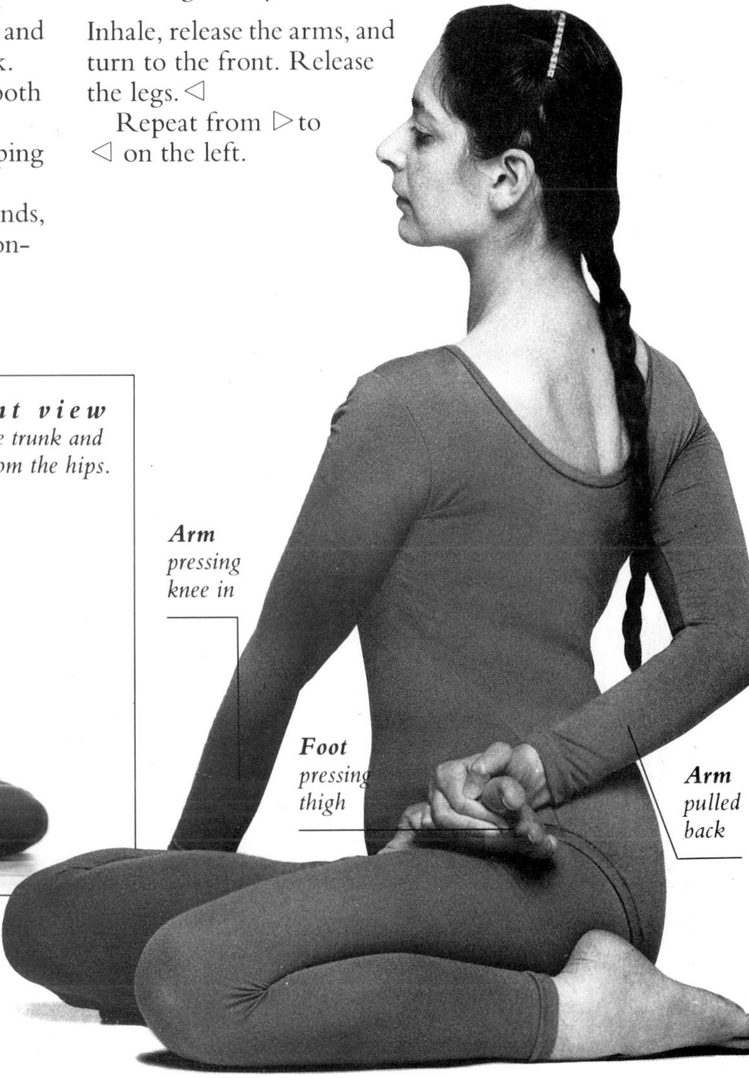

अर्ध मत्स्येन्द्रासन २

Ardha Matsyendrāsana II

ARDHA = half; *MATSYENDRA* = Lord of the fishes

THE STRONG grip of the hands makes the trunk lift and turn freely.♦♦♦

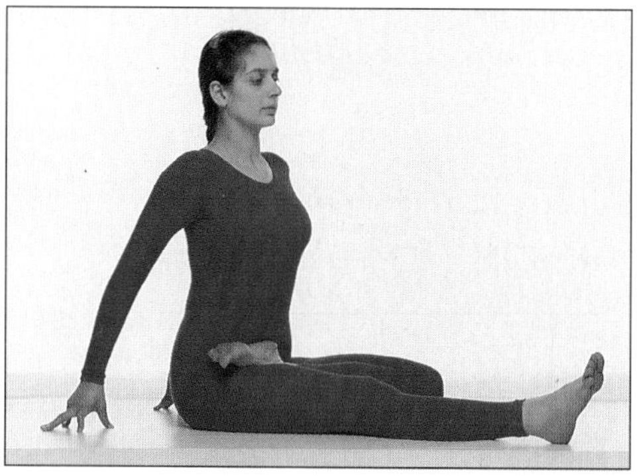

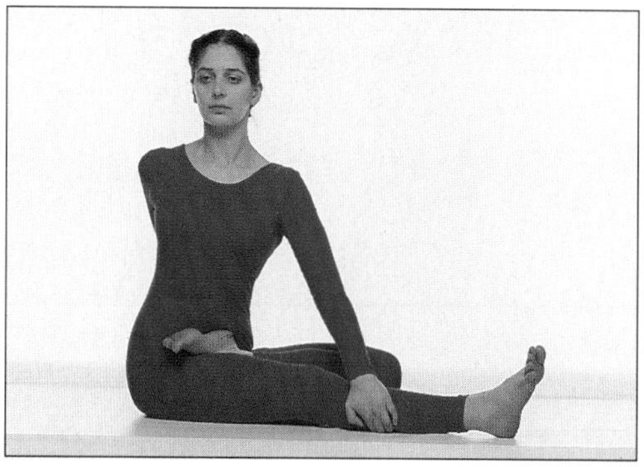

WAYS OF PRACTICING

Use a belt around the bent leg.
Support the bent knee.

1 Sit in Daṇḍāsana (p. 52). ▷Bend the left leg and place the foot against the right side of the groin. Press the fingertips into the floor beside the hips to stretch the trunk up.

2 Turn to the right, placing the left hand on the right outer calf. Take the right arm back. Move the coccyx and sacrum in, take the back ribs in, and stretch the spine up. Pull up the front of the body from the pubis, stretch the abdomen up, and lift the chest. Open the shoulders outward.

WORK IN THE POSTURE

Maintain the grip of the hands. Pull the shoulders back.

Turn the hips and extend the trunk.

Squeeze the abdomen to the right.

Lift the rib cage and breathe well.

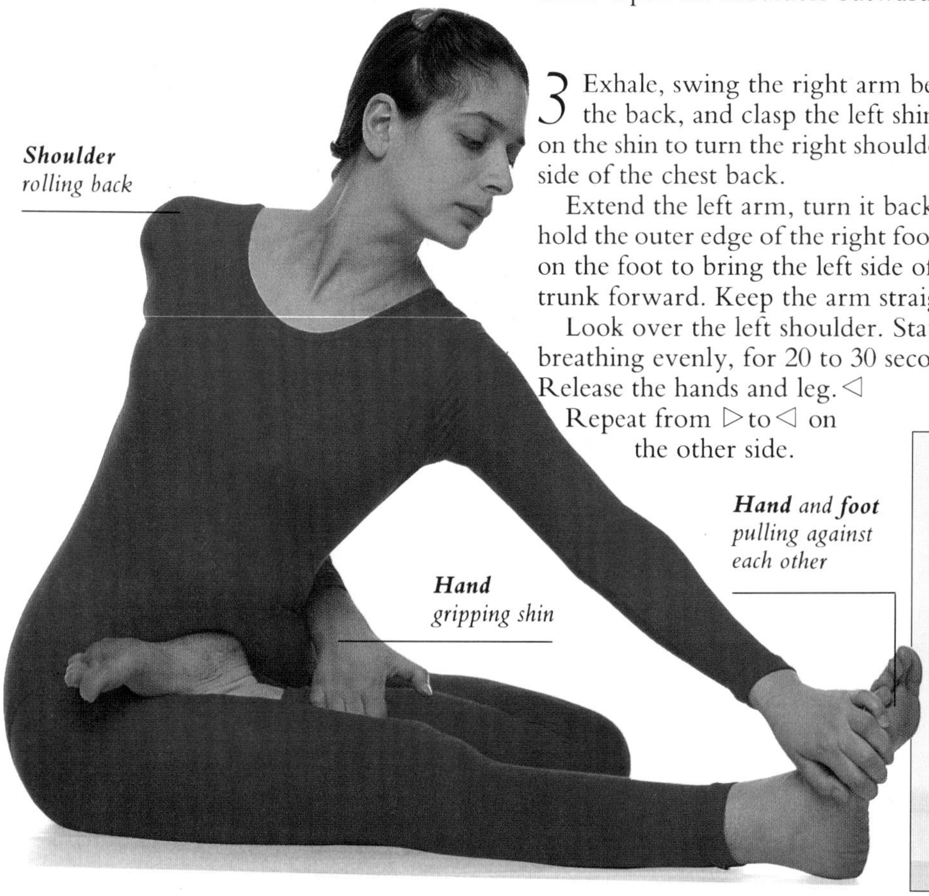
Shoulder
rolling back
Hand
gripping shin
Hand and foot
pulling against
each other

3 Exhale, swing the right arm behind the back, and clasp the left shin. Pull on the shin to turn the right shoulder and side of the chest back.

Extend the left arm, turn it back, and hold the outer edge of the right foot. Pull on the foot to bring the left side of the trunk forward. Keep the arm straight.

Look over the left shoulder. Stay, breathing evenly, for 20 to 30 seconds. Release the hands and leg.◁

Repeat from ▷to◁ on the other side.

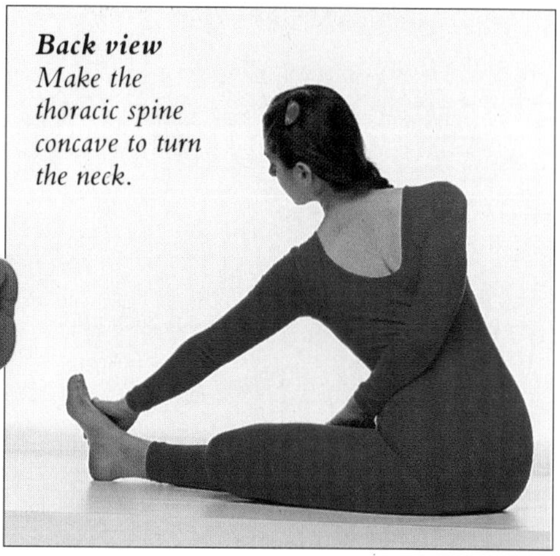

Back view *Make the thoracic spine concave to turn the neck.*

SUPINE & PRONE POSES

After acting, reflect on what you have done. If you do not reflect, there is confused action. Pause between each movement. The self has to find out whether the posture has been done well or not.

B. K. S. IYENGAR

This section includes two categories of posture. They stretch the abdomen, increase the mobility of the spine and hips, and open the groin. Some strengthen the back, arms, and legs. Others are restful.

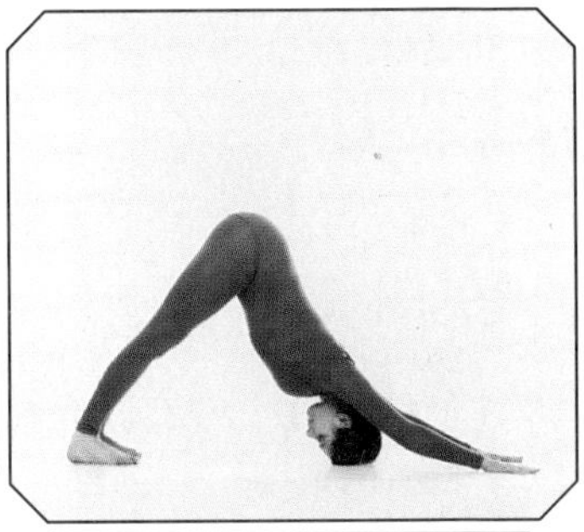

GUIDELINES FOR PRACTICE

The supine postures may be practiced intensively or quietly. When practicing quietly, with a bolster or blankets for support, time should be spent on getting into a comfortable position so that the back can relax fully.

In the back arches there is a tendency for the lumbar spine to contract. The legs and trunk should be stretched well before beginning them.

Adho Mukha Śvānāsana (p. 90) is an important posture as it accustoms the body to being in an inverted position. This inversion is of great benefit in helping to relax the brain.

As with the sitting poses, care should be taken to avoid straining the knees (see the advice given in the postures on pp. 50-51, 54-5).

CAUTIONS: Do not do supine and prone poses after abdominal operations.

During menstruation or in pregnancy, only Supta Baddha Koṇāsana (p. 81), Supta Vīrāsana (p. 82) and Lying on Bolsters (p. 80) may be practiced.

Lying with legs up

THIS REMOVES fatigue in the legs.♦

1 Sit sideways near a wall. Take the legs up the wall one at a time; at the same time lever the trunk around and lie down. Keep the trunk in line with the legs and the buttocks against the wall. Take the shoulders down, stretch the arms to the sides, and relax them, palms up. Relax the feet. If necessary, support the head. Stay for 2 to 5 minutes. Bend the knees and turn to the side, then get up.

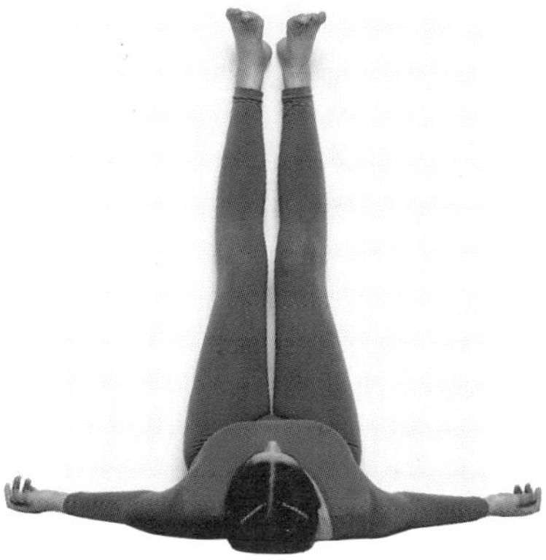

2 As an alternative method, spread the legs apart.

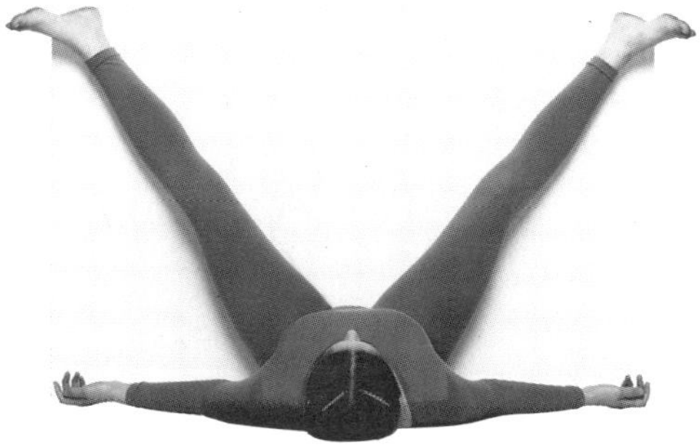

Lying on cross bolsters

THE SUPPORT under the chest facilitates breathing. This is a tonic to the system.♦

1 Lay a bolster or thick rolled blanket on the floor. Across the center lay another bolster lengthwise. Sit on the front of the top bolster and lie back over it with the shoulders on the floor. Place a folded blanket under the head if necessary. If the back is not comfortable, slide slightly up or down to find a good position. Stretch the legs away from the trunk, and then relax them. Take the arms over the head and relax them. Stay for 5 to 15 minutes, breathing evenly.

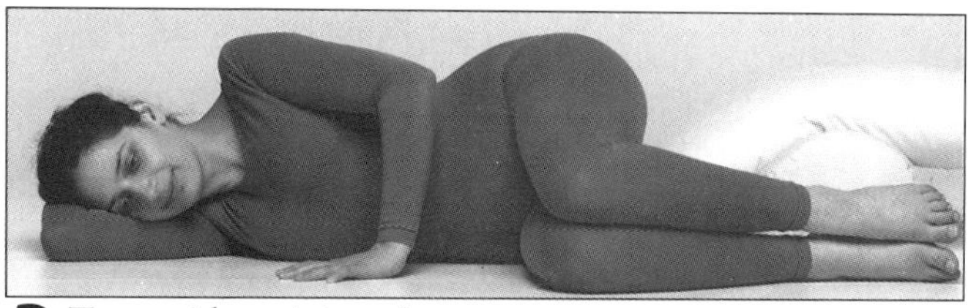

2 To avoid straining the back when coming up, roll to one side, then get up.

WAYS OF PRACTICING

If the lower back feels strained, raise the feet onto a brick or bolster.

WORK IN THE
POSTURE

Feel the chest opening and the breath deepening because of the support under the rib cage.

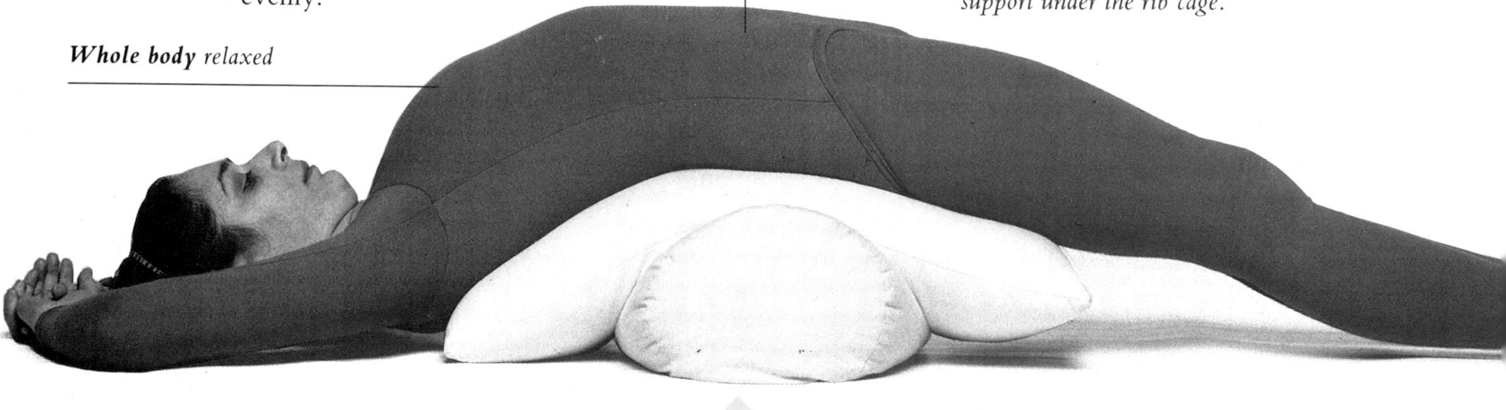

सुप्त बद्ध कोणासन

Supta Baddha Koṇāsana

SUPTA = supine, lying down; BADDHA KOṆA = bound angle

THIS IS a resting pose which is also helpful during menstruation.♦

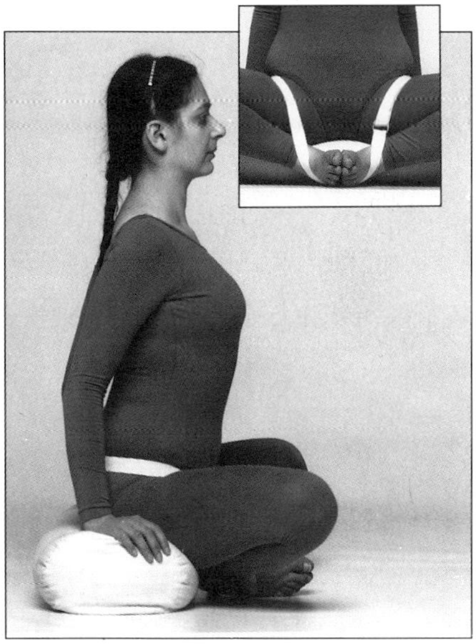

1 Sit in Baddha Koṇāsana (p. 57) on a bolster placed horizontally. Take a long belt (or two belts tied together). Pass it behind the sacrum, over the thighs and shins, and under the feet. Make sure the belt goes across the base of the sacrum. Tie it so that the buckle goes between one thigh and calf; pull on the belt to bring the feet close to the trunk.

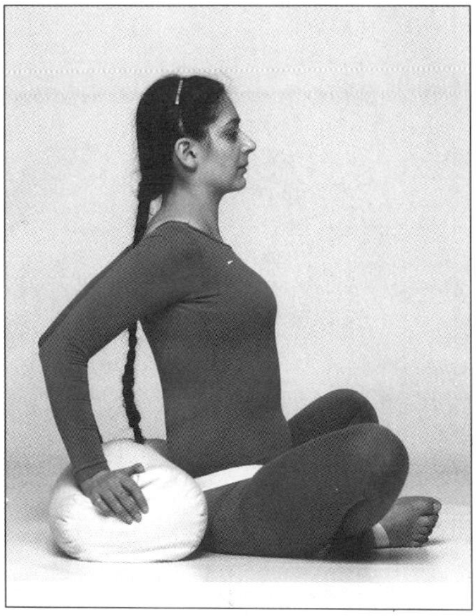

2 Slide forward off the bolster and hold it firmly.

3 Lie back over it, with the shoulders on the floor. If necessary, support the head. Tighten the belt, without creating strain. Take the arms over the head.

Stay for 5 to 10 minutes, breathing evenly.

Inhale, come up; untie the belt.

Ways of Practicing

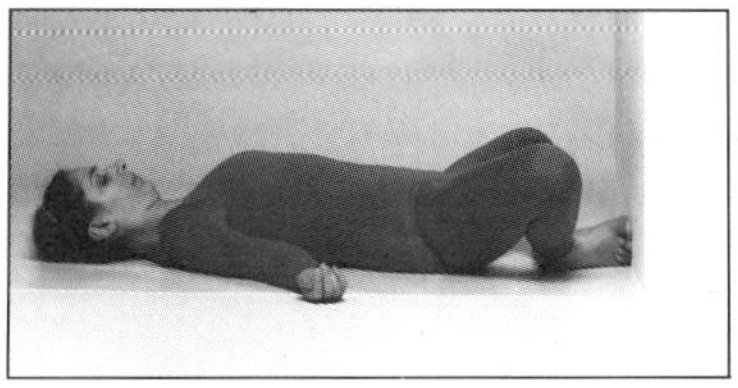

If the lower back is stiff or aches, lay the bolster lengthwise and support the head.

Use two belts; tie each leg separately around the top thigh and bottom shin.

Lie with the toes curling back against a wall. Bring the trunk close to the feet.

Rest the arms beside the trunk or over the head.

WORK IN THE POSTURE

Allow the back to settle over the bolster. Feel the extension of the inner organs. Feel the front ribs and the collarbones opening outward.

♦

Relax completely.

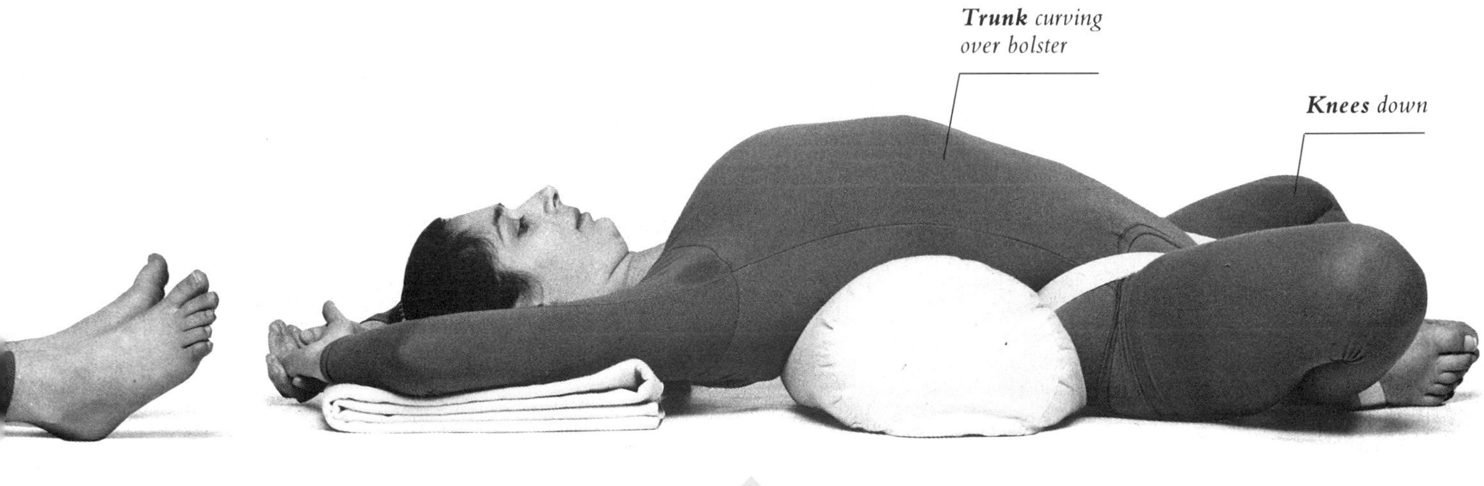

सुप्त वीरासन

Supta Vīrāsana

SUPTA = supine; *VĪRA* = hero

THIS POSE rests the legs and is good for the digestion.♦♦

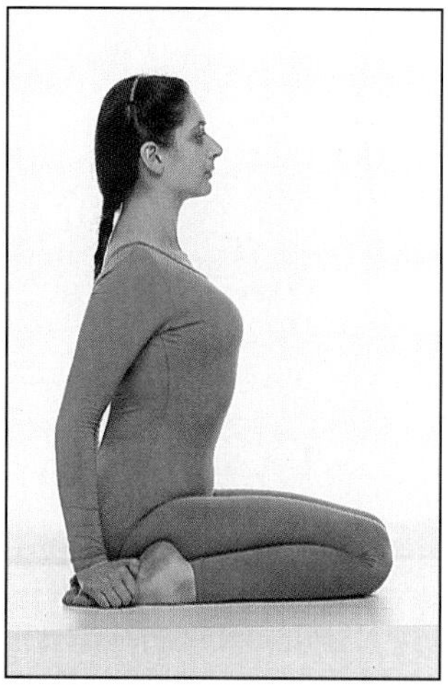

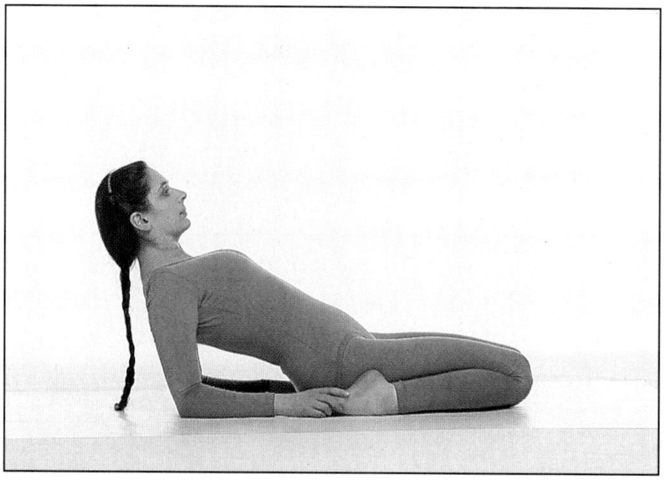

1 Sit in Vīrāsana (p. 50), with the hands on or behind the feet.

2 Move the buttock bones slightly forward; lean back, place the elbows on the ground, and lower the trunk onto the floor.

WAYS OF PRACTICING

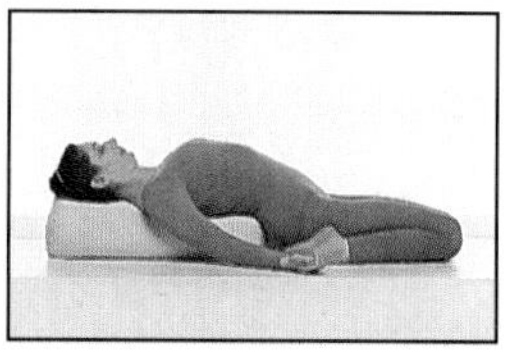

To avoid strain in the knees, place a thin pad behind them or a cushion under them.

Lie back on a bolster.

If necessary, support the head and place an additional blanket under the buttocks.

3 Stretch the arms over the head and lengthen the trunk. Press the thighs and knees down and keep the knees together, without straining them.

Stay for 30 seconds or longer, up to 20 minutes. Breathe evenly.

Inhale, come up. Bend forward in Vīrāsana.

WORK IN THE
POSTURE

Keep the lumbar extended. Stretch the front of the body up from the pubis.

♦

Revolve the thighs outward and draw the shins and feet closer to them.

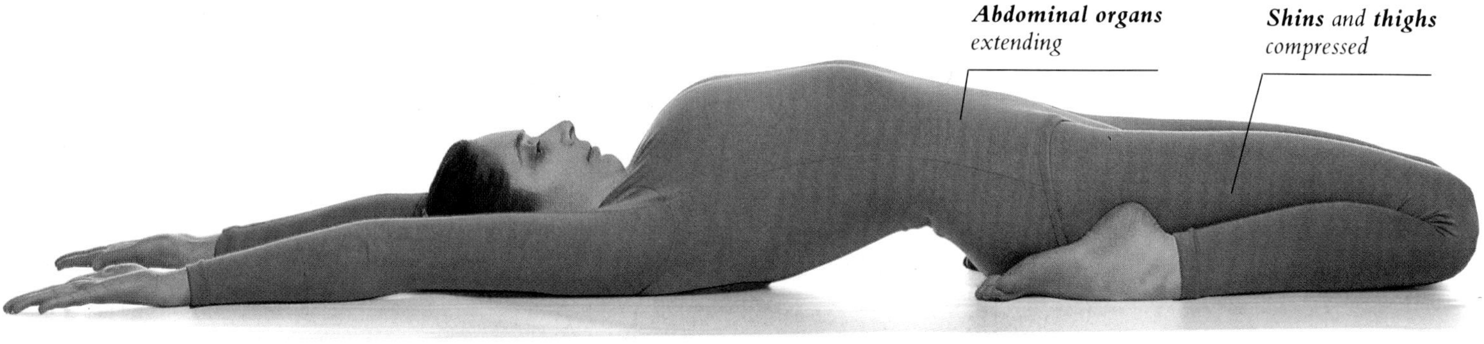

मत्स्यासन

Matsyāsana

MATSYA = fish

THE DOWNWARD action of the legs creates space in the pelvic region.♦♦♦

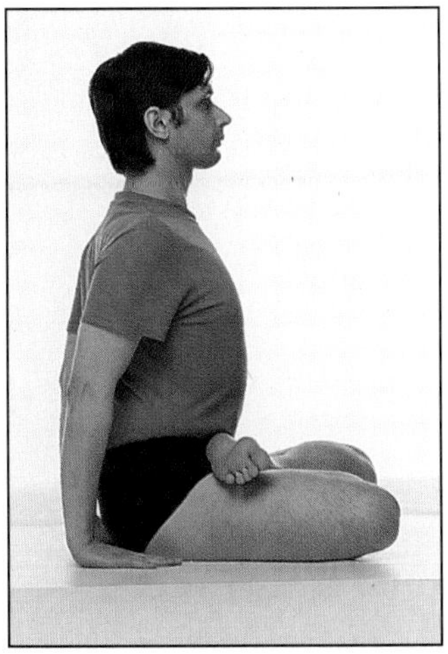

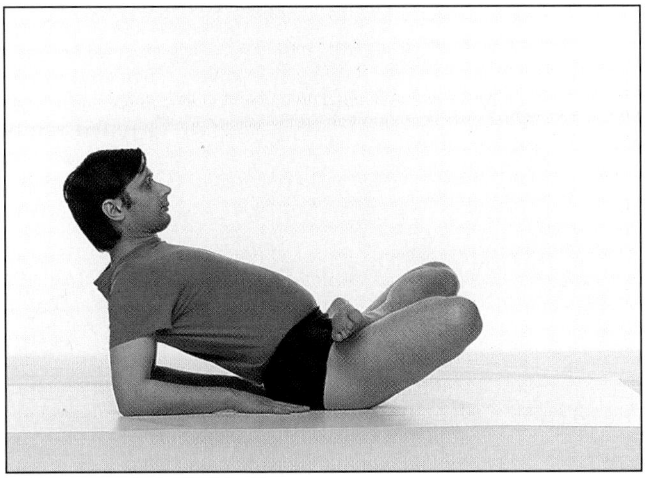

1 ▷Sit in Padmāsana (p. 54) with the right leg crossed first, hands beside the hips. Extend the trunk up.

2 With an exhalation, lean back onto the elbows.

3 Lie back. For a moment pull on the feet to make the crossed legs more compact. Then stretch the arms over the head. Open both sides of the groin and take the knees down.

Stay for 30 seconds or longer, up to 5 minutes, without straining the knees. Breathe evenly.

Inhale and come up with the help of the hands. Release the legs.◁

Repeat from ▷to◁ on the left.

WAYS OF PRACTICING

Lie on a bolster as in Supta Vīrāsana (opposite).

Support the knees with a cushion.

Keep the arms beside the trunk.

WORK IN THE POSTURE

Go on stretching the thighs away from the trunk.

♦

Draw the knees closer together. Press them down on an exhalation.

♦

Keep the lumbar down.

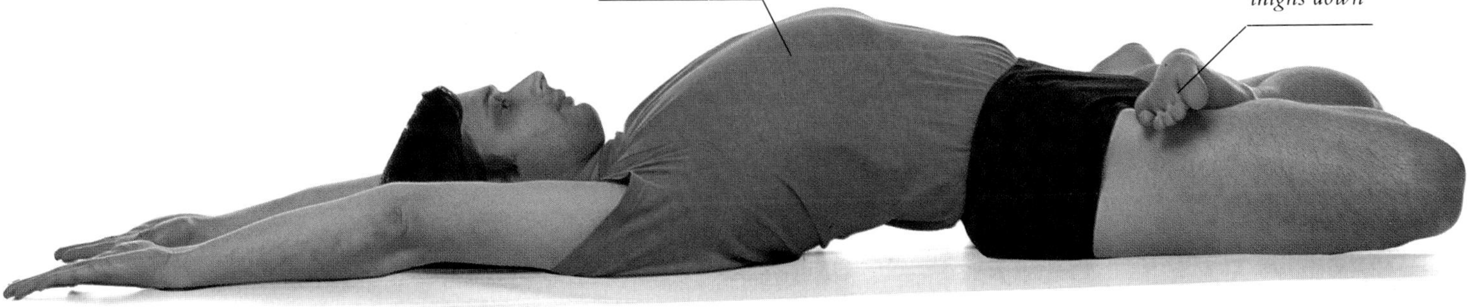

ऊर्ध्व प्रसारित पादासन

Ūrdhva Prasārita Pādāsana

ŪRDHVA = upward; PRASĀRITA = spread out; PĀDA = foot

HERE THE legs are raised to 30°, 60°, and 90°, developing strong abdominal muscles.♦♦♦

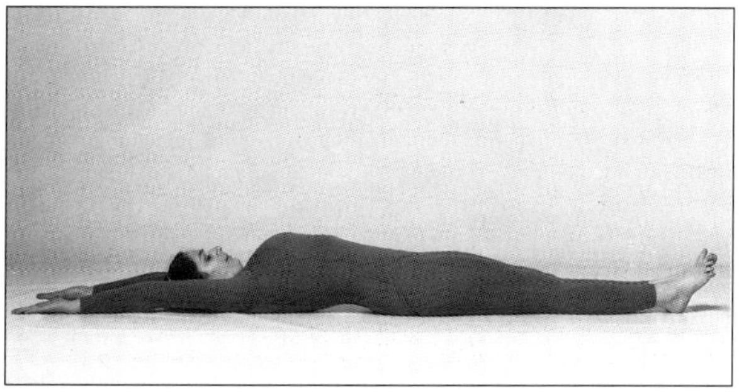

1 Lie in a straight line, arms beside the trunk. Keep the knees facing the ceiling. Extend the arms over the head, palms up and elbows locked. Stretch from the hips to the finger-tips. Tighten the kneecaps and stretch the legs and the feet.

2 Exhale and raise the legs to 30°. Extend the lumbar away from the waist and press it down. Stretch the backs of the legs toward the heels. Stay for a few seconds, without holding the breath.

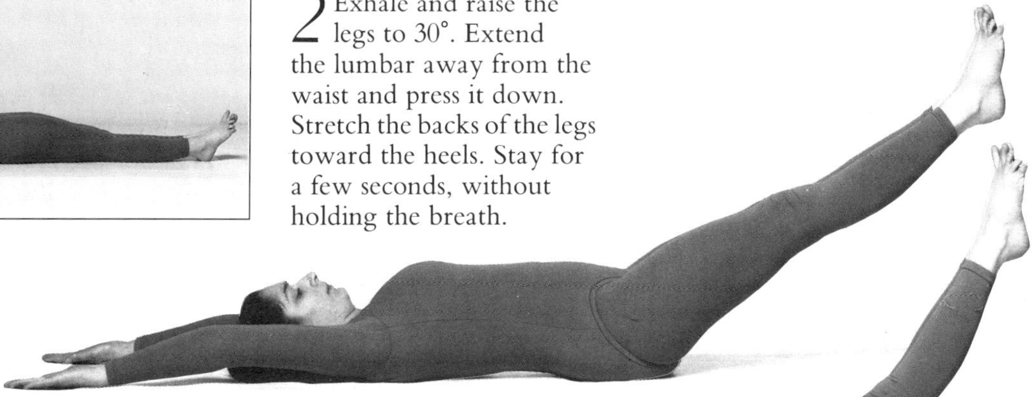

3 Exhale, and raise the legs to 60°, extending as above. Stay for a few seconds.

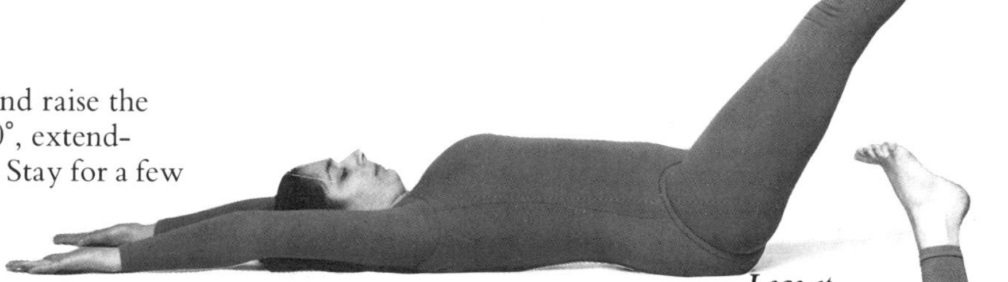

4 Exhale and raise the legs to 90°. Keep the backs of the legs strong, and the abdomen relaxed. Stretch the arms more. Stay for 30 to 60 seconds, breathing evenly.

With an exhalation, lower the legs slowly to the ground, without jerking them. In going down, stretch the arms and legs away from each other.

Bring the arms down, let the feet drop to the sides, and relax.

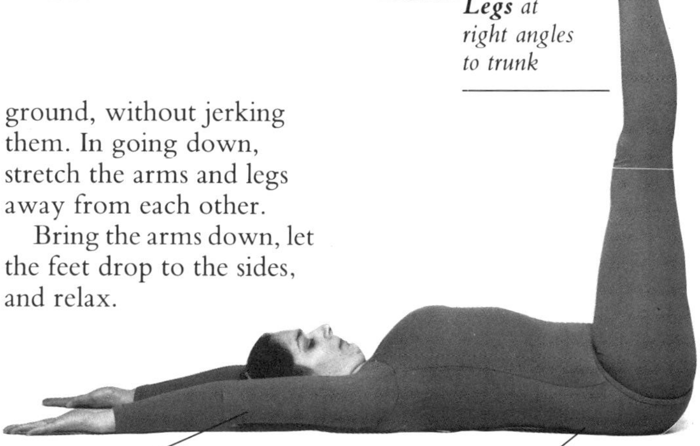

WAYS OF PRACTICING

To avoid straining the back or legs, bend the legs over the abdomen, then straighten them up to 90°.

Hold the feet with a belt (in step 4) to straighten the legs.

Lie with the legs against a wall. Raise the legs to 90° and lower them, 8 to 12 times in quick succession.

WORK IN THE POSTURE

Do not hold the breath.

Press the outer hips down.

Keep the abdomen passive. Do not let the chest collapse.

जठर परिवर्तनासन

Jaṭhara Parivartanāsana

JAṬHARA = stomach, abdomen; *PARIVARTANA* = turning around

THE ABDOMEN gets an internal massage as the legs swing down from one side to the other.♦♦

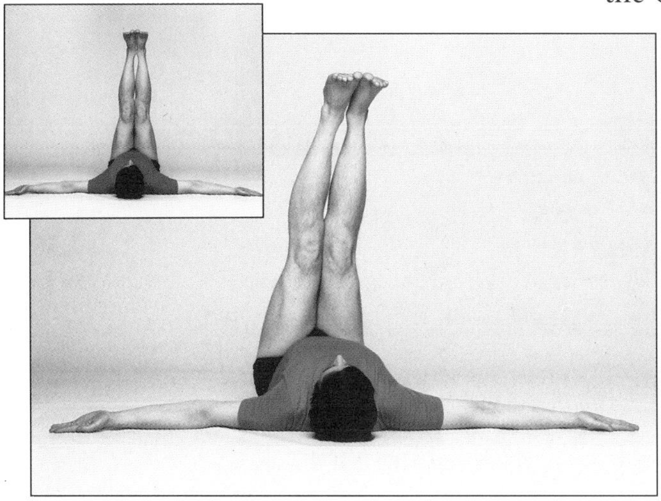

1 Lie with the arms stretched sideways at shoulder level, palms up.

With an exhalation raise the legs to 90°, keeping the hips down and the legs straight. Take one or two breaths. ▷Move the hips 5 to 10° to the left. Keep the legs together.

2 Simultaneously press the left shoulder down and extend the left arm to the left, revolve the abdomen to the left, and take the legs diagonally down toward the right hand. Go down until the feet are about 3 in above the floor.

Stay for 20 to 30 seconds. Do not hold the breath.

Inhale, raise the legs.◁ (If necessary, bend the legs for a moment.)

Repeat from ▷ to ◁ on the left, then bring the legs and the arms down, and relax.

WAYS OF PRACTICING

In Step 1, bend the legs over the abdomen and then straighten them.

Place a weight on the left hand while going to the right.

Take the legs halfway down.

VARIATION

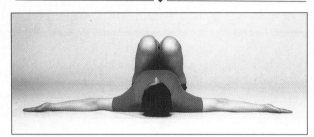

This is useful for relieving backache.

1 Lie down with the arms stretched out to the sides. Bend the knees over the abdomen.

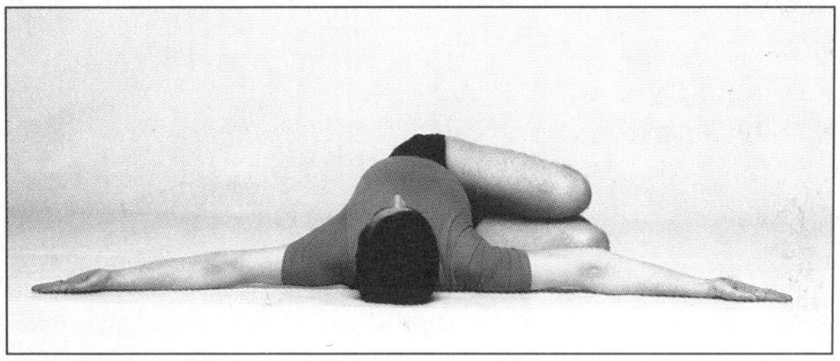

2 Take the knees down to the right. Repeat on the left.♦

WORK IN THE POSTURE

Do not shorten the body. Do not let it roll to the side when the legs go down.

♦

Keep the top of the right leg tucked in toward the hip.

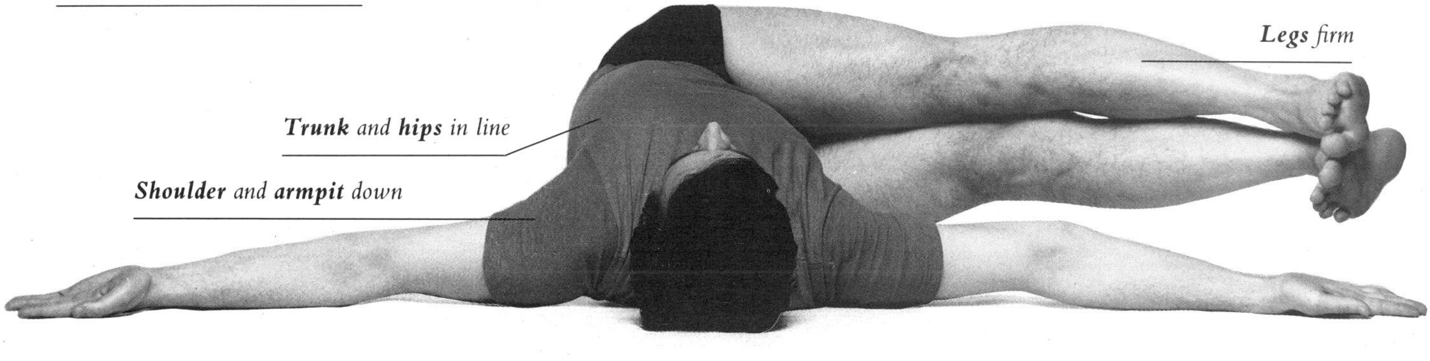

भेकासन

Bhekāsana

BHEKA = frog

STRENGTH in the arms helps to develop flexibility in the legs. ♦♦

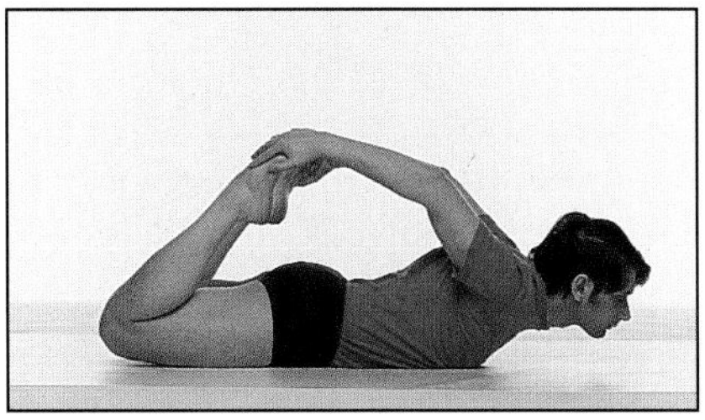

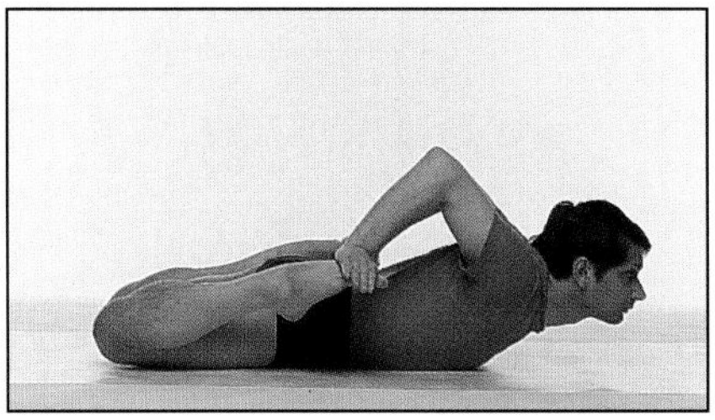

1 Lie face down on the floor, with the arms stretched back beside the trunk. Stretch the tops of the thighs away from the trunk, then bend the legs back. One at a time, bend the arms with the elbows pointing up and place the hands on top of the feet.

2 Swivel the wrists in and turn the hands outward.

3 Continue turning the hands until the fingers point toward the head. With the heels of the hands just above the toes, press the feet down beside the hips. Keep the feet in line with the shins. Exhale and raise the head and chest. Stay for 10 to 15 seconds, breathing evenly.

Release the hands and legs.

Ways of Practicing

Work with one leg at a time, repeating several times.

Reflection

Flexibility in the joints is important for circulation and energy to flow in the body healthily. Where a joint does not straighten or cannot bend, circulation and energy are blocked, inviting disease. Flexibility assists movement so that the postures can be completed and their full benefit experienced.

WORK IN THE POSTURE

Use the pressure of the hands on the metatarsals to curve the feet down. Do not let the knees splay out too much.

♦

Press the coccyx down, lift the upper chest, and take the shoulders back. Keep the elbows in.

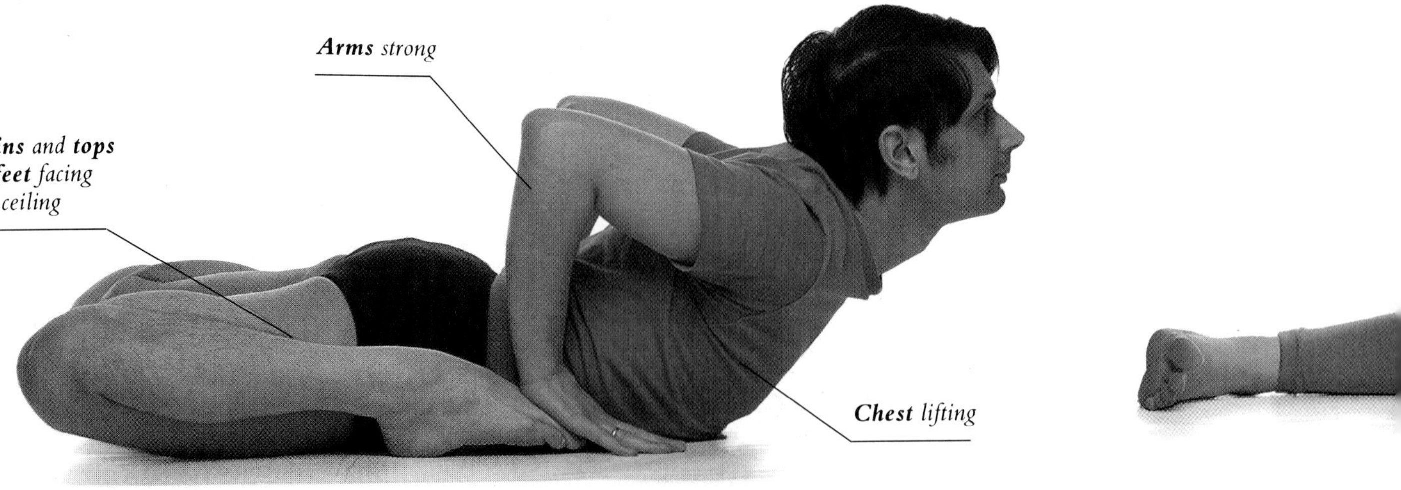
Arms *strong*
Shins *and* **tops of feet** *facing the ceiling*
Chest *lifting*

अनंतासन

Anantāsana

ANANTA = the Eternal One; serpent couch of Lord Vishnu

THE BODY reclines on the side, one leg extending up toward infinity.♦♦

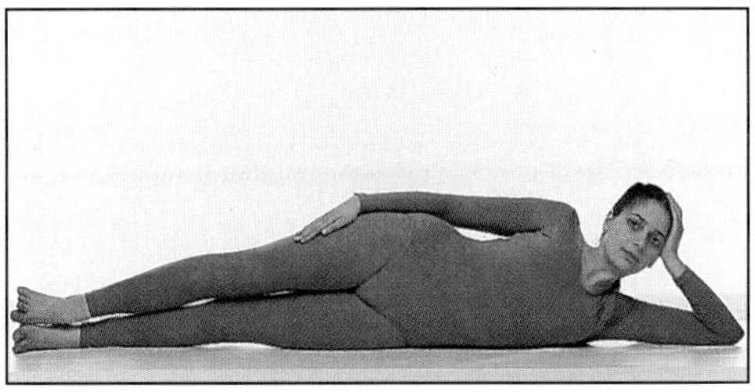

1 ▷Lie on the back. Turn onto the left side. Keep the knees straight, feet and legs together. Extend the left arm along the floor beyond the head. Bend the elbow, take the head slightly back, and support it. Press the armpit down. Extend the right arm along the right side and balance. Squeeze the buttocks lightly together to move the sacrum in. Press the outer edge of the left foot down.

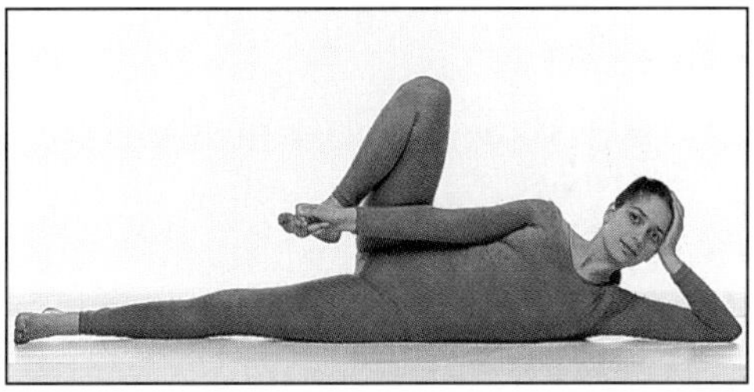

2 Inhale, turn, and bend the right leg up, knee facing the ceiling. Take the right arm in front of the leg and catch the big toe with the thumb, index, and middle fingers.

3 Straighten the leg up, turning it outward in its socket so that the inner leg faces the same way as the front of the body. Turn the buttock with the leg.

Stretch the back of the knee and the heel up; tuck the kneecap in. Pull on the big toe and let the toe pull the leg upward. Keep the right elbow straight and stretch the arm up.

Balance for 20 to 30 seconds, breathing evenly, keeping the head facing forward.

Release the arm and leg.◁ Repeat from ▷to◁ on the right.

WAYS OF PRACTICING

Use a belt to catch the foot.

Lie with the back against a wall to understand alignment.

WORK IN THE POSTURE

Extend the front of the body from the groin to the shoulders. Bring the left hip and side of the trunk forward and make the dorsal spine concave.

Extend both legs to the heels. Keeping the left leg firm, pull the right leg toward the head, without letting the right hip drop forward or backward.

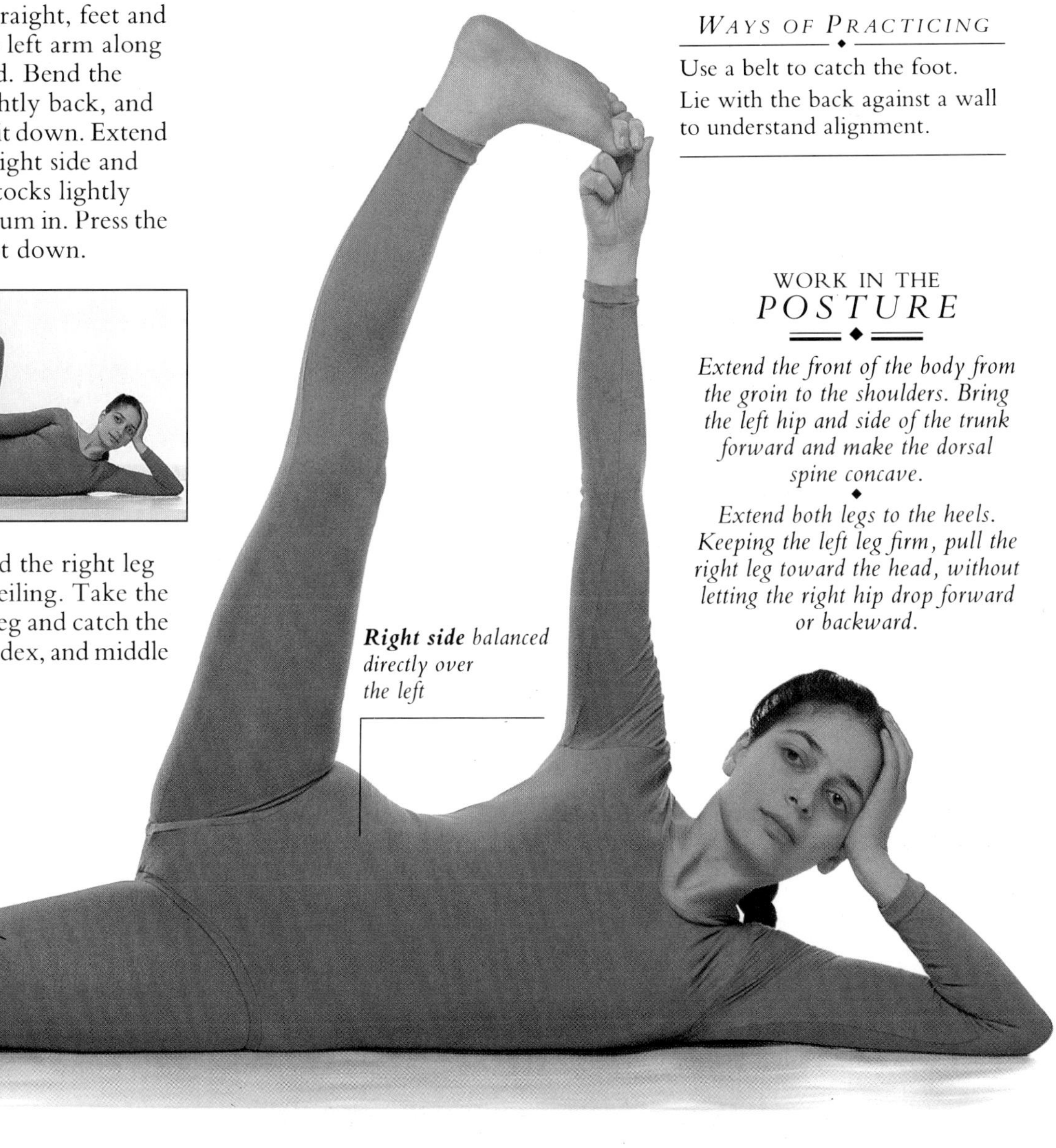
Right side balanced directly over the left
Leg, trunk, and **upper arm** in line

सुप्त पादांगुष्ठासन

Supta Pādāṅguṣṭhāsana

SUPTA = supine, lying down; *PĀDĀṄGUṢṬHA* = the big toe

THIS POSE is useful for releasing the lower back.♦♦

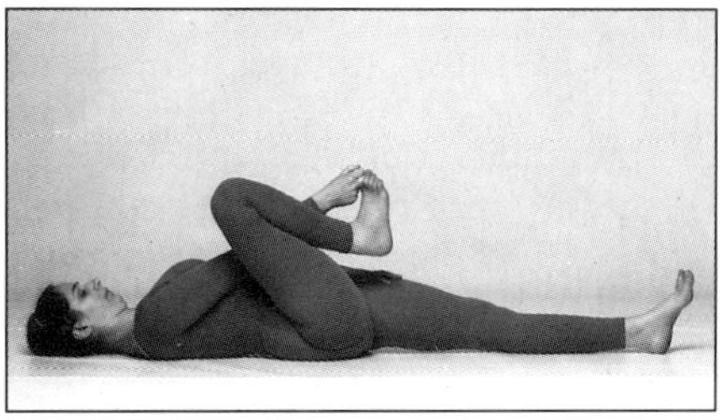

1 Lie on the back, with the knees straight and the feet together. Stretch the legs. Lengthen the lumbar and sacrum away from the waist. Keep the head straight.

▷Keep the left leg firm and place the left hand on top of the thigh. Bend the right leg over the abdomen and hold the big toe between the right thumb, index, and middle fingers.

WAYS OF PRACTICING

Use a belt to catch the foot.

Practice step 2 against a door frame or column, with the vertical leg supported from the buttock bone.

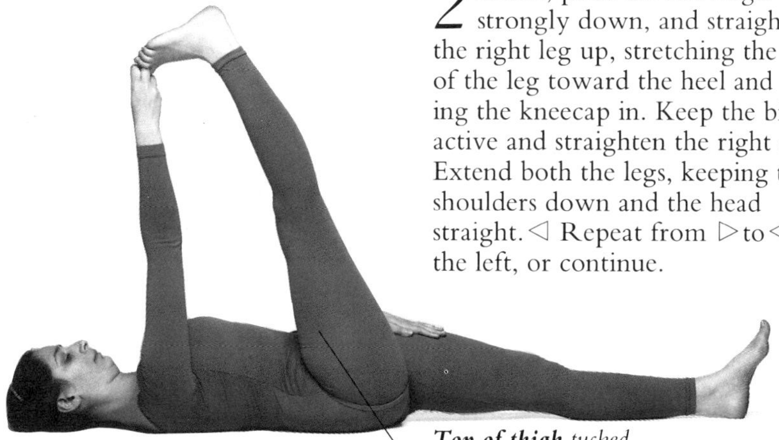
Top of thigh *tucked in toward hip*

2 Inhale, press the left thigh strongly down, and straighten the right leg up, stretching the back of the leg toward the heel and tucking the kneecap in. Keep the big toe active and straighten the right arm. Extend both the legs, keeping the shoulders down and the head straight.◁ Repeat from ▷to◁ on the left, or continue.

3 ▷▷Keep the left side of the trunk firmly on the floor. Revolve the right thigh bone outward in its socket; exhale and take the leg down to the right. Do not pull the trunk over to the right. Keep the arm and the leg straight. Stay for 20 to 30 seconds, breathing evenly.

Inhale and raise the right leg up. ◁◁ Repeat from ▷to◁◁ on the left, or continue.

- *Do not proceed if the hamstrings are pulling.*

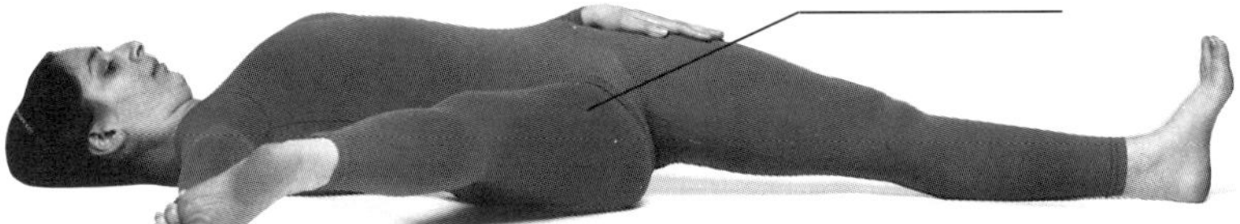
Inner leg *stretching toward heel*

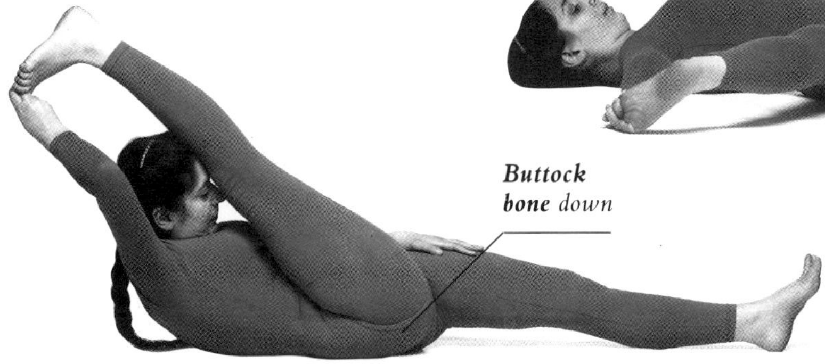
Buttock bone *down*

4 With an exhalation, bend the right elbow outward, and draw the leg toward the head. Simultaneously raise the head and chest toward the leg, until the head touches the shin. Stay for 15 to 20 seconds.

Exhale, lower the head and trunk; bring the arms and the right leg down.◁◁◁ Repeat from ▷▷to ◁◁◁ on the left.

WORK IN THE
POSTURE

Go on extending the backs of the legs; keep the heels strong. Keep the thigh muscles gripping the bones.

Elongate the trunk and open the chest.

चतुरंग दंडासन

Caturaṅga Daṇḍāsana

CATUR = four; *AṄGA* = limb; *DAṆḌA* = stick, rod

THE BODY is held parallel to the ground by the strength of the legs and arms.♦♦

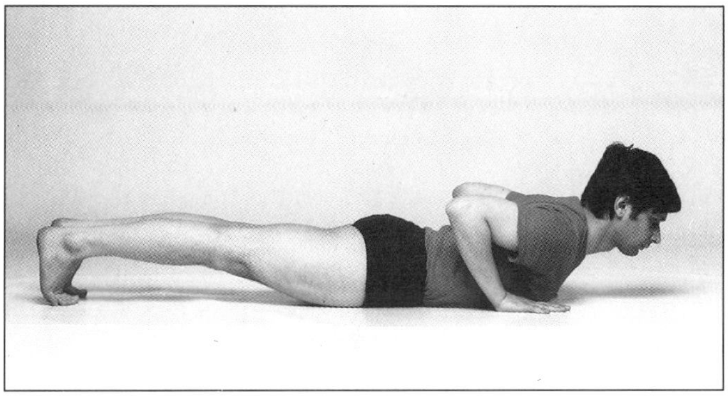

1 Lie prone on the floor, arms beside the trunk. Take the feet about 1ft apart and extend the legs away from the trunk. Bend the elbows, place the palms on the floor beside the chest, and spread the fingers. Bring the elbows in. Tuck the toes under and keep the soles of the feet perpendicular. Straighten the knees. Raise the head. Take a deep breath.

2 With a sharp exhalation raise the legs and the trunk a few inches above the ground, parallel to it. Extend the spine and the trunk forward and take the shoulders up and back, keeping the coccyx and sacrum slightly tucked in. Do not raise the hips higher than the legs and trunk.

Stay for 15 to 20 seconds, looking ahead and breathing evenly.

Exhale and come down.

Focus *Opening the backs of the legs.*
Extend from the heels to the buttocks. Broaden the calf muscles near the knees. Stretch the backs of the knees and open them horizontally; stretch the back thigh muscles. Project the skin and flesh of the backs of the legs (calves, knees, and thighs) up toward the ceiling. Puff the muscles toward the skin; do not let them sag.

WORK IN THE POSTURE

Keep the legs straight and stretch them back slightly.

♦

Press the heels of the hands down. Move the shoulder blades into the rib cage. Keep the chest open.

WAYS OF PRACTICING

To help lift the trunk, place the hands on bricks.

Press the soles of the feet against a wall.

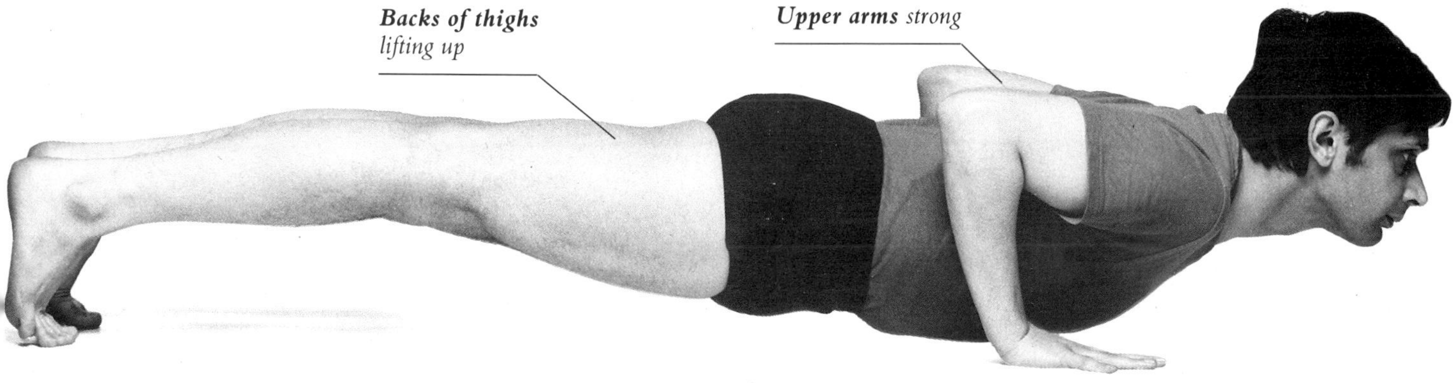

अधो मुख श्वानासन

Adho Mukha Śvānāsana

ADHO = downward; *MUKHA* = face; *ŚVĀNA* = dog

THIS POSTURE imitates a dog stretching downward. It rests the heart.♦

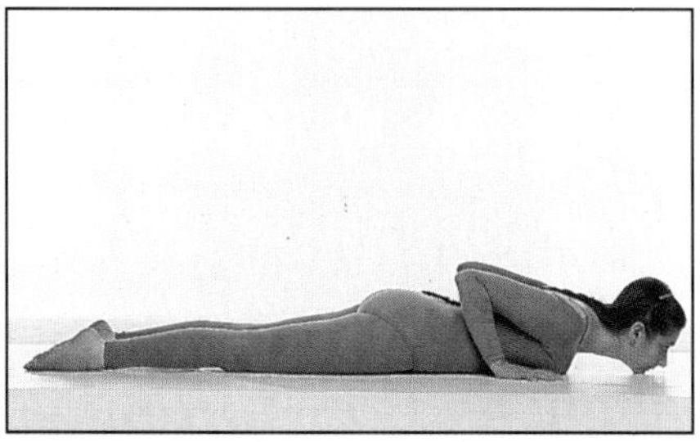

1 Lie face down on the floor. Take the feet about 1ft apart. Bend the elbows and place the hands beside the rib cage. Open the palms and spread the fingers, with the middle fingers pointing forward.

Keep the hands in line with each other and also in line with the feet. This is the base of the posture.

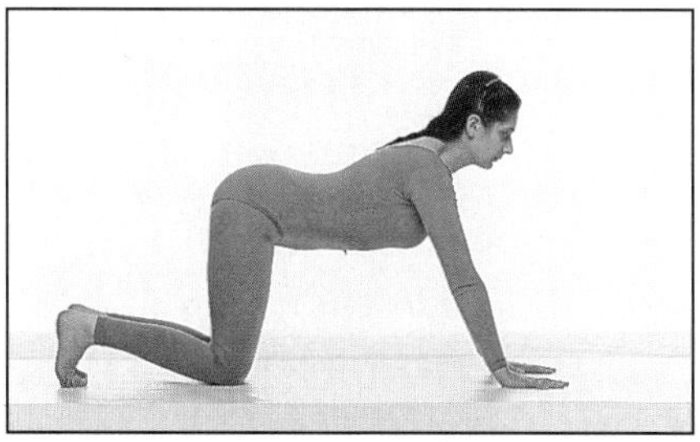

2 Tuck the toes under, raise the head and trunk; bend the legs to raise the hips. Straighten the arms. Check alignment of feet and hands.

Alternative Method

From Uttānāsana (p. 44), place the hands on the floor and walk the feet back until body forms a right angle.

3 Straighten the legs, lift the hips higher, and take the head and trunk down. Make the knees firm.

Press the heels of the hands into the floor, stretch the fingers, and extend the arms up.

Raise the shoulders and move the shoulder blades into the back ribs and up. Lift the pelvis. Keep the coccyx and the bottom of the pubis pointing up.

Without losing the height of the hips, stretch the heels down. Move the thighs and shins back to bring the weight onto the backs of the legs and the heels.

Relax the head and neck. If possible, rest the head on the floor. Stay for half to one minute, or longer, breathing evenly.

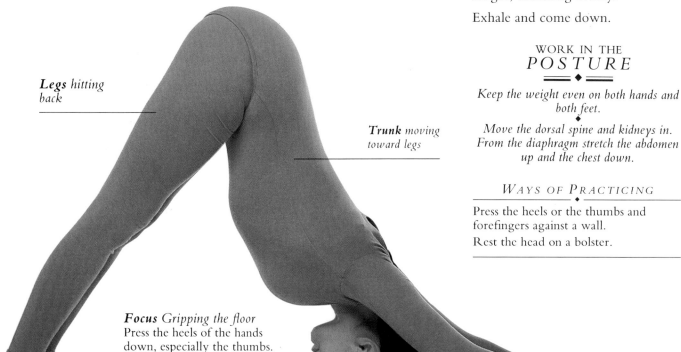

Exhale and come down.

WORK IN THE
POSTURE

Keep the weight even on both hands and both feet.

Move the dorsal spine and kidneys in. From the diaphragm stretch the abdomen up and the chest down.

WAYS OF PRACTICING

Press the heels or the thumbs and forefingers against a wall.

Rest the head on a bolster.

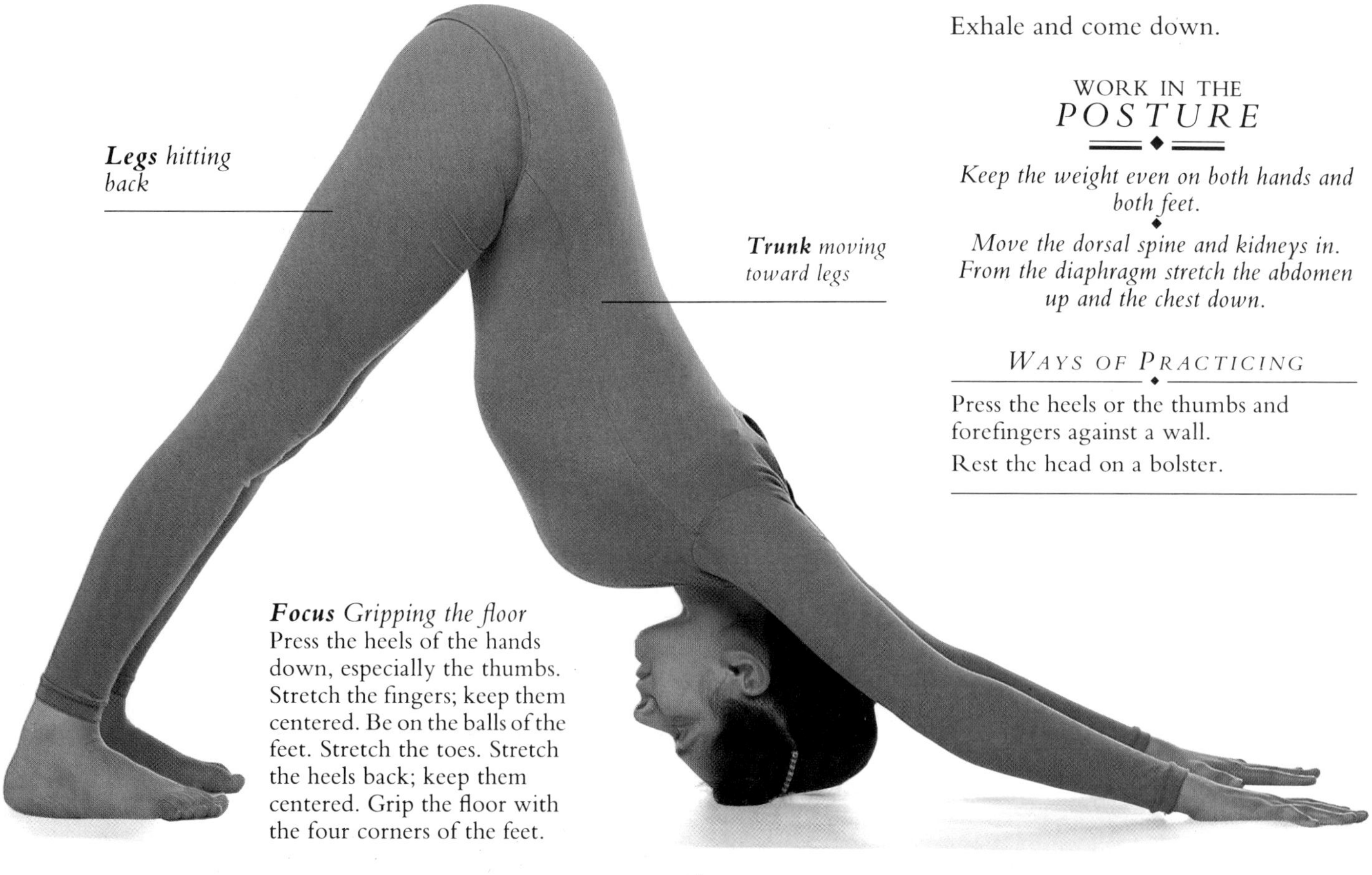
***Legs** hitting back*
***Trunk** moving toward legs*
***Focus** Gripping the floor*
Press the heels of the hands down, especially the thumbs. Stretch the fingers; keep them centered. Be on the balls of the feet. Stretch the toes. Stretch the heels back; keep them centered. Grip the floor with the four corners of the feet.

ऊर्ध्व मुख श्वानासन

Ūrdhva Mukha Śvānāsana

ŪRDHVA = upward; *MUKHA* = face; *ŚVĀNA* = dog

THIS IS a vigorous upward stretch of the trunk.♦

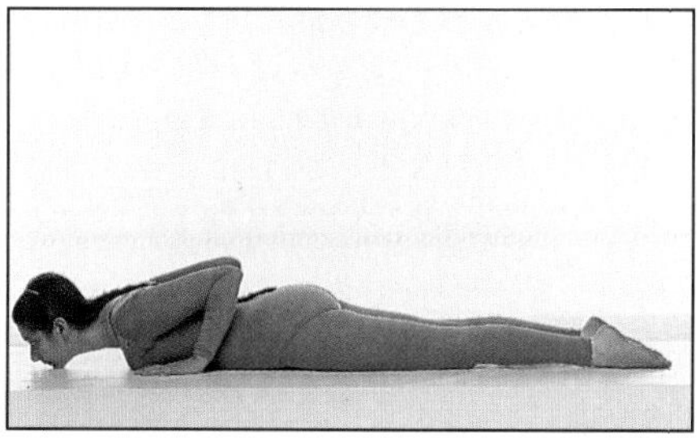

1 Lie face down on the floor. Take the feet about 1ft apart. Stretch the toes back. Bend the elbows and place the palms on the floor beside the chest, fingers apart and middle fingers pointing forward. Straighten the knees and stretch the legs.

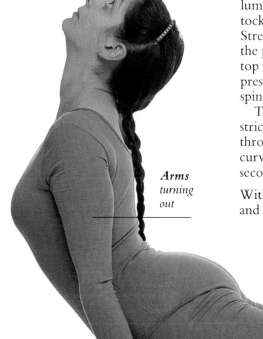

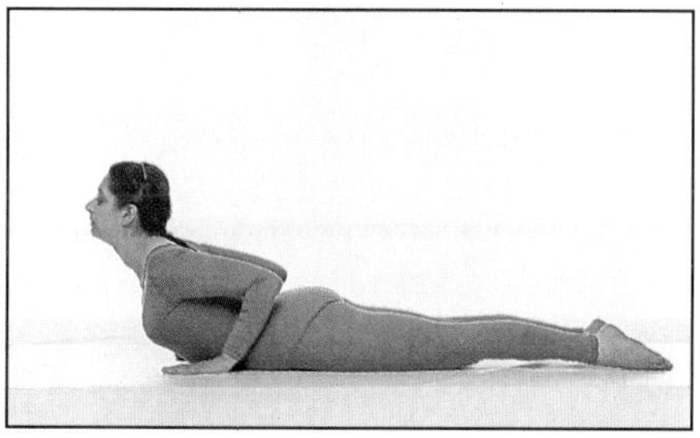

2 With an inhalation press the tops of the feet and the palms into the floor. Raise the head and chest.

3 Straighten the arms and lift the waist, hips, and knees a few inches above the floor. Pull the trunk and legs forward. Turn the arms out and curve the trunk back between them. Bring the coccyx, sacrum, and lumbar forward. Contract the buttocks lightly and take them down. Stretch the front of the body from the pubis. Raise the sternum and the top ribs. Take the shoulders back and press the shoulder blades and dorsal spine in.

Take the head back, without constricting the neck or straining the throat. Gaze back to intensify the curve of the trunk. Stay for 20 to 30 seconds, breathing evenly.

With an exhalation bend the arms and come down.

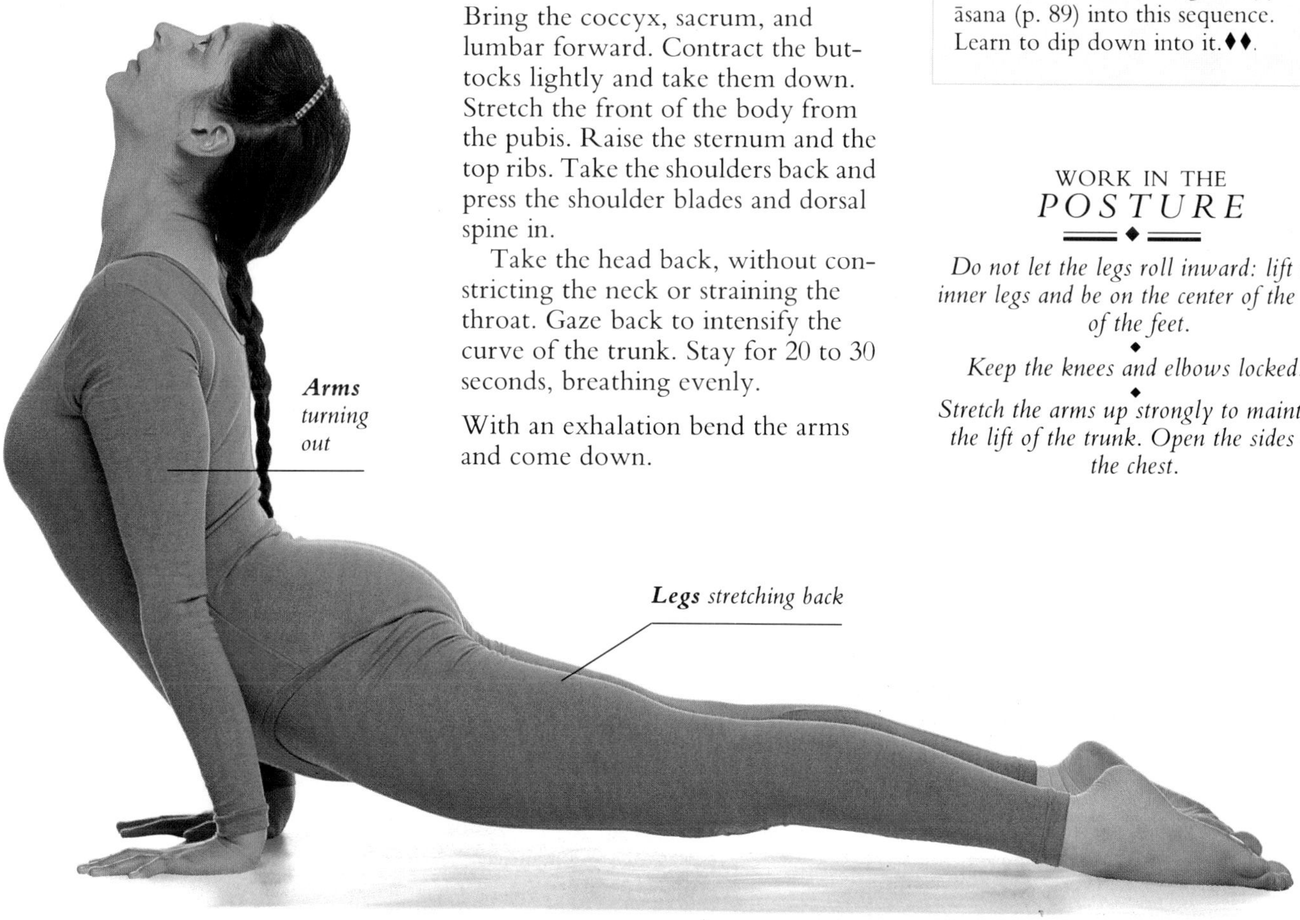
Arms *turning out*
Legs *stretching back*

WAYS OF PRACTICING

To get a better lift, place the hands on a brick.

Place a chair against a wall; rest the tops of the thighs on it, grip the chair firmly and curve back.

SIMPLE JUMPING SEQUENCE

Combine Adho Mukha Śvānāsana with Ūrdhva Mukha Śvānāsana, alternating them in quick succession. First learn to flick or roll the feet over the toes from one posture to the other. Later jump from one to the other.

Then insert Caturaṅga Daṇḍāsana (p. 89) into this sequence. Learn to dip down into it.♦♦.

WORK IN THE POSTURE

Do not let the legs roll inward: lift the inner legs and be on the center of the tops of the feet.

Keep the knees and elbows locked.

Stretch the arms up strongly to maintain the lift of the trunk. Open the sides of the chest.

शलभासन १

Śalabhāsana I

ŚALABHA = locust

THE CHEST and legs lift and extend, giving the pose a tensile strength.♦

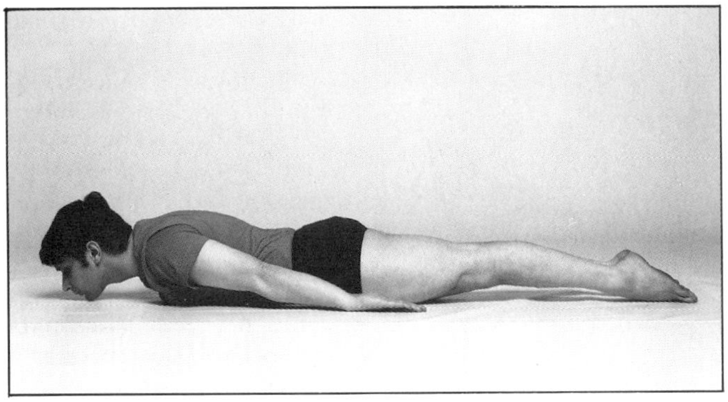

1 Lie on the front with the feet together, toes stretching back, arms beside the trunk. Straighten the knees.

2 Turn the palms up. Raise the arms parallel to the floor and stretch them back. Contract the buttock muscles and press the sacrum down. Inhale and raise the head, chest, and legs as high as they will go, without straining the back.

Stretch the trunk forward and the legs back. Balance on the lower abdomen. Look forward. Stay for 20 to 30 seconds, breathing evenly.

Exhale and come down.

WAYS OF PRACTICING

Raise the chest and the legs separately.

ŚALABHĀSANA II

Do the posture with the legs bent back. Raise the legs higher and higher.♦♦

Focus *Good pain and bad pain*

During the postures, muscles (or parts of the body unaccustomed to moving) experience the pain of stretching. This is healthy pain. It disappears the moment that action stops.

Unhealthy pain is a sign of overstrain to the point of injury. It is long-lasting and easily aggravated. To gain relief, work on surrounding areas, keeping the injured part passive.

WORK IN THE POSTURE

Keep the legs together; do not bend the knees. Make the feet strong. Open the backs of the legs (see Focus, p. 89).

Raise the chest more, move the dorsal spine in, and stretch the shoulders back together with the arms.

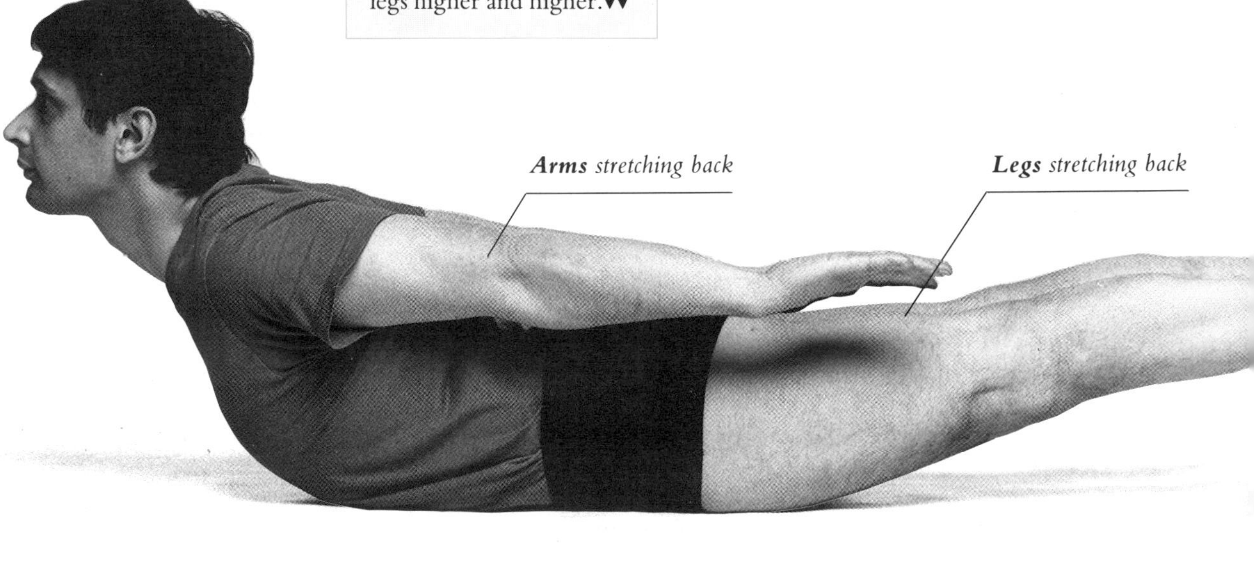

भुजंगासन

Bhujaṅgāsana

BHUJAṄGA = a snake, cobra

THE BODY resembles a cobra poised to strike. ♦♦

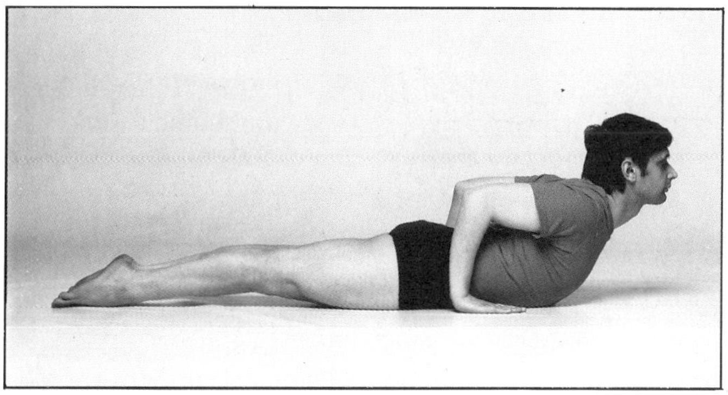

1 Lie face down with the feet together and the toes pointing back. Bend the elbows and place the hands on the floor in front of the hips, fingers apart. Draw the shoulders back and lift the head.

2 Keeping the legs on the floor and the knees straight, inhale, and raise the head, chest, and abdomen and straighten the arms. Press the sacrum and pubis down. Extend the front of the body toward the chin, and coil the spine backward. Do not strain.

Take the head further back and look back, without constricting the neck. Stay for 20 to 30 seconds, breathing evenly.

Exhale and come down.

Focus *Avoiding pain in the spine*

The whole spine must be involved in stretching, otherwise pain will occur in the weak areas. Where there is a pinching feeling, that part of the spine is contracted, with the intervertebral discs rubbing against each other. To avoid this, create space in the spine: extend and curve it vertebra by vertebra.

WAYS OF PRACTICING

Begin by placing the hands beside the rib cage, then take the hands further back while curving.

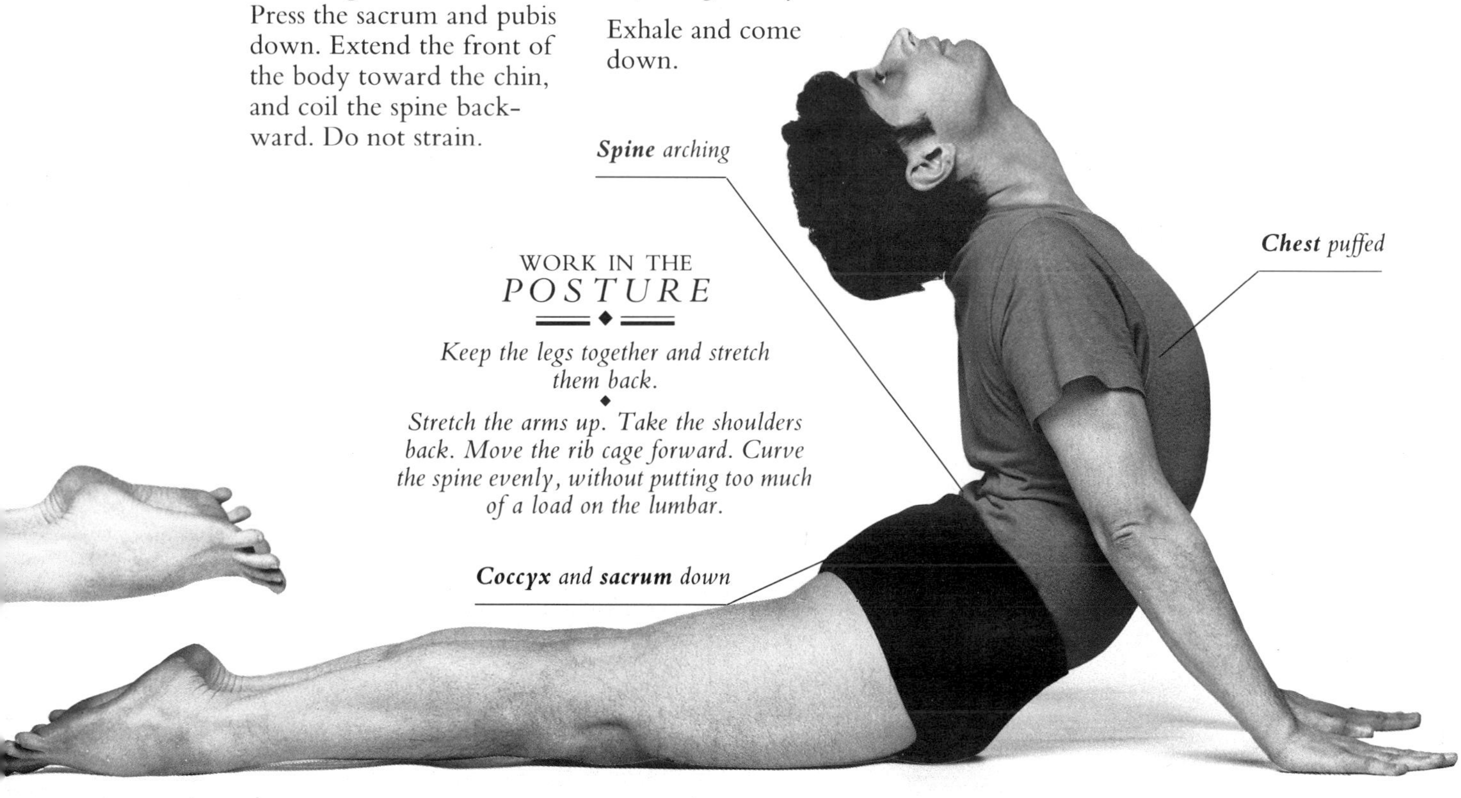

WORK IN THE POSTURE

Keep the legs together and stretch them back.

♦

Stretch the arms up. Take the shoulders back. Move the rib cage forward. Curve the spine evenly, without putting too much of a load on the lumbar.

धनुरासन

Dhanurāsana

DHANURA = a bow

IN THIS posture the body arches like a strung bow.♦♦

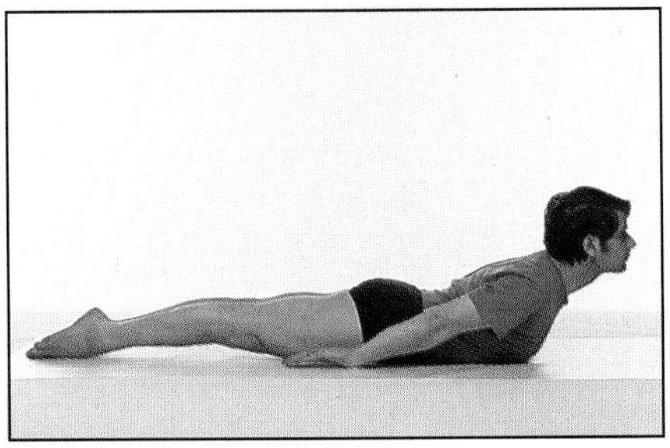

1 Lie prone, with the arms beside the trunk and palms down. Keep both sides of the body even. Stretch the legs and toes back; move the thighs away from the trunk.

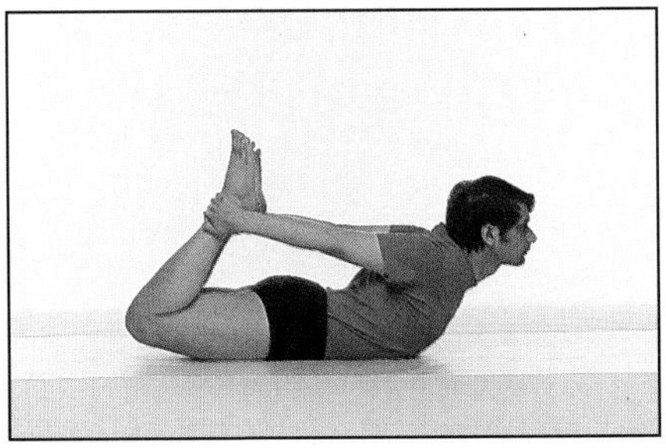

2 Bend the legs back. Press the coccyx and sacrum down, flatten the back, and stretch the arms back. Hold the ankles or shins and raise the head.

3 Inhale, pull firmly on the shins, and raise the chest, waist, and thighs. Take the shoulders back and the shoulder blades in. Keep the arms straight. Extend the front of the body up. Contract the buttocks and lift the legs and trunk higher, without straining. Move the body weight forward onto the abdomen.

Take the head back and look up without constricting the back of the neck or straining the throat. Stay for 15 to 20 seconds, breathing evenly.

Exhale, release the legs, and come down.

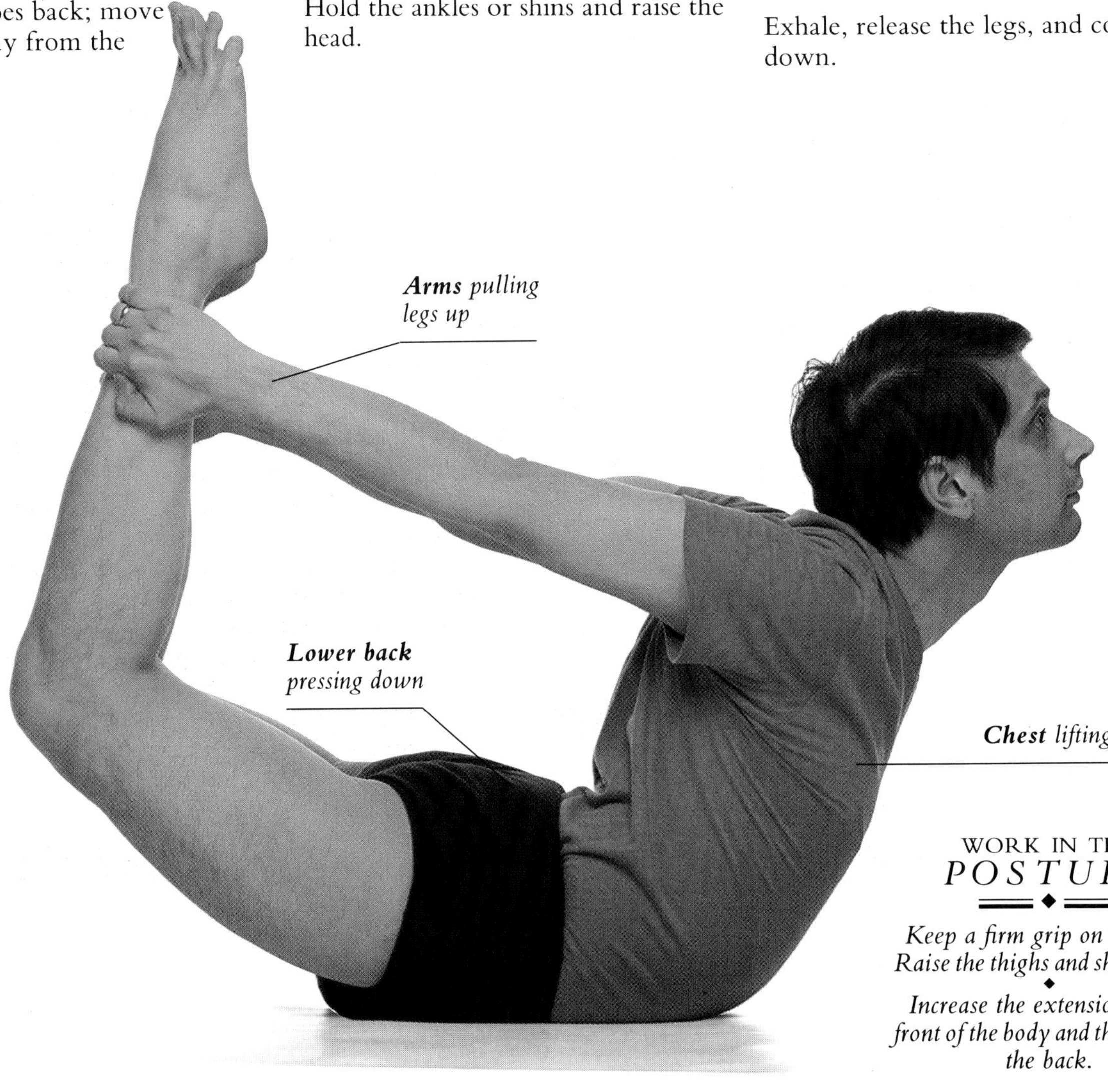
Arms *pulling legs up*
Lower back *pressing down*
Chest *lifting*

WORK IN THE
POSTURE

Keep a firm grip on the legs. Raise the thighs and shins more.

♦

Increase the extension of the front of the body and the curve of the back.

INVERTED POSES

You must savor the fragrance of a posture. Until you are relaxed, you cannot savor the fragrance.

B. K. S. IYENGAR

The inverted poses revitalize the whole system. They take the weight off the legs, relieving strain. By inverting the inner organs, they activate parts that are sluggish. They improve circulation and tone the glandular system. They help concentration as blood is brought to the brain, and are a marvelous aid to sleep. Śīrṣāsana in particular activates the pituitary gland. Sarvāṅgāsana strengthens the nervous system and the emotions; it activates the thyroid and parathyroid glands.

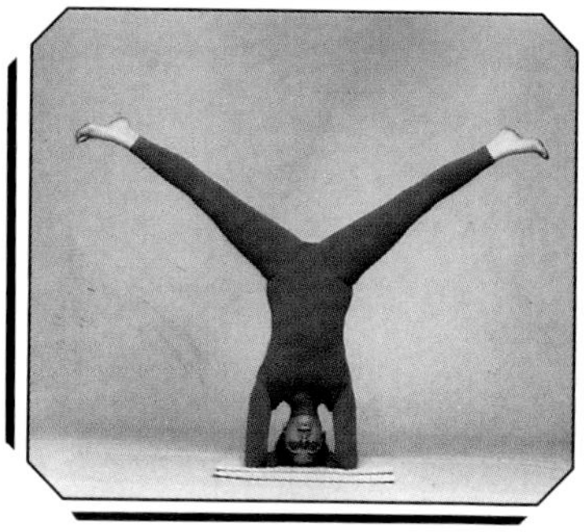

GUIDELINES FOR PRACTICE

There should be no strain in the head, eyes, ears, neck, or throat.

As the head is delicate, Śīrṣāsana (p. 98) should always be done on a blanket. The blanket should be firm, not spongy.

It is not advisable to repeat Śīrṣāsana as this irritates the brain and nerves.

The variations may be learned once the balance is steady.

In Sarvāṅgāsana (p. 108), the neck should always be soft and relaxed. If the posture is done flat on the floor, there is a tendency for the neck to collapse and to feel pressure. To avoid this, the shoulders and elbows should be supported on folded blankets, the height of which should be varied according to the length and suppleness of the neck.

The above arrangement may not be suitable for those with neck injuries or conditions such as cervical spondylosis. Other methods need to be tried, after consultation with a teacher.

Sarvāṅgāsana variations (pp. 112-5) are easier if the blankets are not too high.

Although Sarvāṅgāsana is learned before Śīrṣāsana, once the latter is learned it is practiced first: Śīrṣāsana after Sarvāṅgāsana could injure the neck.

Śīrṣāsana, if practiced by itself, can produce a feeling of irritability, which is soothed by Sarvāṅgāsana, so should always be followed by it.

CAUTIONS: Do not do inverted postures during menstruation.

Do not do inverted postures if suffering from high blood pressure, heart problems, detached retina, or ear problems.

If suffering from neck injuries, seek advice.

During pregnancy, Śīrṣāsana, Sarvāṅgāsana, and Ardha Halāsana (p. 110) may be done with support, provided there is no discomfort or medical contraindication.

Remove contact lenses.

अधो मुख वृक्षासन

Adho Mukha Vṛkṣāsana

ADHO MUKHA = face down; *VṚKṢA* = tree

THIS IS the full-arm balance, which gives tremendous energy. (Do not attempt this posture if the arms are not strong.)♦♦♦

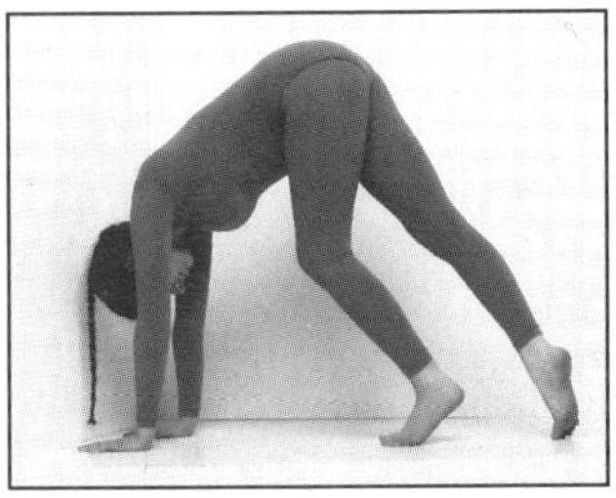

1 Stand about 3ft away from a wall, facing it. Bend down and place the hands on the floor, 3 to 5in away from the wall, a shoulder's-width apart. Straighten the elbows and stretch the arms and shoulders up. Open the chest. Walk in. Prepare to jump up: bring the left leg forward and bend it; keep the right leg straight.

2 Exhale and kick up with the right leg, keeping it straight, and follow quickly with the left leg. Lock the elbows and stretch the trunk up. Straighten both legs, stretch the heels up the wall; extend the soles of the feet and the toes. Take the coccyx and sacrum in (see Focus, opposite).

Relax the neck and head. Stay for 20 to 30 seconds or longer, breathing evenly.

Exhale and come down, without collapsing the arms. Keep the head down for a few moments.

WORK IN THE POSTURE

Press the heels of the hands down and stretch the fingers forward. Keep the arms strong.

♦

Stretch the trunk vertically up. Lift the shoulders, take the shoulder blades in, and open the armpits. Stretch the waist, lumbar, and hips up.

♦

Stretch from the forearms to the feet.

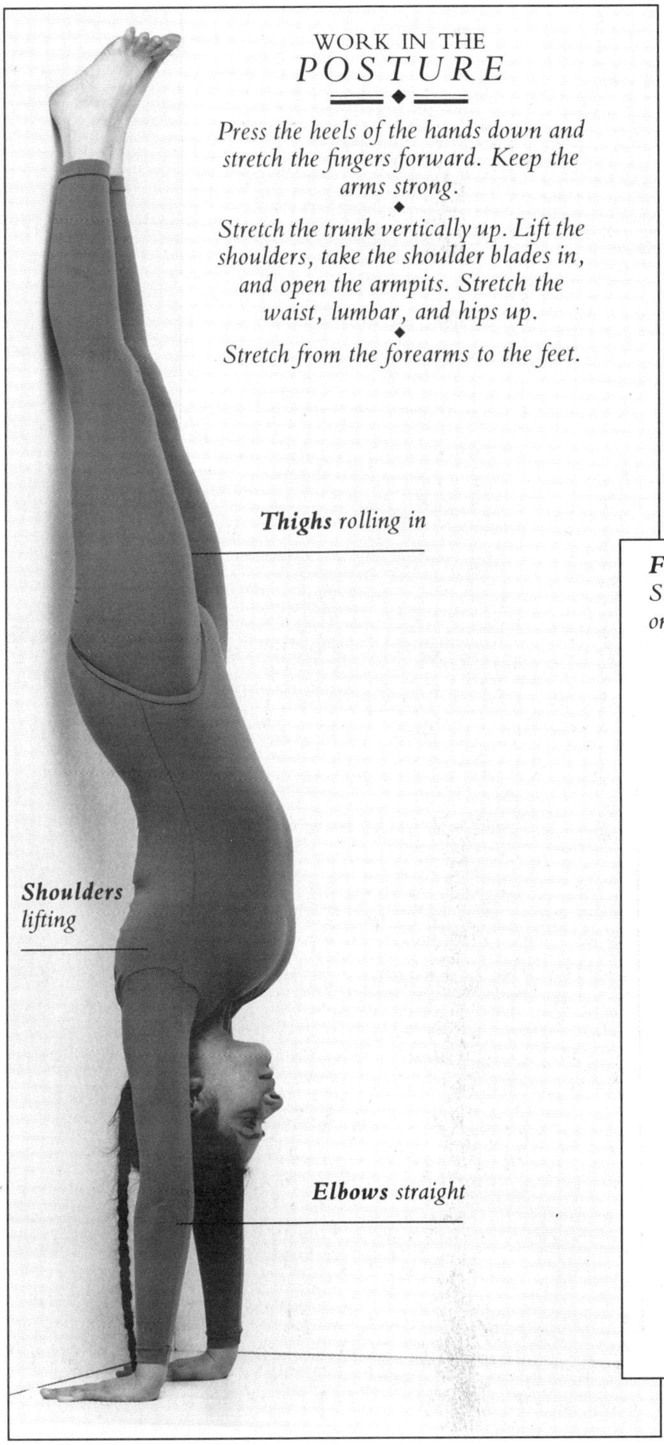

WAYS OF PRACTICING

To keep the arms straight, tie them with a belt, just above the elbows.

Practice Adho Mukha Śvānāsana (p. 90) until the arms are strong; then practice jumping repeatedly until the legs go up.

Raise the head and look back to stretch the neck.

Take the feet off the wall and balance.

Learn to jump with the other leg, then with both legs together.

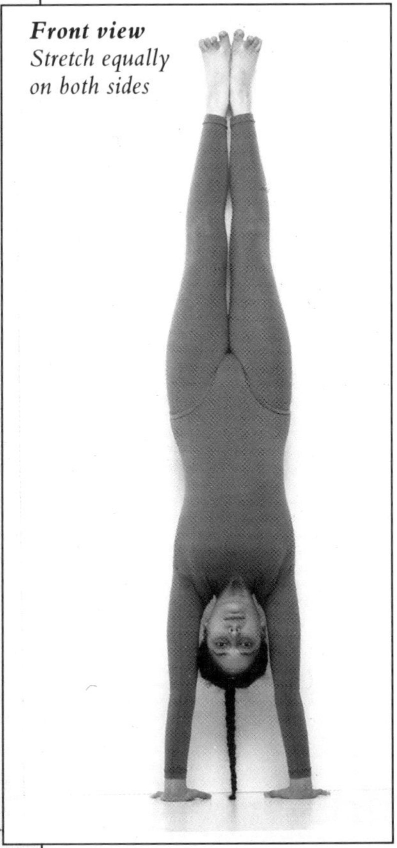

***Front view** Stretch equally on both sides*

पिञ्च मयूरासन

Piñca Mayūrāsana

PIÑCA = tail feather; *MAYŪRA* = a peacock

THE TRUNK and legs resemble the fanlike tail of a peacock.♦♦♦

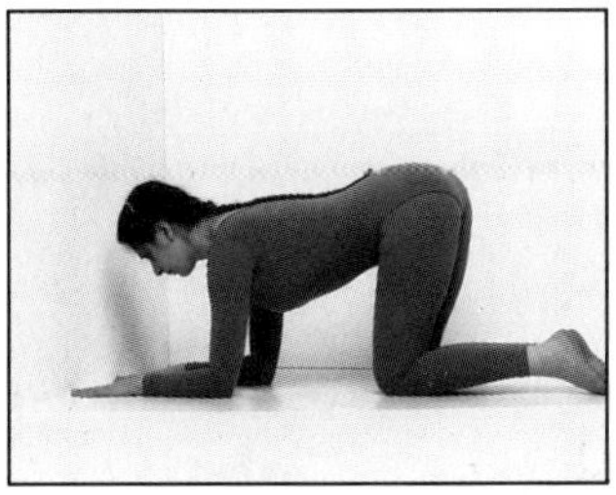

1 Kneel facing a wall. Place the forearms and palms on the floor, a shoulder's-width apart, fingers spread. Press the index and middle fingers against the wall. Keep the upper arms perpendicular. Raise the shoulders and head; look up.

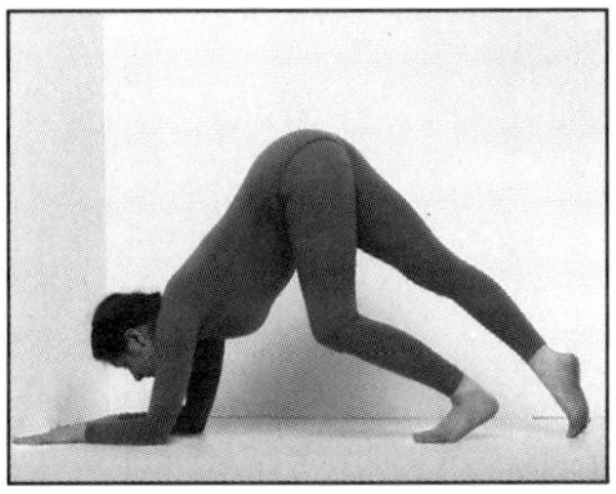

2 Straighten the legs and walk in, raising the trunk and hips. Keep the left leg bent and slightly forward, the right leg straight and slightly behind. Prepare to jump.

3 Keep the head and shoulders lifted. Exhale and kick up with the right leg, following quickly with the left. Keep the feet together on the wall. Move the dorsal spine in. Stretch the trunk and the legs up. Look back. Stay for 20 to 30 seconds or longer, breathing evenly.

Exhale and come down. Stay for a few moments with the head down.

WAYS OF PRACTICING

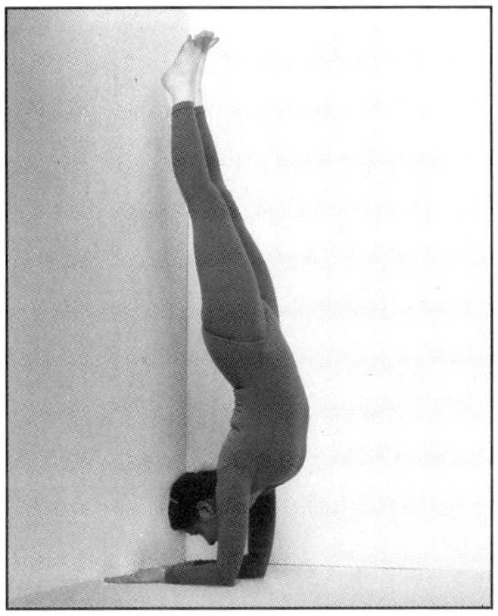

Tie a belt just above the elbows to keep the arms in.

Hold a brick between the thumbs and index fingers to keep the wrists apart.

Balance with the feet away from the wall for a more vertical stretch.

Focus *Taking the coccyx and sacrum in*
After going up, take the legs slightly apart, move the coccyx and sacrum in, and tighten the buttocks. Join the legs, rolling the thighs from the outside in.

WORK IN THE POSTURE

Keep the elbows in and the wrists apart. Press the palms down.

♦

Go on lifting the upper arms and shoulders. Extend the lumbar up and take the sacrum and coccyx in (see Focus, below left).

♦

Stretch the heels firmly to raise the hips.

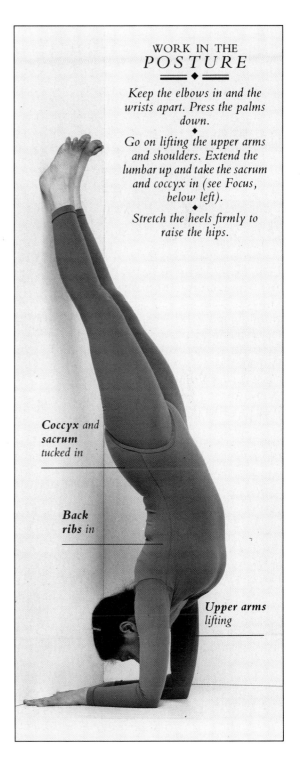

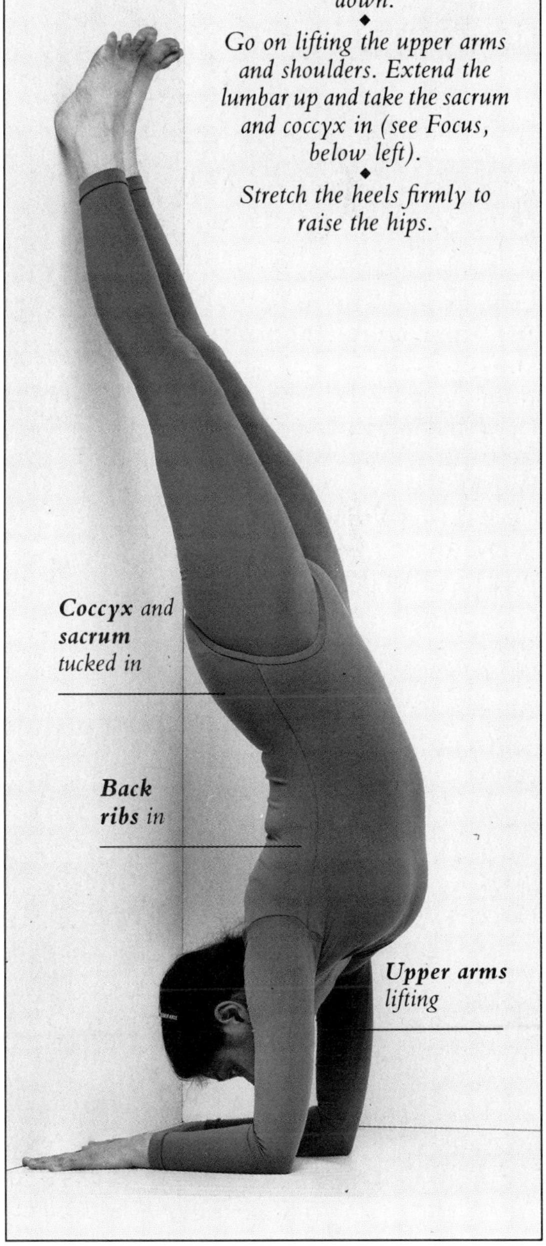

सालंब शीर्षासन १

Sālamba Śīrṣāsana I

SĀLAMBA = supported; *ŚĪRṢA* = head

THE HEAD-BALANCE is called the king of the postures. It develops poise and lightness, and stimulates the brain.♦♦

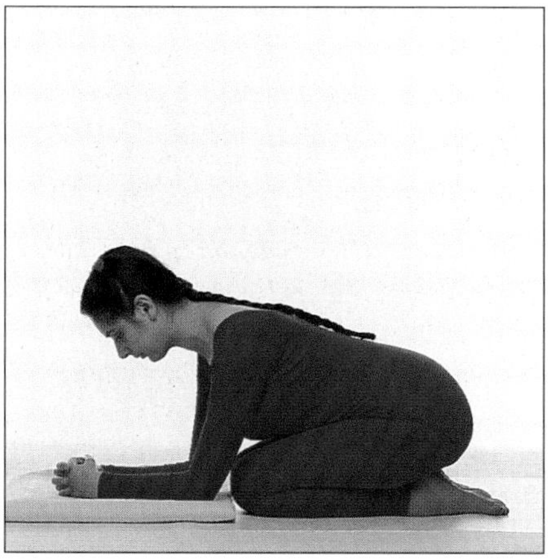

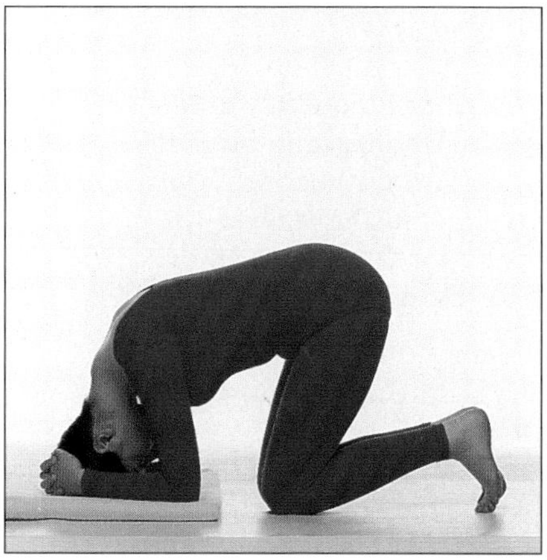

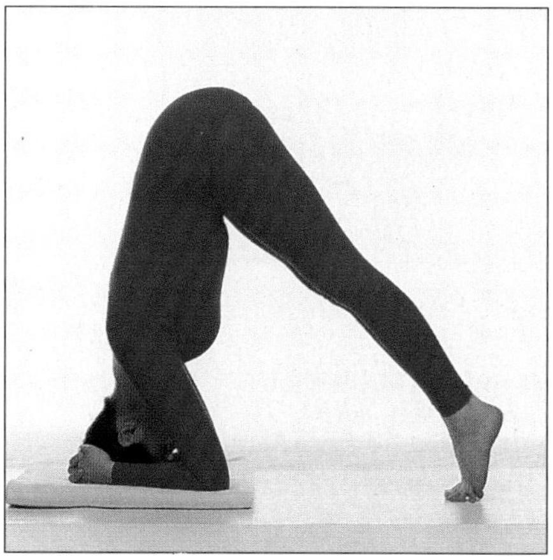

1 Place a folded blanket on the floor, square to the room (see Focus, p. 101). Kneel in front of the blanket, with the feet and knees together and in line. Line up the trunk with the legs. Bend down, interlock the fingers (see Focus, below right), and place the outer elbows, forearms, and hands on the blanket. Keep the elbows directly under the shoulders. Keep the inner and outer edges of the forearms, wrists, and hands parallel. Bring the wrists slightly in and cup the hands.

Cautions

- *Do not attempt Śīrṣāsana until Sarvāṅgāsana and Halāsana (pp. 108-110) can be held for 8 to 10 minutes.*
- *If there is pressure or discomfort in the head, eyes, ears, or neck, come down. Try again another day. If the problem persists, do restful forward bends (p. 63) and seek advice.*

2 Extend the neck and place the crown of the head down. Be on the center of the crown and keep the elbows equidistant from the head. Raise the upper arms and shoulders.

Focus *Arm support in head-balance*
Place the elbows in line with each other. Be on the outer edges of the forearms and stretch them toward the wrists. Go into the base of the fingers to clasp the hands, with the knuckles loosely bent. Keep the hands relaxed, the skin of the palms and fingers sensitive.

Make the forearms and hands symmetrical, forearms slightly diagonal. Keep the wrists and hands rounded, to make room for the head. Once balance is steady, change the interlock every now and then.

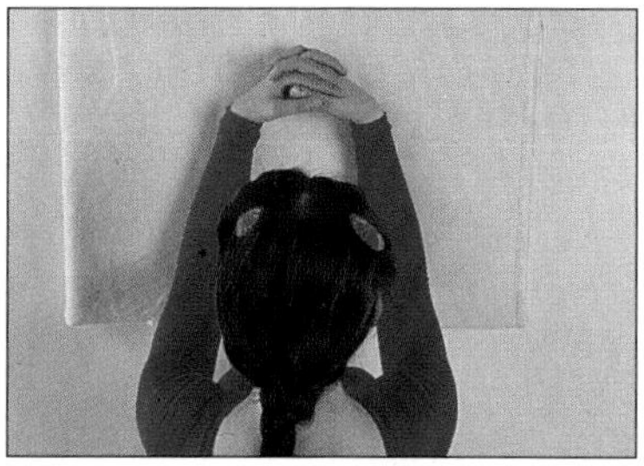

3 Straighten the legs, raise the hips, and walk in until the trunk is almost perpendicular. Open the chest.

Reflection
Whichever part of the body is on the ground, that is the base of the posture. The base is the guideline for correct practice. It should be accurately aligned to give the posture its direction. In head-balances the crown of the head and the forearms form the base, the crown being the center over which the body balances. This equilibrium is the foundation of Yoga.

4 Exhale and swing the legs up until they are vertical.

Lift the shoulders, stretch the neck, and take the dorsal spine in. Extend the trunk and the legs up. Tuck the sacrum and coccyx in (see Focus, p. 97). Keep the knees straight and facing forward. Extend the heels, soles of the feet, and toes.

Stay for 5 to 10 minutes or longer, keeping the face and eyes relaxed. Do not stare. Breathe evenly.

Continue the cycle, or exhale and come down with straight legs. Bend the legs and rest the head, until it clears, on the floor.

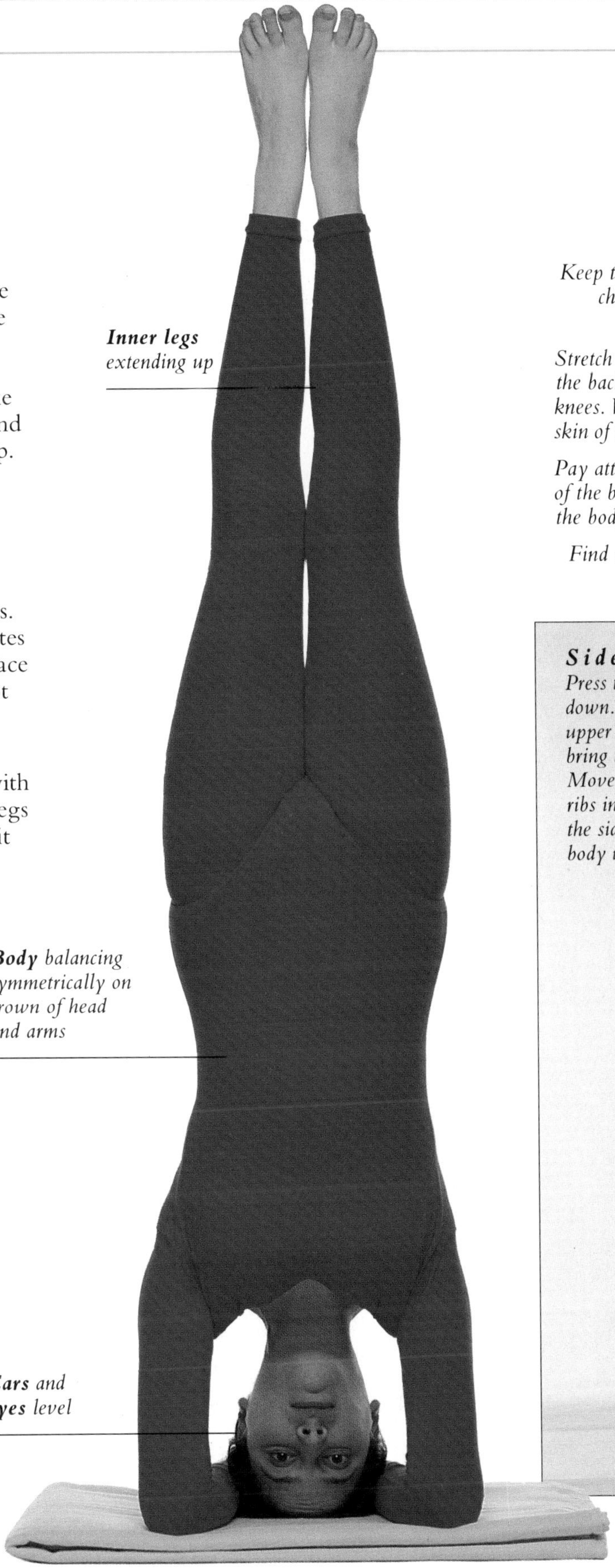

***Inner legs** extending up*

***Body** balancing symmetrically on crown of head and arms*

***Ears** and **eyes** level*

WORK IN THE POSTURE

Keep the arms and head steady. Move the chest forward, without collapsing the lumbar.

◆

Stretch the legs away from the hips. Stretch the backs of the legs. Open the backs of the knees. While extending the legs up, draw the skin of the front of the legs toward the trunk.

◆

Pay attention to alignment. Keep both sides of the body level and working evenly. Keep the body centered. Do not lean on one side.

◆

Find repose and lightness in the posture.

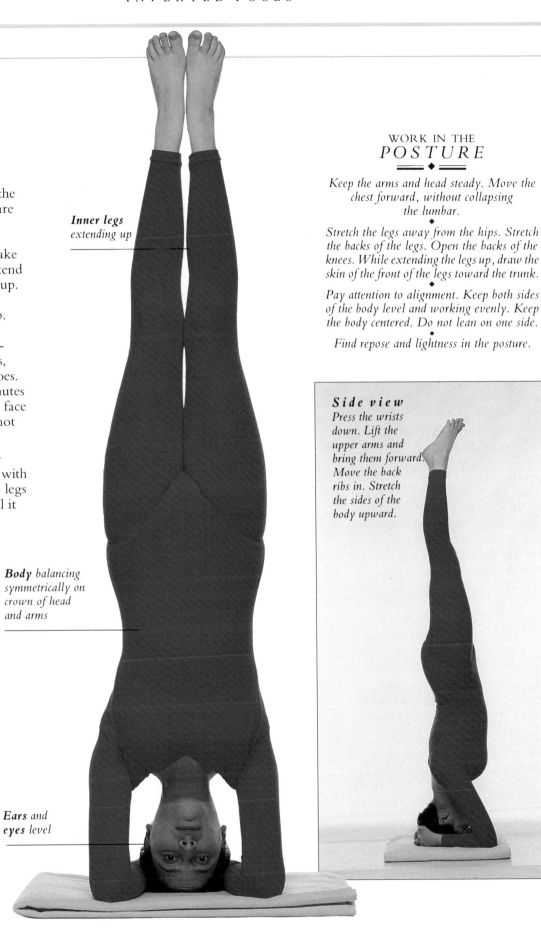

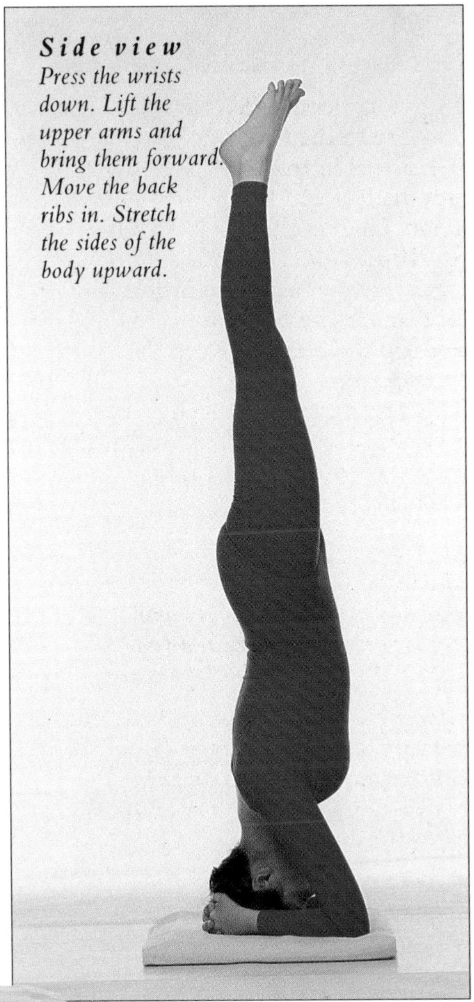

Side view
Press the wrists down. Lift the upper arms and bring them forward. Move the back ribs in. Stretch the sides of the body upward.

सालम्ब शीर्षासन

Śīrṣāsana (with bent legs)

ŚĪRṢA = head

GOING UP into Śīrṣāsana with the legs bent requires less strength in the lumbar. ♦♦

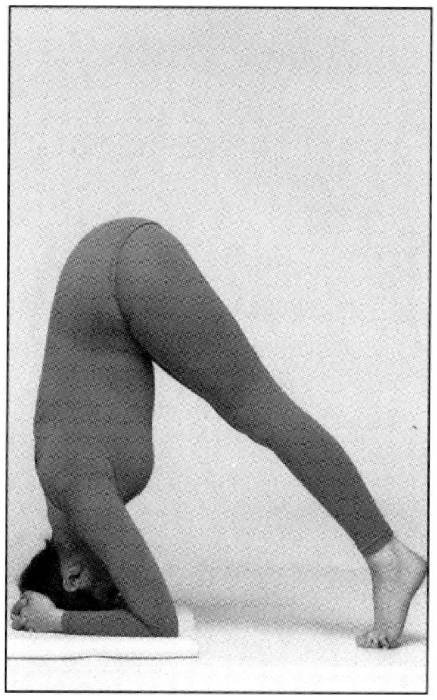

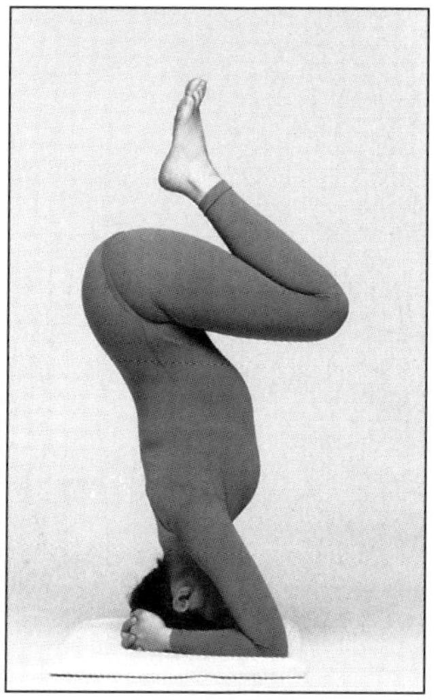

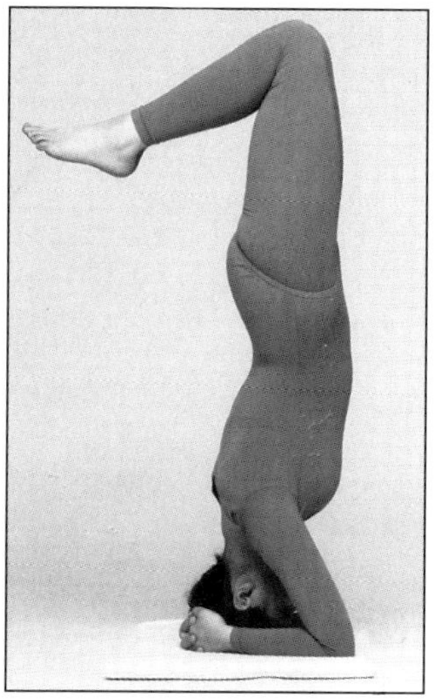

1 Follow steps 1 and 2 of Śīrṣāsana (p. 98). Straighten the legs and walk the feet in.

2 Exhale, bend the legs, and jump up. If unable to go up with both legs together (or if suffering from a bad back), jump with one leg. Keep the legs bent over the abdomen.

3 Take the bent legs up and over, with the knees facing the ceiling. Lift the shoulders and take the sacrum firmly in.

Focus *Stages in going up*

1 Start practicing near a wall or corner of a room, using the methods described on p. 98.

2 Go up 9 to 12 in away from the wall; as confidence comes, increase the distance.

3 Go up in the middle of the room with bent legs.

4 Go up with straight legs.

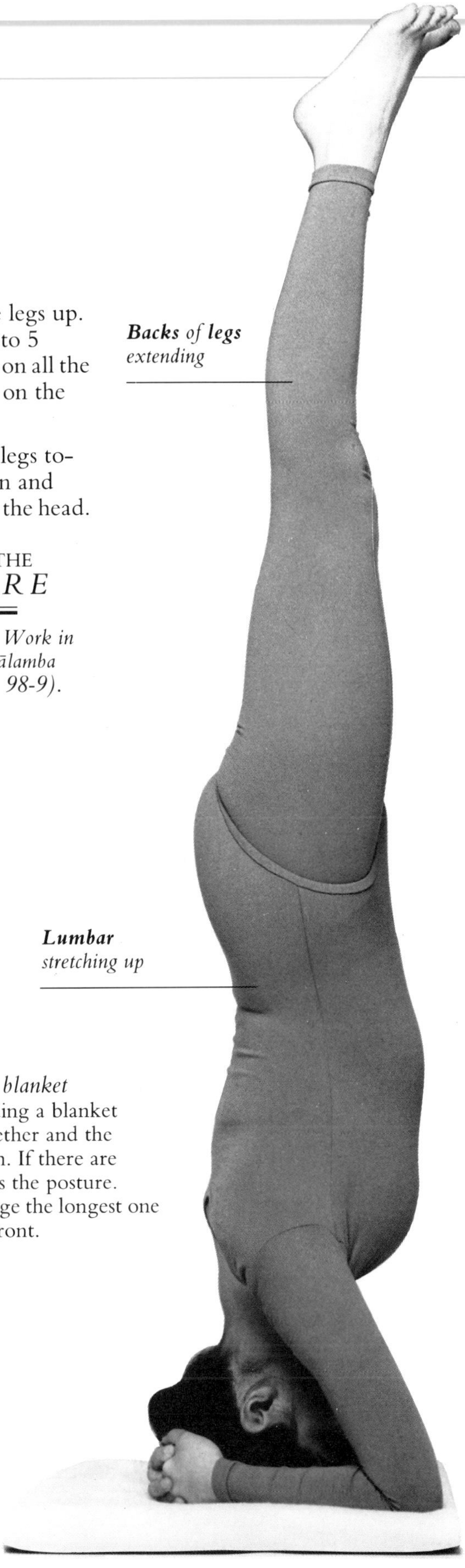

4 Straighten the legs up. Balance for 1 to 5 minutes, working on all the points mentioned on the previous pages.

Exhale. Bend the legs toward the abdomen and come down. Rest the head.

WORK IN THE POSTURE

See instructions for Work in the Posture for Sālamba Śīrṣāsana I (pp. 98-9).

Focus *Folding a blanket*
At all stages of folding a blanket keep the edges together and the folded parts smooth. If there are creases, this disturbs the posture. Make the folded edge the longest one and keep it at the front.

WAYS OF PRACTICING

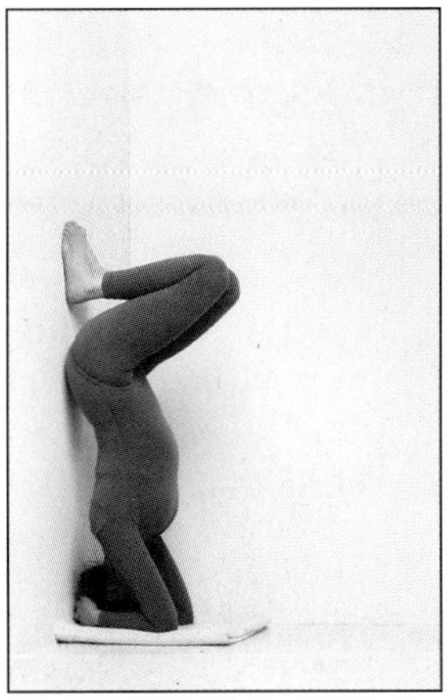

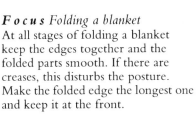

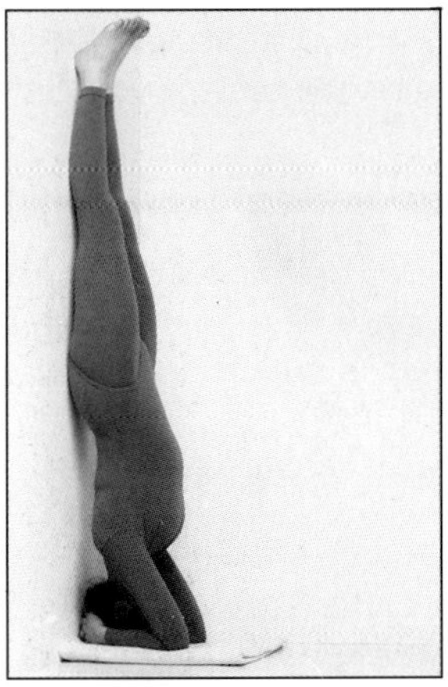

Śīrṣāsana near a wall

1 Place a folded blanket near a wall. Kneel and clasp the hands as in step 1 of Śīrṣāsana (p. 98), with the knuckles touching the wall. Place the crown of the head down, straighten the legs, and walk in. Exhale, bend the legs, and jump them up. Rest the feet on the wall.

2 Straighten the legs up, keeping the buttocks and heels on the wall.

Then bring the coccyx and sacrum forward and stretch up. Learn to balance by taking the feet, one at a time, 2 or 3in away from the wall.

Come down with bent legs.

Śīrṣāsana in a corner
Keep the interlocked fingers centered and touching the corner. Keep the arms equidistant from the two walls. With the heels, measure the distance from the corner, and make it equal on both sides.

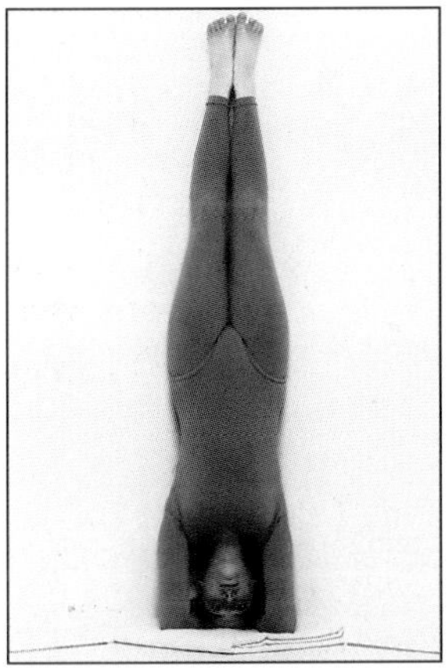

सालम्ब शीर्षासन

Śīrṣāsana cycle

ŚĪRṢĀSANA variations develop strength in the arms as well as balance and a sense of line.

Pārśva Śīrṣāsana

PĀRŚVA = side, flank; ŚĪRṢA = head
The trunk and legs lift and turn strongly.♦♦

Be in Śīrṣāsana (p. 98). Keep the base of the posture firm. Lift the upper arms and shoulders and stretch the legs.

▷Exhale and turn to the right, taking the left side of the body forward and the right side back. Turn the rib cage, waist, hips, and legs. Compress the hips, thighs, and shins. Tuck in the abdomen. Stay for 15 to 20 seconds, breathing evenly. Exhale and turn to the front. Center the head and trunk.◁

Repeat from ▷to◁ on the left.

Continue the cycle, or exhale and come down.

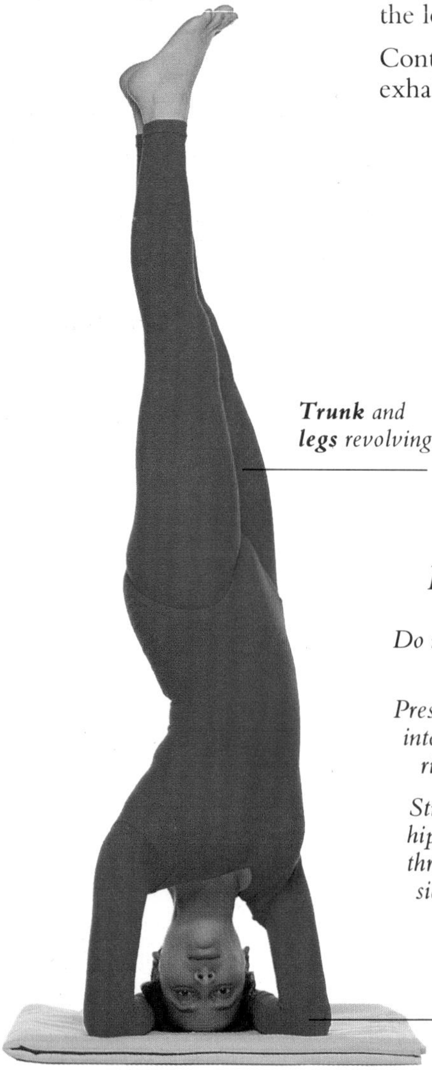
Trunk and **legs** revolving
Arms stable

WORK IN THE
POSTURE

Do not disturb the elbows or the head.

♦

Press the left shoulder blade into the back ribs. Lift the right side of the trunk.

♦

Stretch from shoulders to hips, hips to feet. Do not throw the hips out to one side. Turn the spine on its axis.

Parivṛtta Eka Pāda Śīrṣāsana

PARIVṚTTA = revolved; EKA PĀDA = one leg; ŚĪRṢA = head
As the trunk turns, the legs spread apart.♦♦♦

Be in Śīrṣāsana (p. 98).

▷Stretch the hips up. Take the left leg forward and the right leg back. Keep the knees straight. Exhale and turn to the right. Keep the head and neck facing forward, the shoulders lifted. Keep the pubis pointing up. Make the heels strong and stretch the backs of the legs and feet without disturbing the line of the legs. Stay for 15 to 20 seconds, breathing evenly. Exhale, turn to the front. Join the legs.◁

Repeat from ▷to◁, changing the legs.

Continue the cycle or exhale and come down.

WAYS OF PRACTICING

Use a wall: do Pārśva Śīrṣāsana, then take the legs apart.

WORK IN THE
POSTURE

Stretch the back of the left leg from the lumbar to the heel. Stretch the front of the right leg from the waist to the toes.

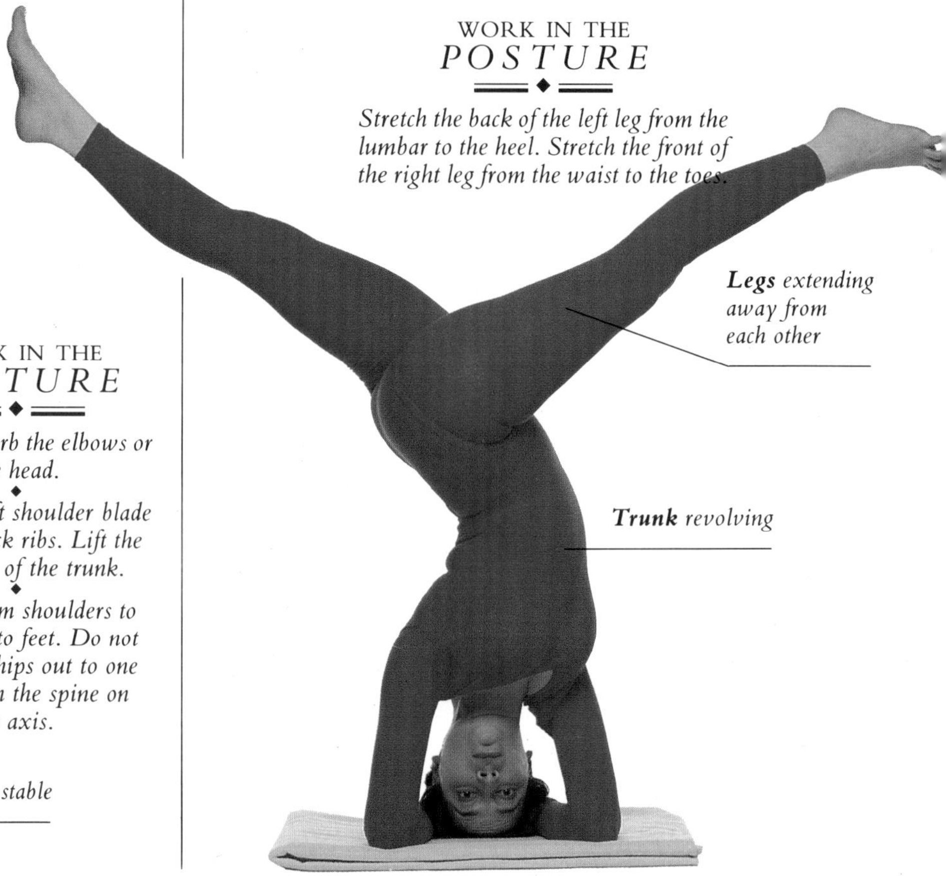
Legs extending away from each other
Trunk revolving

सालम्ब शीर्षासन

Eka Pāda Śīrṣāsana

EKA PĀDA = one leg; *ŚĪRṢA* = head

The trunk balances, with one leg stretching up and the other reaching down.♦♦♦

Be in Śīrṣāsana (p. 98).

▷Extend the left leg up, simultaneously lower the right leg to the floor directly in front of the trunk. Pull the right side of the groin back and do not allow the left leg and hip to lean forward. Keep the legs straight and in line; this is more important than reaching the floor.

Stay for 15 to 20 seconds, breathing evenly. Inhale and bring the right leg up.◁

Repeat from ▷to◁ on the left.

Continue the cycle or exhale and come down.

Ways of Practicing

Use a wall for support.

Take the leg down onto a chair.

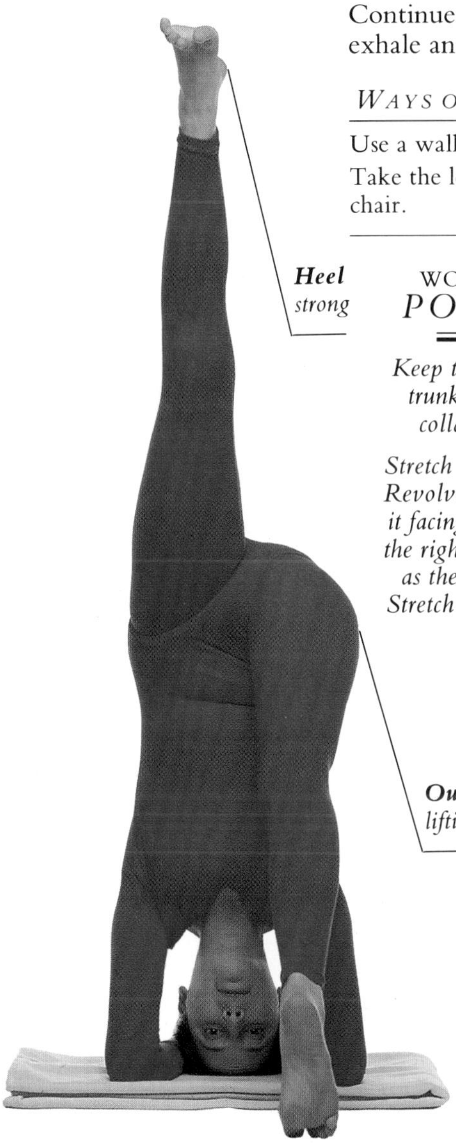

WORK IN THE POSTURE

Keep the shoulders and trunk lifting; do not collapse the chest.

♦

Stretch the left inner leg. Revolve the leg in to keep it facing forward. Move the right buttock forward as the leg goes down. Stretch the feet and toes.

Pārśvaika Pāda Śīrṣāsana

PĀRŚVA = sideways; *EKA PĀDA* = one leg; *ŚĪRṢA* = head

One leg descends to the side, without disturbing the vertical extension of the pose.♦♦♦

Be in Śīrṣāsana (p. 98).

▷Stretch the left leg up. Turn the right leg outward in its socket and take it sideways down to reach the floor. Do not lean to the side. Keep the foot in line with the leg, and the back of the leg facing the ceiling.

Stay for 15 to 20 seconds, breathing evenly.

Inhale, bring the right leg up and turn it forward.◁

Repeat from ▷to◁ on the left.

Continue the cycle or exhale and come down.

Ways of Practicing

Use a wall for support.

Take the leg down onto a chair.

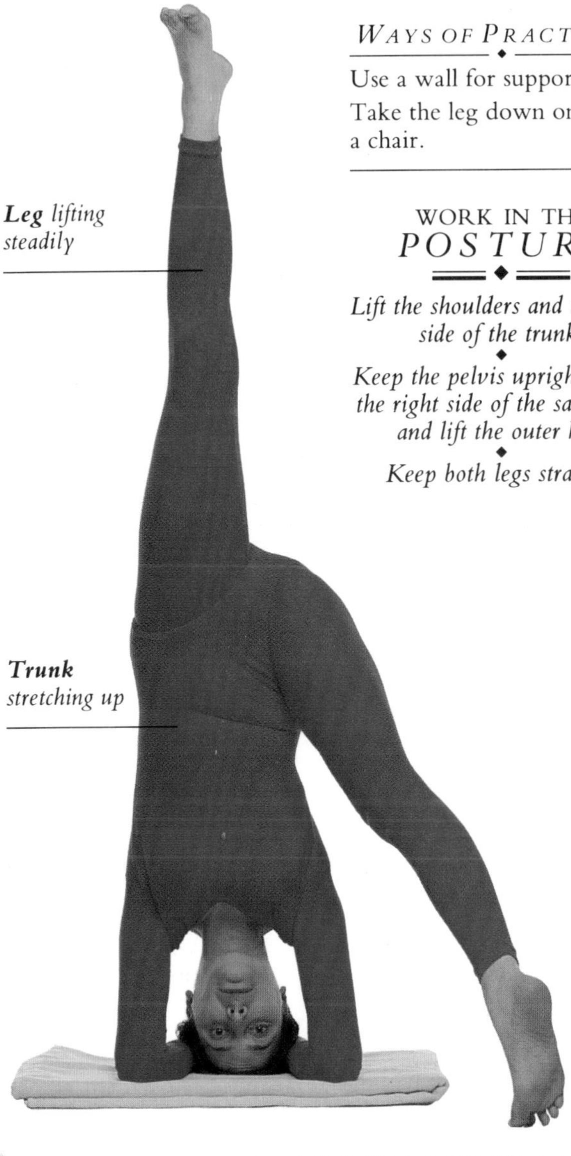

WORK IN THE POSTURE

Lift the shoulders and the right side of the trunk.

♦

Keep the pelvis upright: move the right side of the sacrum in and lift the outer hip.

♦

Keep both legs straight.

सालम्ब शीर्षासन

Śīrṣāsana cycle

Baddha Koṇāsana in Śīrṣāsana

BADDHA = bound; KOṆA = angle; ŚIRṢA = head
The pelvic opening of this posture is especially beneficial for women.♦♦

Be in Śīrṣāsana (p. 98).

With an exhalation bend the knees to the sides. Bring the heels close to the perineum, soles together, toes pointing up.

Open the thighs outward to keep the knees in line with the hips. Stay for 15 to 20 seconds, breathing evenly.

Straighten the legs up. Continue the cycle or exhale and come down.

Ways of Practicing

Use a wall for support.

WORK IN THE *POSTURE*

Stretch the trunk up and raise the hips. Keep the coccyx and the back of the pelvis tucked in. Move the knees further back.

Relax the abdomen. Balance steadily.

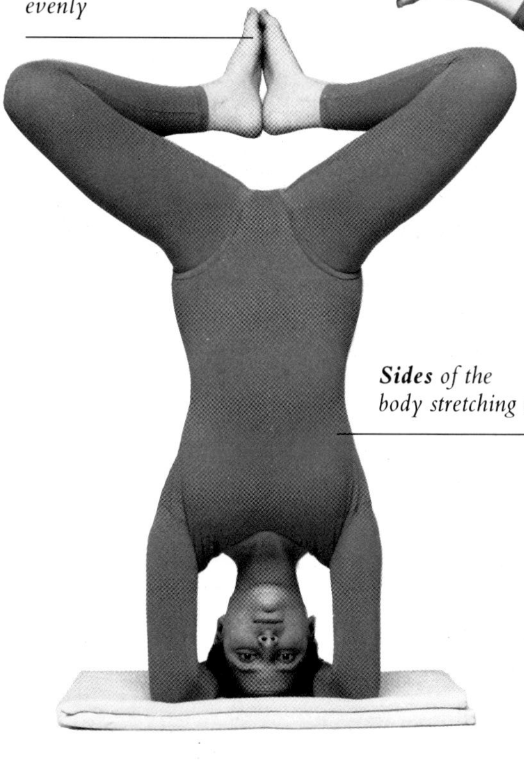
Feet pressing evenly
Sides of the body stretching up

Upaviṣṭa Koṇāsana in Śīrṣāsana

UPAVIṢṬA = settled; KOṆA = angle; ŚĪRṢA = head
The wide spread of the legs lifts and opens the pelvic area.♦♦

Be in Śīrṣāsana (p. 98).

Spread the legs wide apart, opening the inner thighs away from each other. Keep the feet in line with the hips, not in front of them.

Stay, breathing evenly, for 15 to 20 seconds.

Bend the legs back into Baddha Koṇāsana, then straighten the legs up. Continue the cycle or exhale and come down.

Ways of Practicing

Use a wall for support.

Spread the legs from Baddha Koṇāsana in Śīrṣāsana.

WORK IN THE *POSTURE*

Stretch the spine and back of the body up. Move the sacrum and lumbar forward.

Keeping the hips up, take the legs further apart. Be strong in the heels and inner legs.

Do not drop the shoulders.

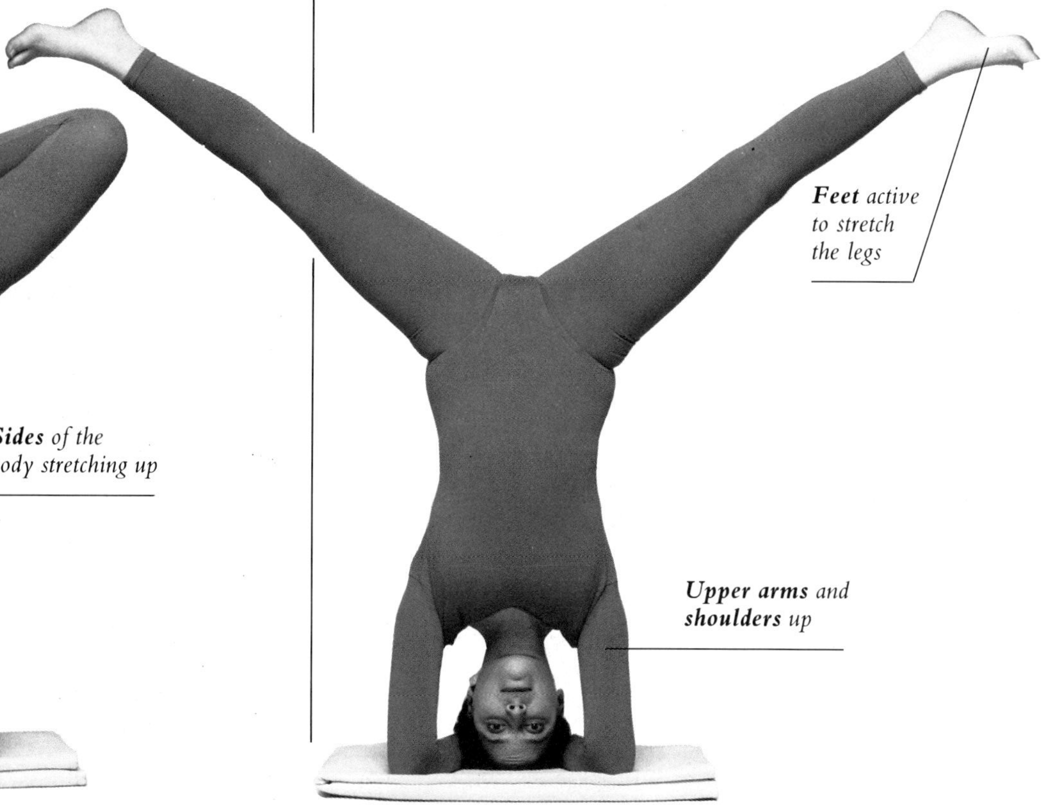
Feet active to stretch the legs
Upper arms and **shoulders** up

Pārśva Vīrāsana in Śīrṣāsana

PĀRŚVA = sideways; VĪRA = hero; ŚĪRṢA = head
The pelvis is brought forward strongly for the legs to turn.♦♦

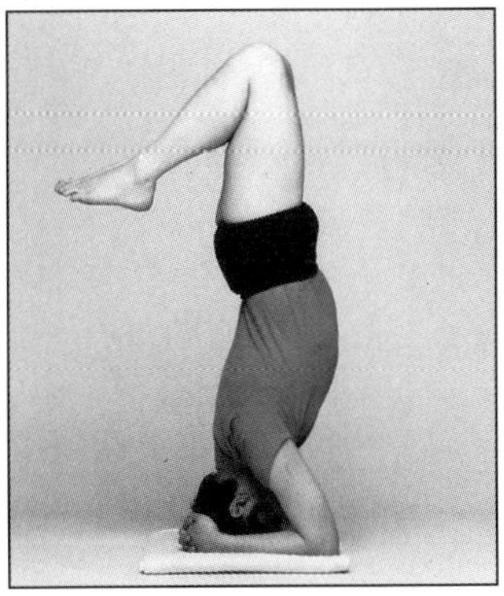

1 Be in Śīrṣāsana (p. 98). Lift the hips. Bend both legs back with the thighs perpendicular, knees pointing up. Move the coccyx and sacrum forward. Join the legs and feet; stretch the heels and toes.

2 Turn to the right. Keep the upper arms and shoulders lifted and the shoulder blades pressed in. Keep the coccyx and sacrum tucked in. Stretch the thighs up.

Breathe evenly and stay for 15 to 20 seconds. Turn to the front. ◁ Repeat from ▷ to ◁ on the left.

Straighten the legs up. Continue the cycle or exhale and come down.

WAYS OF PRACTICING

Keep the knees apart to bring the coccyx forward.

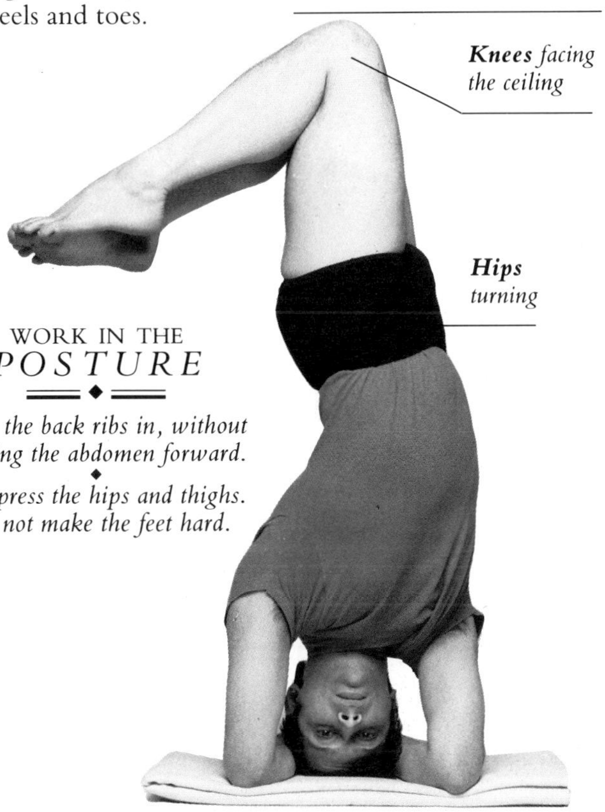
Knees *facing the ceiling*
Hips *turning*

WORK IN THE POSTURE

Press the back ribs in, without pushing the abdomen forward.

Compress the hips and thighs. Do not make the feet hard.

Ūrdhva Daṇḍāsana

ŪRDHVA = upward; DAṆḌA = stick, staff
The legs are lowered from Śīrṣāsana to make a right angle with the trunk.♦♦♦

Be in Śīrṣāsana (p. 98).

Lift the shoulders. With an exhalation draw the thighs together and take the legs down until they are parallel to the ground. Keep them straight. Stretch the trunk up as the legs descend.

Stay for 15 to 20 seconds, breathing evenly.

Inhale and return to Śīrṣāsana with straight legs.

Continue the cycle or exhale and come down.

WAYS OF PRACTICING

Face a wall in Śīrṣāsana and keep the feet on it.

Take the feet down onto a table.

WORK IN THE POSTURE

Do not compress the neck. Extend both sides of the body.

Keep the lumbar strong and the knees locked. Draw the tops of the thigh muscles toward the hips. Hit the fronts of the legs toward the bones, and the backs of the legs toward the ceiling.

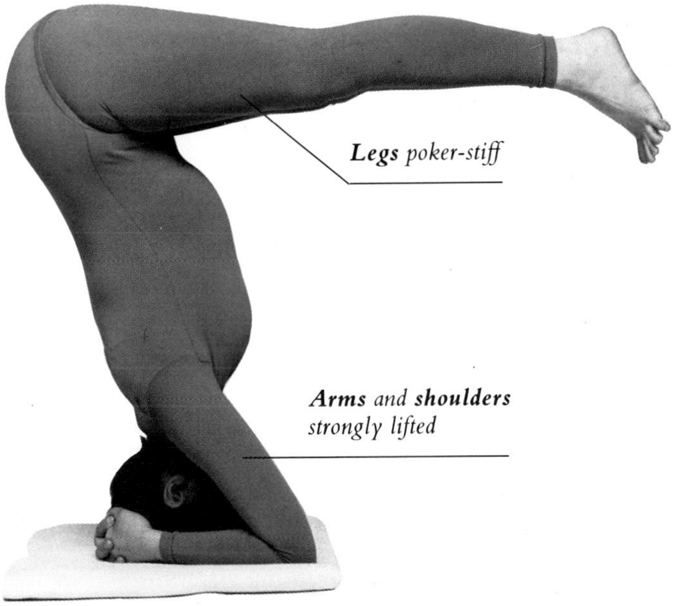
Legs *poker-stiff*
Arms *and* **shoulders** *strongly lifted*

सालम्ब शीर्षासन

Śīrṣāsana cycle

Ūrdhva Padmāsana in Śīrṣāsana

ŪRDHVA = upward; PADMA = lotus; ŚĪRṢA = head
Strength, lightness, and flexibility combine in this posture.♦♦♦♦

1 Be in Śīrṣāsana (p. 98). ▷Exhale, bend the right leg vigorously, and place the foot into the left side of the groin.

2 Bend the hips forward. Take the left foot into the right side of the groin. Stretch the thighs up. Tuck in the coccyx and sacrum. Press the knees back. Stay, breathing evenly, for 10 to 15 seconds.

Inhale and release the legs.◁

Repeat from ▷ to◁ with the left leg bent first.

Continue the cycle or exhale and come down.

PĀRŚVA ŪRDHVA PADMĀSANA

PĀRŚVA = sideways
From Ūrdhva Padmāsana in Śīrṣāsana turn to the right. Keep the coccyx and sacrum tucked in and press the knees back.

Stay for 10 to 15 seconds.

Turn to the front and then to the left. Change the legs and repeat.♦♦♦

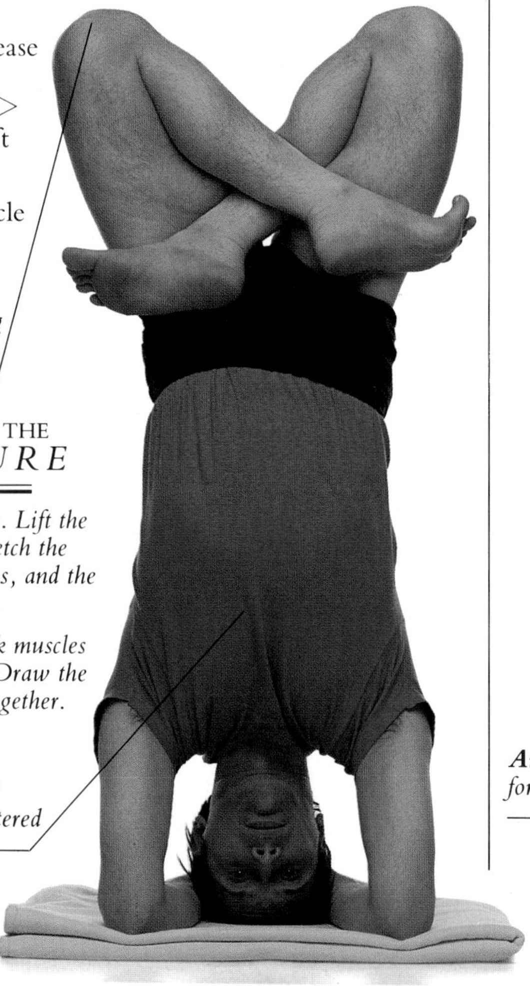

***Knees** facing the ceiling*

***Head** and **trunk** centered*

WORK IN THE
POSTURE

Learn to balance. Lift the shoulders. Stretch the abdomen, the hips, and the lumbar.

♦

Tuck the buttock muscles into the pelvis. Draw the knees closer together.

Piṇḍāsana in Śīrṣāsana

PIṆḌA = a ball, globe; ŚĪRṢA = head
The trunk and folded legs form a compact ball.♦♦♦♦

▷From Ūrdhva Padmāsana in Śīrṣāsana, exhale and bend the legs over the abdomen, keeping the shoulders and trunk well lifted. Do not collapse the neck or trunk when the legs bend down. If the neck is strong, bend further, and take the knees close to the armpits. Stay for 10 to 15 seconds, breathing evenly.

Inhale and come up.

Release the legs.◁

Repeat from ▷to◁ with the left leg bent first.

Exhale and come down.

WORK IN THE
POSTURE

Lift the upper arms strongly and move them forward. Extend the neck.

♦

Allow the back to curve when taking the legs down. Move the chest toward the legs. Draw the knees closer together.

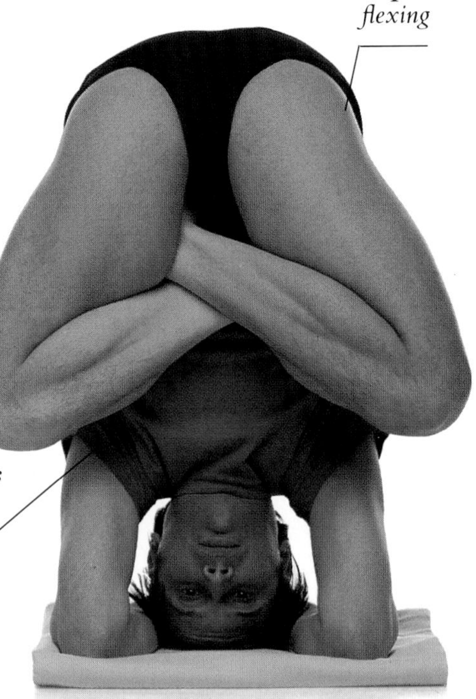

***Hips** flexing*

***Armpits** forward*

सालम्ब शीर्षासन २

Sālamba Śīrṣāsana II

SĀLAMBA = supported; *ŚĪRṢA* = head

WITH ONLY the palms for support this three-point head-balance gives a feeling of lightness. ♦♦♦

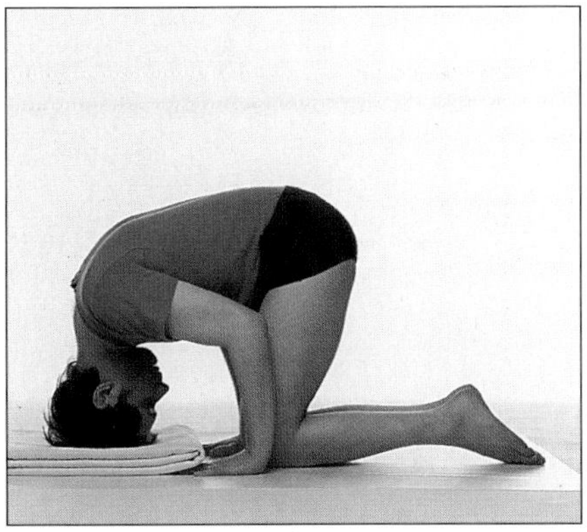

1 Place a folded blanket on the floor and kneel in front of it. Place the head on the blanket and the palms under it. Spread the fingers and keep the hands and elbows a shoulder's-width apart. Keep the forearms perpendicular. Make the arms steady and raise the shoulders.

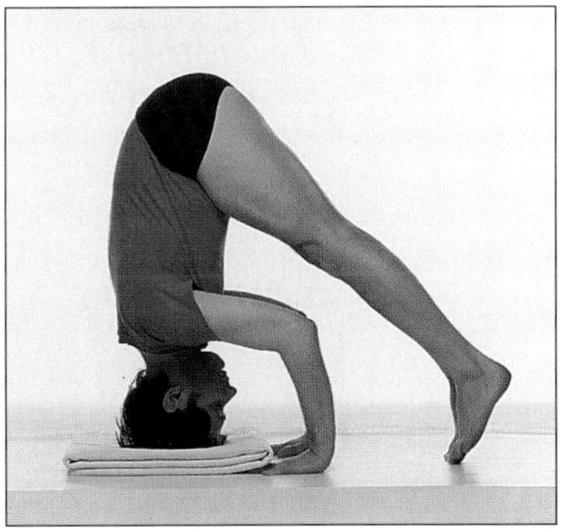

2 Straighten the legs, raise the hips, and walk in until the trunk is almost perpendicular.

3 Exhale and go up into head-balance with straight or bent legs. Extend the trunk and legs and balance.

Stay for 5 minutes or longer.

Exhale and come down. Keep head down for a few moments.

WAYS OF PRACTICING

Use a wall for support.

WORK IN THE POSTURE

Adjust the weight on the hands from moment to moment to keep the body balanced. Press the inner palms down and bring the elbows in. Lift the forearms, upper arms, and shoulders, and also the shoulder blades.

♦

Take the dorsal spine and the sacrum in.

♦

Stretch the thighs away from the hips.

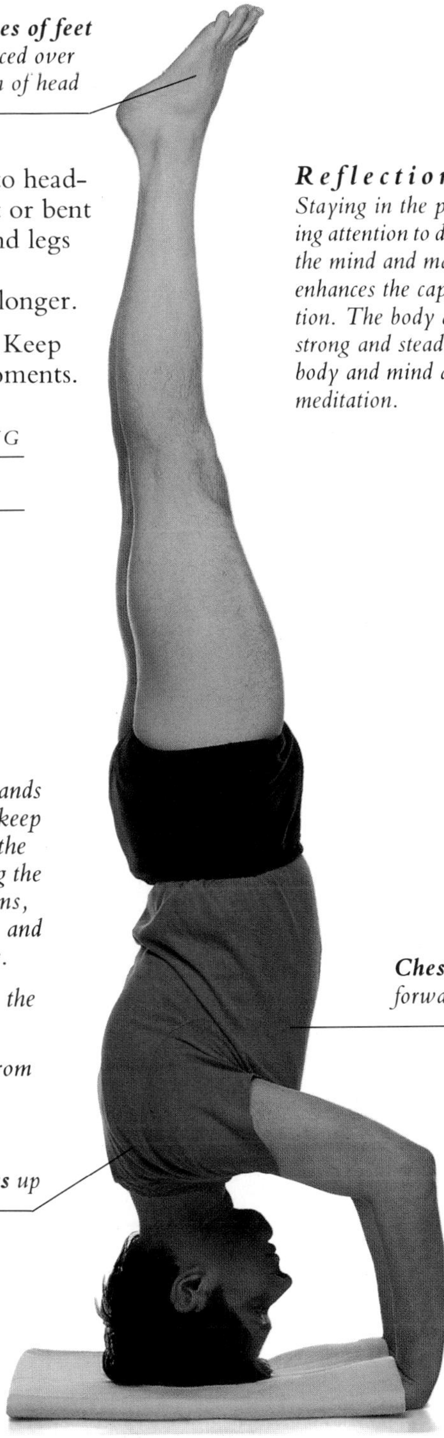

***Arches of feet** balanced over crown of head*

***Chest** moving forward*

***Shoulders** up*

Reflection

Staying in the postures and paying attention to detail concentrates the mind and makes it calm. It enhances the capacity for reflection. The body also becomes strong and steady. Firmness of body and mind are necessary for meditation.

सालम्ब सर्वांगासन

Sālamba Sarvāṅgāsana

SĀLAMBA = supported; *SARVĀṄGA* = all parts of the body

THIS IS called the queen or mother of the āsanas. It soothes and nourishes the whole body.♦

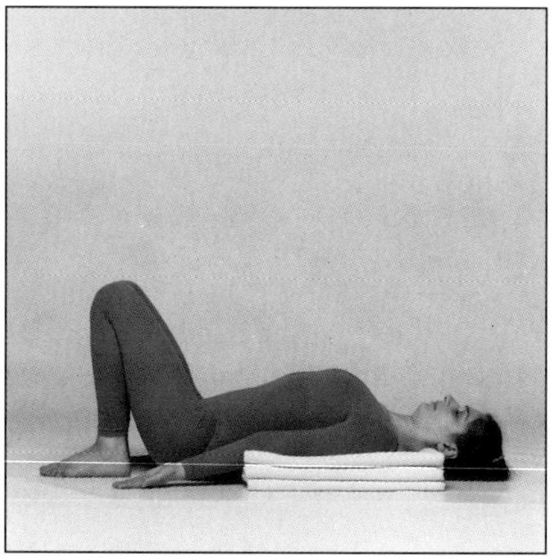

1 Place 3 to 5 folded blankets exactly above each other on the floor (see Focus, p. 101). Lie with the shoulders and arms on the blankets and the head on the floor. Press the shoulders down and draw the shoulder blades toward the waist. Turn the upper arms out and extend them toward the legs; bring the elbows close to the trunk. Move the back ribs in. Bend the legs, with the feet close to the buttocks.

Alternative method

Swing the body up with straight legs.♦♦

Focus *Improving the neck balance*

Be on the tops of the shoulders: move the shoulders away from the neck. One at a time release the hands, lengthen the upper arms, and turn them out, palms facing up. Replace the hands on the back and bring the elbows in. Press the hands, especially the thumbs and index fingers, into the ribs to lift the trunk.

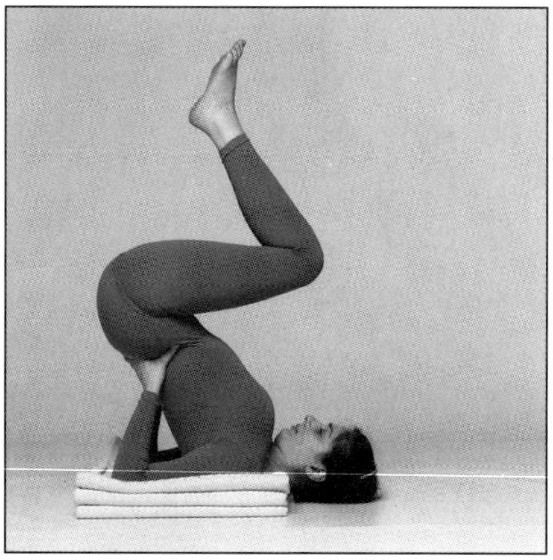

2 With the palms up, press the elbows into the floor. Exhale and lift the trunk, bending the legs over the abdomen. Support the back with the hands.

WAYS OF PRACTICING

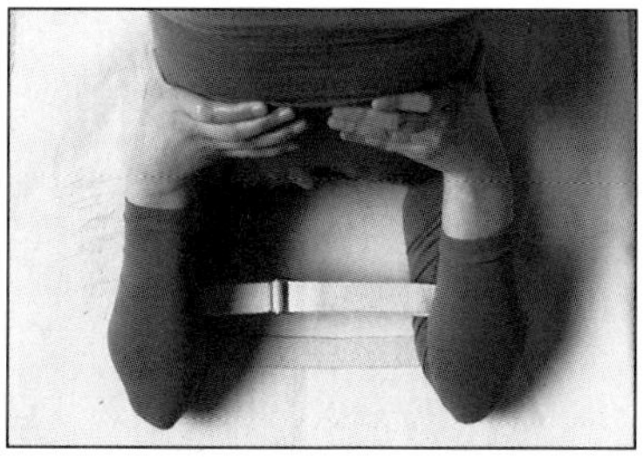

Tie a belt just above the elbows to keep them in.

Use a chair for support (see p. 118).

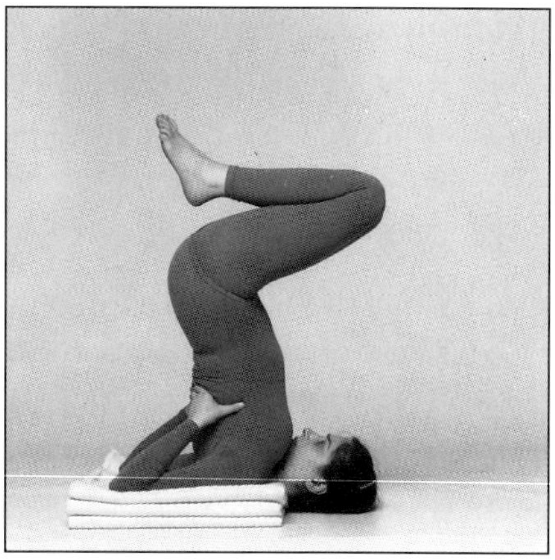

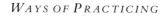

3 Raise the trunk and legs higher, bringing the chest toward the chin. Take the hands lower down and press the back ribs forward.

Caution

• *Do not stay in the posture if there is pressure in the head, ears, eyes, or throat. This may happen if the body jerks when going up, or if the support under the neck and shoulders is not correct. Relax, re-arrange the support if necessary, then go up again, more correctly. If the problem persists, do Adho Mukha Śvānāsana (p. 90) and restful forward bends (p. 63) for some weeks, until the problem disappears.*

सालम्ब सर्वांगासन

4 Straighten the legs up until they are vertical. With the help of the hands raise the shoulder blades and extend the trunk up. Lift the hips and stretch the legs.

Stay for 5 to 20 minutes or longer. Keep the head relaxed. Continue into Halāsana (p. 110) or exhale and slide down carefully, releasing the hands.

If the back aches after coming down, bend the knees over the abdomen and clasp the hands around them.

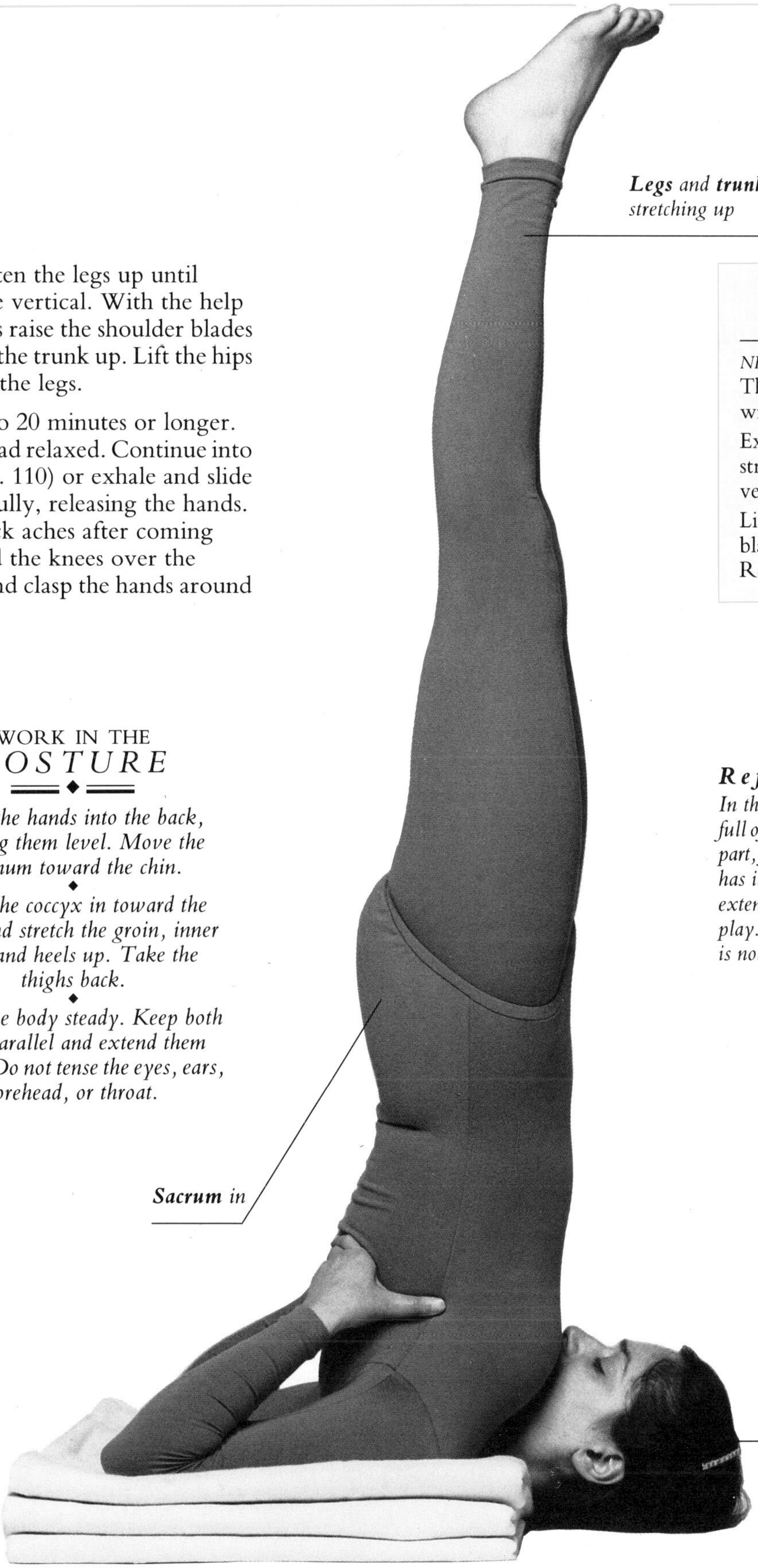

NIRĀLAMBA SARVĀṄGĀSANA

NIRĀLAMBA = without support

The body stretches up and balances without the help of the arms.

Extend the arms, with elbows straight, (a) beyond the head or (b) vertically up, palms facing the hips.

Lift the upper back and shoulder blades. Extend the abdomen up. Relax the head. ♦♦♦

WORK IN THE POSTURE

Press the hands into the back, keeping them level. Move the sternum toward the chin.

♦

Tuck the coccyx in toward the pubis and stretch the groin, inner legs, and heels up. Take the thighs back.

♦

Make the body steady. Keep both sides parallel and extend them evenly. Do not tense the eyes, ears, forehead, or throat.

Reflection

In the āsanas every cell of the body becomes full of life. This makes the body vibrant. Each part, from the toes to the fingers, is active. Each has its own job to do – lifting, turning, extending, or pressing – in a complex interplay. If one part is not sensitive, the posture is not complete. This total action is Yoga.

हलासन

Halāsana

HALA = plow

WITH THE trunk and legs taken over the head, the brain relaxes.♦

Be in Sarvāṅgāsana (p. 108).

Keeping the legs straight, exhale and take them over the head; rest the tips of the toes on the floor.

Raise the hips and take them over the head to curve the trunk slightly. Tuck the kneecaps in and lift the thighs, shins, and ankles. Keep the feet vertical, the heels stretching away from the trunk.

Stay, breathing evenly, for 3 to 5 minutes or longer.

Continue the Sarvāṅgāsana cycle or exhale and slide down. Sit and bend forward.

WAYS OF PRACTICING

To avoid straining the back, go down with bent legs.

Release the hands and take the arms over the head.

Rest the toes on a stool.

VARIATION

For a more intense stretch, clasp the hands behind the back. Keep the palms facing in, or turn them out. Straighten the elbows. Press the arms down. Move the thoracic spine in and lift the hips.♦♦

ARDHA HALĀSANA

ARDHA = half; *HALA* = plow

Before doing Sarvāṅgāsana (p. 108), place a chair over where the head will be and put two or three blankets on it. Then, from Sarvāṅgāsana, exhale and bring the legs onto the chair.

Move the legs forward to support the tops of the thighs. Take the arms over the head and relax completely.

Stay for 5 to 10 minutes or longer, breathing evenly.♦

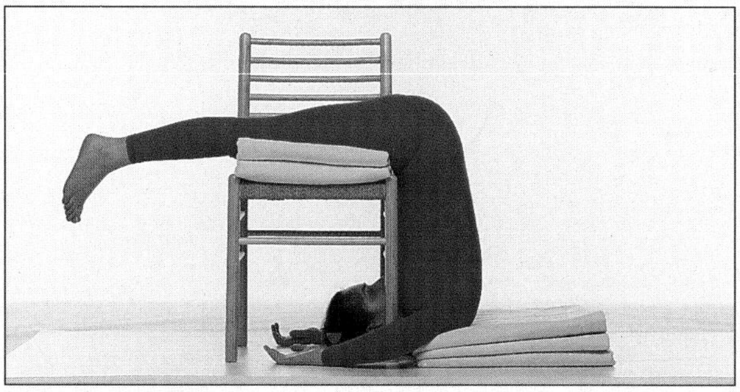

WORK IN THE *POSTURE*

With the hands, press the back ribs forward. Lift the front and sides of the body up. Stretch the lumbar.

♦

Open the backs of the legs (see Focus, p. 89).

♦

Learn to relax.

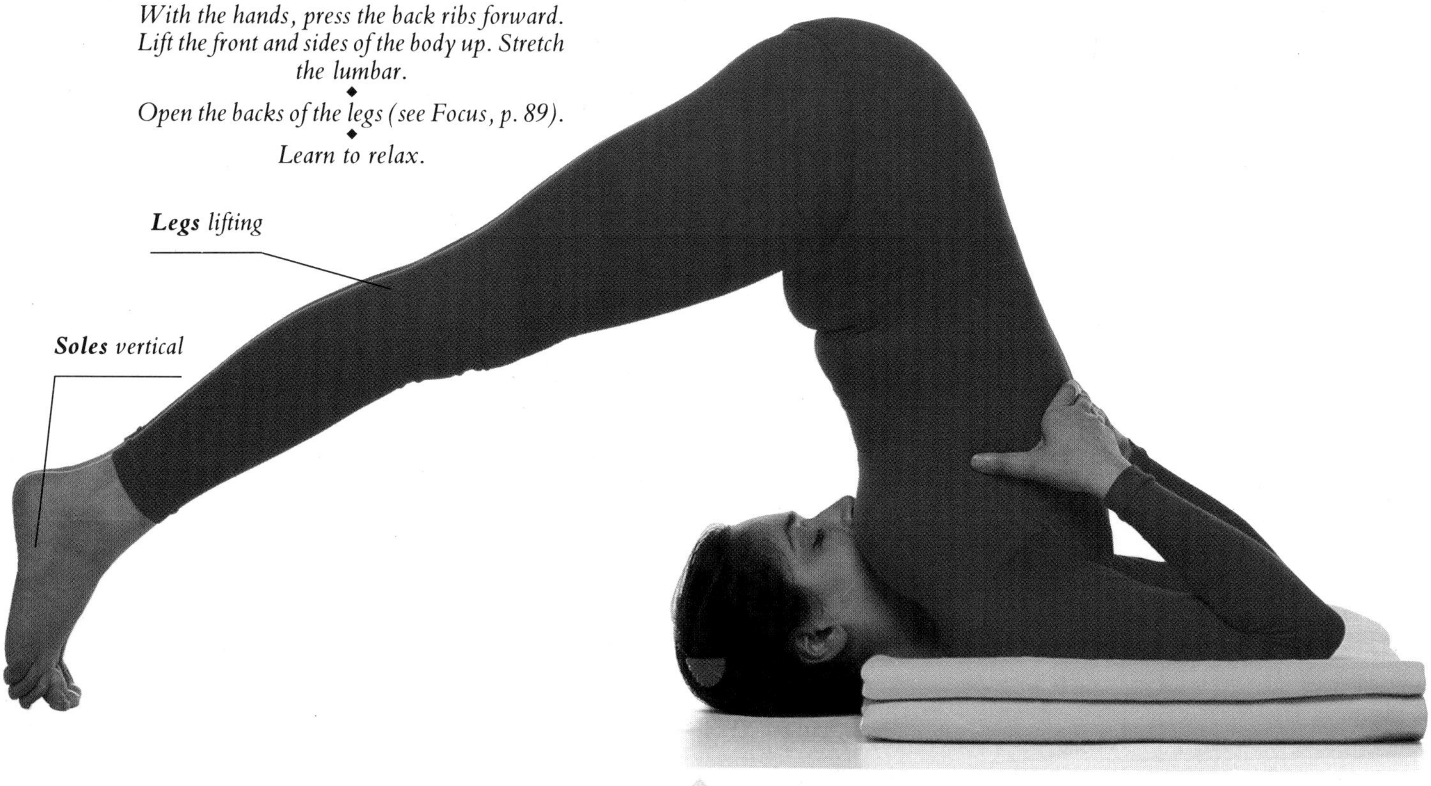

सालम्ब सर्वांगासन

Sarvāṅgāsana cycle

SARVĀṄGĀSANA variations refresh the legs and strengthen the back.

Eka Pāda Sarvāṅgāsana

EKA PĀDA = one leg;
SARVĀṄGĀSANA = neck-balance

The upward and downward stretches of the legs counterbalance each other.♦♦

Be in Sarvāṅgāsana (p. 108). ▷Keep the left leg stable. Exhale and take the right leg down, with the big toe resting on the floor. Lift the right outer thigh. Do not turn either leg when going down, but stay in line. Keep the legs straight rather than reaching for the floor.

Stay for 10 to 15 seconds, breathing evenly.

Inhale, take the right leg up.◁ Repeat from ▷to◁ on the left.

Continue the cycle or exhale and come down.

WAYS OF PRACTICING

Take the leg down onto a chair.

Go halfway down.

WORK IN THE POSTURE

Do not disturb the elbows or the head.

Stretch the left leg and the right side of the trunk up, as the right leg goes down.

Open the inner thighs away from each other. Keep both kneecaps locked.

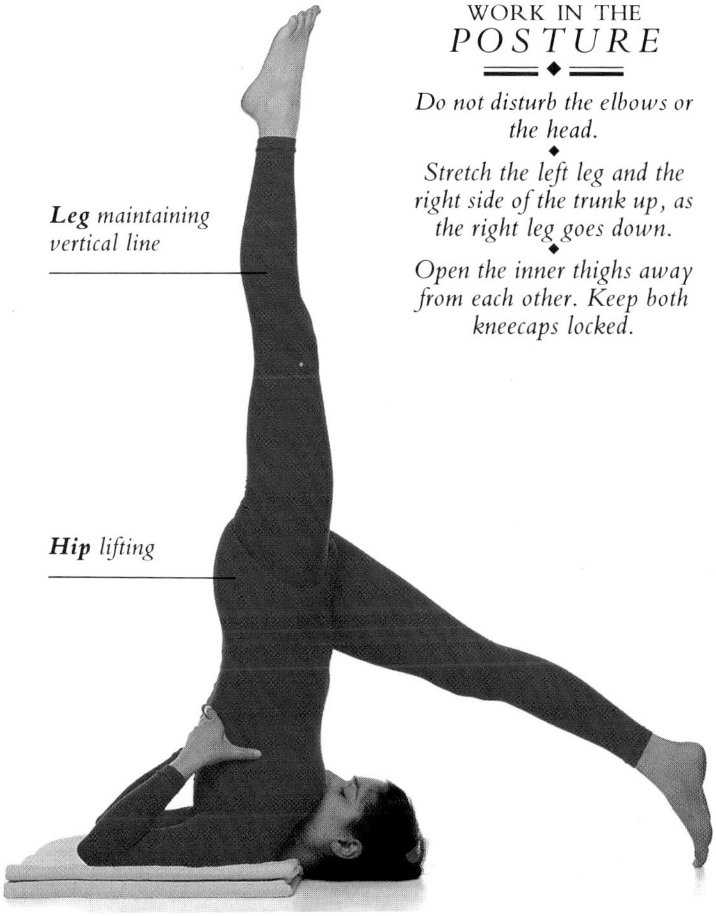

***Leg** maintaining vertical line*

***Hip** lifting*

Pārśvaikapāda Sarvāṅgāsana

PĀRŚVA = sideways; *EKA PĀDA* = one leg;
SARVĀṄGĀSANA = neck-balance

The strong rotation of the leg gives mobility to the hip.♦♦

Be in Sarvāṅgāsana (p. 108). ▷Keep the left leg straight, do not turn it. Turn the right leg outward in its socket; exhale and take it down sideways to the ground, placing the foot in line with the right shoulder. Lift the right hip.

Stay for 10 to 15 seconds, breathing evenly.

Inhale and raise the right leg.◁ Repeat from ▷to◁ on the left.

Continue the cycle or exhale and come down.

WAYS OF PRACTICING

Take the leg halfway down or onto a chair.

WORK IN THE POSTURE

Move the right side of the trunk forward when turning the leg.

Extend both legs to the heels and keep them straight.

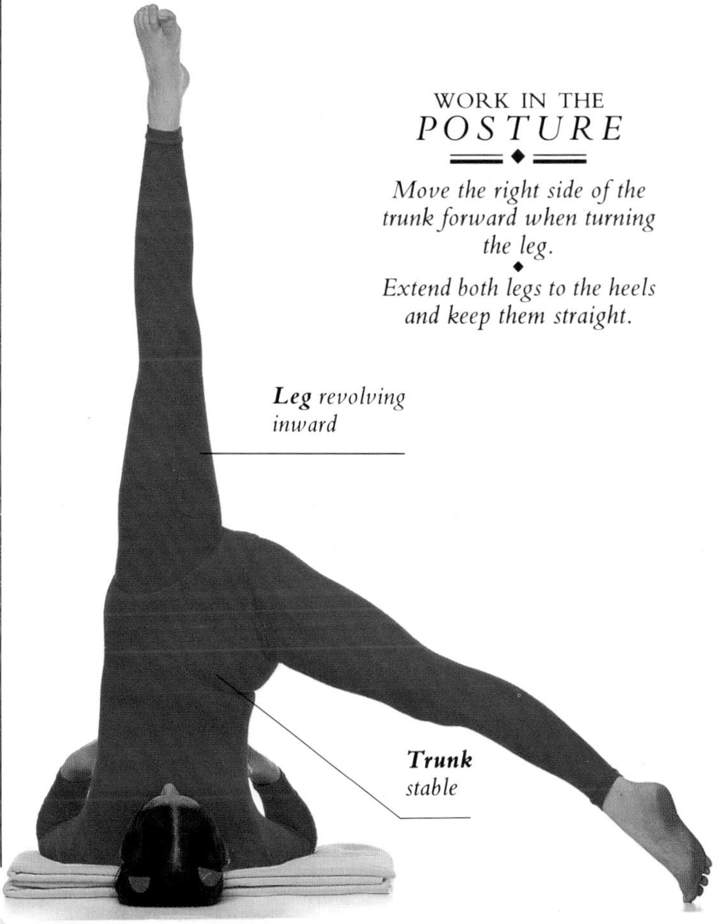

***Leg** revolving inward*

***Trunk** stable*

सालम्ब सर्वांगासन

Sarvāṅgāsana cycle

Karṇapīḍāsana

KARṆA = ears; PĪḌA = pressure

The senses are shut away from external distractions and the body relaxes.♦♦

Be in Halāsana (p. 110). Exhale and bend the legs. Take the knees to the ground beside the ears, close to the shoulders. Be on the centers of the shins and stretch the feet back. Bring the sternum forward and lift the trunk. Settle into the posture without straining the back and neck. Take the arms around the legs and clasp the hands.

Stay for 10 to 15 seconds, breathing evenly.

Straighten the legs into Halāsana.

Continue the cycle or exhale and come down.

Ways of Practicing

Rest the knees on a bolster.

Keep the hands on the back until the neck can support the weight of the body.

WORK IN THE POSTURE

Do not compress the abdomen.

Extend the shins toward the knees.

Learn to surrender to the pose to become comfortable.

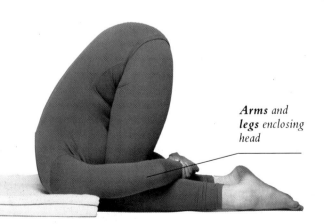

Arms and
legs enclosing
head

Pārśva Halāsana

PĀRŚVA = sideways; HALA = plow

A strong action in the hips is needed for the legs to step to the side.♦♦

Be in Halāsana (p. 110). ▷Raise the hips. Exhale and take a large step to the right with the right leg and bring the left leg toward it. Walk further until the feet are in line with the right shoulder. Keep the knees straight and facing the ground, the backs of the legs facing the ceiling.

Do not move the head and shoulders while taking the legs to one side.

Stay for 10 to 15 seconds, breathing evenly.

Walk the feet to the center.◁ Repeat from ▷to◁ on the left.

Continue the cycle or exhale and come down.

WORK IN THE POSTURE

Keep the left elbow down. Extend the front of the body and the groin up.

Bring the right side of the trunk forward. Raise the left outer thigh and pull the right buttock bone back.

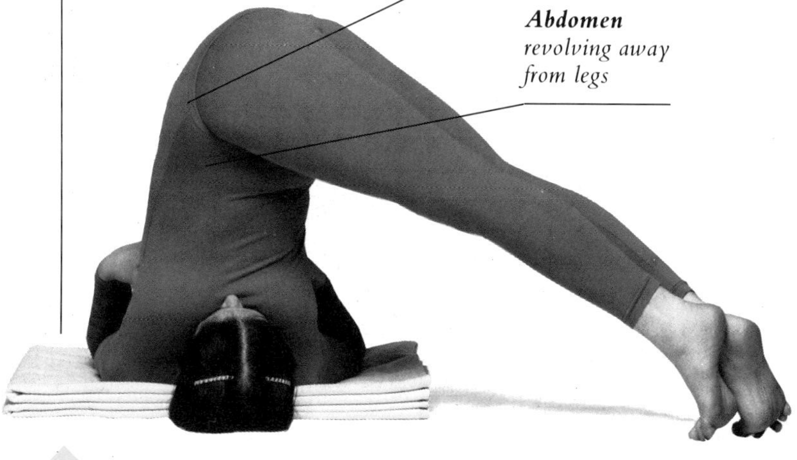
Hips lifting
Abdomen
revolving away
from legs

सालम्ब सर्वांगासन

Supta Koṇāsana

SUPTA = supine; KOṆA = angle
The hands gripping the feet help the legs to spread.♦♦

Be in Halāsana (p. 110). Exhale and spread both legs simultaneously to the sides, as far as they will go. Release the hands from the back and hold the big toes with the thumbs, index, and middle fingers. Raise the hips, lock the kneecaps, and stretch the soles of the feet up. Keep the centers of the backs of the legs facing the ceiling. Do not let the legs roll in.

Stay for 10 to 15 seconds, breathing evenly.

Place the hands on the back. Join the legs.

Continue the cycle or exhale and come down.

WAYS OF PRACTICING

With the hands on the back learn to sweep the legs apart, raising the feet slightly.

Do the posture from Sarvāṅgāsana (p. 108), turning the legs in their sockets, spreading them, and lowering them to the ground.

WORK IN THE POSTURE

With the help of the hands move the legs further apart. Stretch the inner legs to the heels.

Lift the chest, abdomen, and pubis.

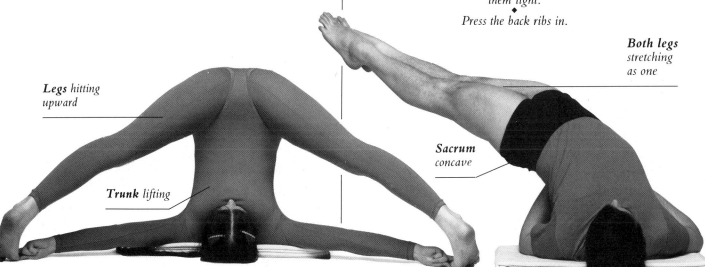

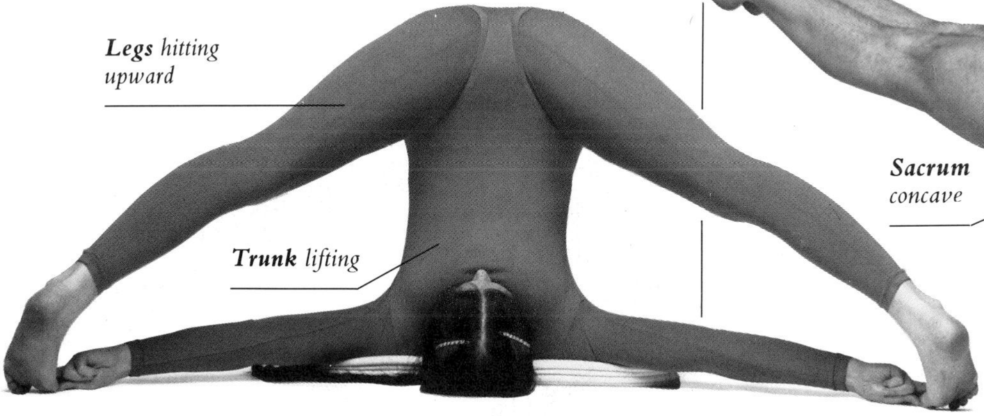

Legs hitting upward
Trunk lifting

Pārśva Sarvāṅgāsana

PĀRŚVA = sideways;
SARVĀṄGĀSANA = neck-balance
The legs are held poker-stiff to balance the sideways arch of the trunk.♦♦♦♦

1 Be in Sarvāṅgāsana (p. 108). ▷ Turn the trunk to the right. Release the left hand and place it on the sacrum, fingers pointing to the coccyx. Replace the elbow on the floor, lowering the sacrum to rest firmly on the hand. The legs now slant forward.

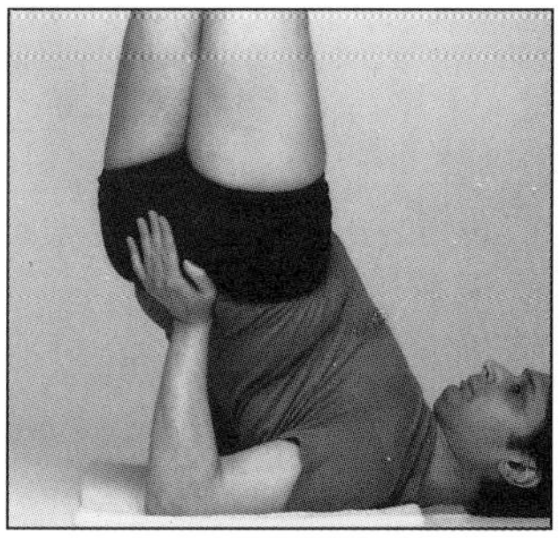

2 Bring the chest forward. Exhale and take the legs diagonally back; keep them extended and tighten the buttocks. Lower the trunk and legs to the maximum.

Stay for 5 to 10 seconds, breathing evenly.

Continue the cycle or exhale and come down.

WORK IN THE POSTURE

Do not move the left elbow. Press the heel of the hand into the sacrum and the fingertips into the area of the coccyx to get a good grip.

Stretch the legs strongly to make them light.

Press the back ribs in.

Both legs stretching as one
Sacrum concave

सालम्ब सर्वांगासन

Sarvāṅgāsana cycle

Ūrdhva Padmāsana in Sarvāṅgāsana

ŪRDHVA = up; *PADMA* = lotus, *SARVĀṄGĀSANA* = neck-balance

With the legs crossed, the body gets a strong upward stretch.♦♦♦

Be in Sarvāṅgāsana (p. 108). Bend in the hips and bring the legs slightly forward. ▷Exhale, bend the right leg, and place the foot into the left side of the groin. Catch the foot with the hands and bring it further down. Exhale and bend the left leg. With the help of the hands, cross it over the right, taking the foot as far down as possible. Tuck the coccyx and sacrum in, and stretch the thighs up so that the knees face the ceiling. Extend the whole trunk up.

Stay for 10 to 15 seconds, breathing evenly.◁

Repeat from ▷to◁ with the left leg first.

Continue the cycle or exhale and come down.

WAYS OF PRACTICING

Cross the legs without the help of the hands.

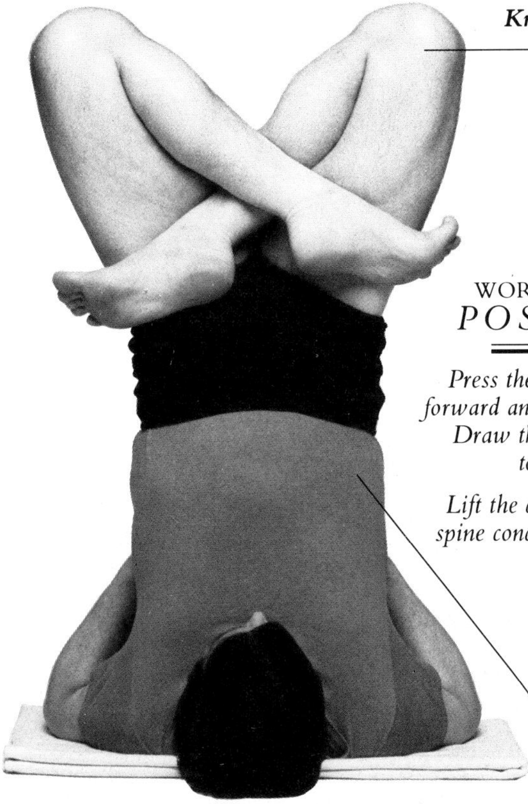

WORK IN THE POSTURE

Press the buttock bones forward and the knees back. Draw the knees closer together.

Lift the chest, make the spine concave, and stretch it up.

Piṇḍāsana in Sarvāṅgāsana

PIṆḌA = a ball; *SARVĀṄGĀSANA* = neck-balance

The body is rolled into a compact ball.♦♦♦

Be in Ūrdhva Padmāsana in Sarvāṅgāsana (left) with the right leg crossed first. ▷With an exhalation bend the legs over the chest. Support the back firmly with the hands.

If possible, bend still more, taking the shins over the head. Draw the knees closer together. Release the arms, lengthen them from the armpits, and clasp them around the legs.

Stay for 5 to 10 seconds. Inhale, bring the legs up, and release them.◁

Repeat from ▷to◁ with the left leg first.

Continue the cycle or exhale and come down.

WAYS OF PRACTICING

Rest the thighs on a stool.

Rest the knees on a bolster.

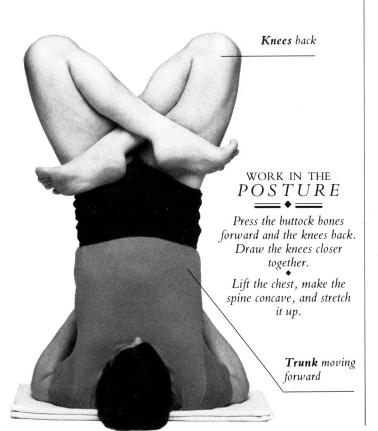

WORK IN THE POSTURE

Learn to balance.

Bend more in the groin.

Keep the head and the back relaxed.

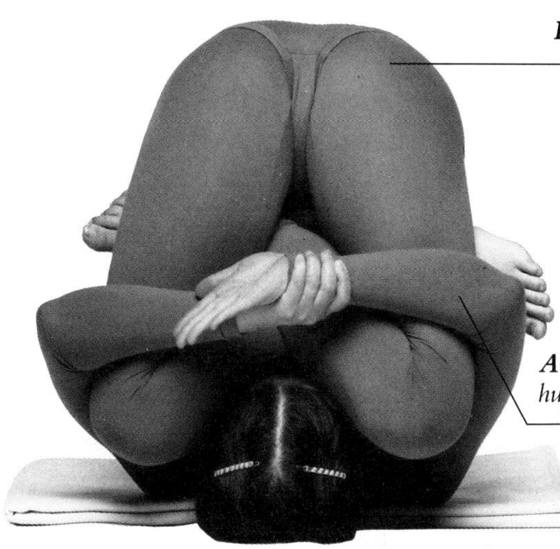

सालम्ब सर्वांगासन

Pārśva Ūrdhva Padmāsana in Sarvāṅgāsana

PĀRŚVA = sideways; ŪRDHVA = up; PADMA = lotus; SARVĀṄGĀSANA = neck-balance

Pliability, strength, and balance are the keys to this posture.♦♦♦♦

Be in Ūrdhva Padmāsana in Sarvāṅgāsana (far left), with the right leg crossed first. ▷Turn the trunk to the left. Place the right palm under the sacrum to support it, fingers pointing to the coccyx. Move the dorsal spine in and arch the chest. Exhale and lower the legs to the right, as far down as possible. Stretch the groin and the crossed legs diagonally away from the trunk, without overbalancing.

Stay for 5 to 10 seconds. Inhale, come up, turn to the center. Repeat on the left. Release the legs.◁ Repeat from ▷to◁, changing the legs.

Continue the cycle or exhale and come down.

WAYS OF PRACTICING

Go into Pārśva Piṇḍāsana on the opposite side before changing the legs.

WORK IN THE POSTURE

Keep the elbows in. Move the back ribs deep in and open the chest.

Dig the heel of the right hand into the sacrum, fingers into the coccyx, to keep the coccyx and sacrum pressed in. Make the lower back concave. Extend the front of the body.

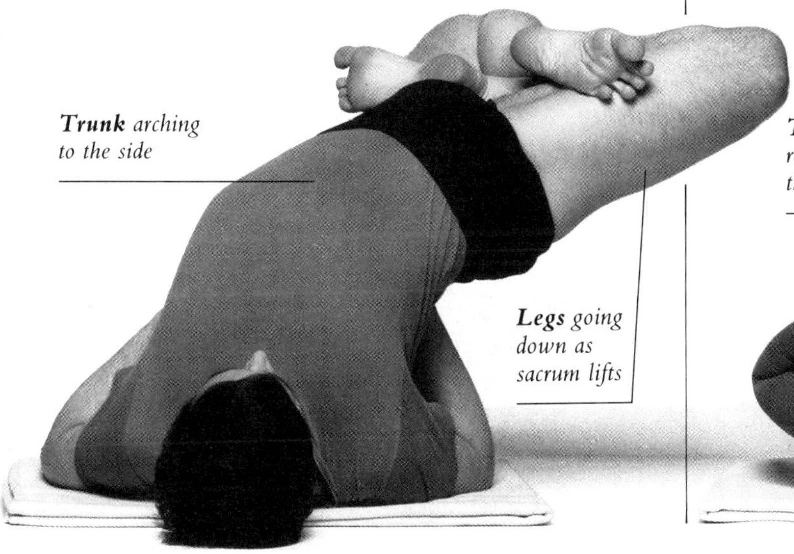

Pārśva Piṇḍāsana in Sarvāṅgāsana

PĀRŚVA = sideways; PIṆḌA = a ball; SARVĀṄGĀSANA = neck-balance

The lower back gets a transverse stretch.♦♦♦♦

Be in Ūrdhva Padmāsana in Sarvāṅgāsana (far left), with the right leg crossed first. ▷Turn the trunk to the right, without disturbing the head and neck. Stretch the sides of the body up.

Exhale, bend the trunk down, and take the crossed legs toward the right ear. Rest first the right knee and then the left on the floor beside the ear. Bring the legs closer to the head.

Press the left elbow down. Stay for 10 to 15 seconds, breathing evenly.

Press the left upper arm down and lift the hips to raise the knees, then come up. Turn to the front and come up. Repeat on the left. Release the legs.◁ Repeat from ▷to◁ with the left leg first.

Exhale and come down. Sit and bend forward to rest the head.

WAYS OF PRACTICING

Grip the blankets with the left hand.

Rest the knees on a bolster.

WORK IN THE POSTURE

Lift the chest. Bring the right side of the chest forward. Extend the left side toward the left knee.

Allow the back to release.

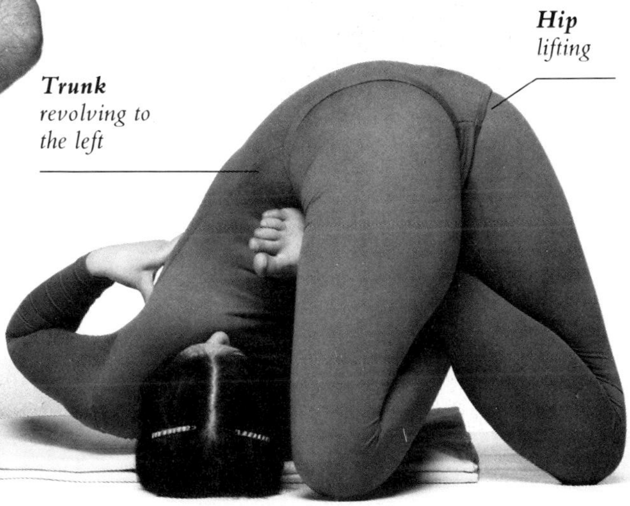

सेतुबन्ध सर्वांगासन

Setu Bandha Sarvāṅgāsana

SETU = bridge; *BANDHA* = formation; *SARVĀṄGĀSANA* = neck-balance

THIS DEVELOPS a supple back and strong wrists.♦♦♦

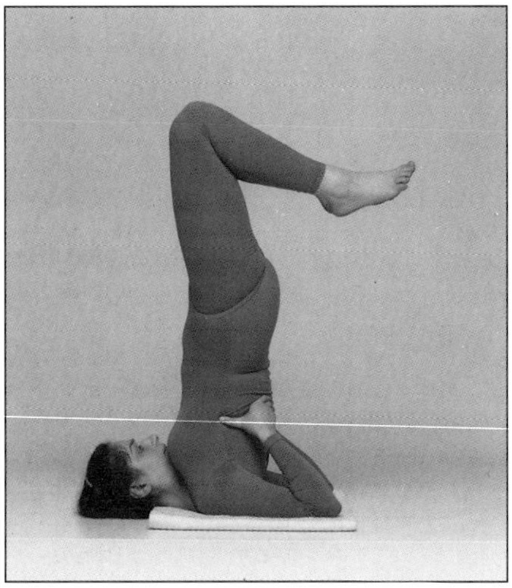

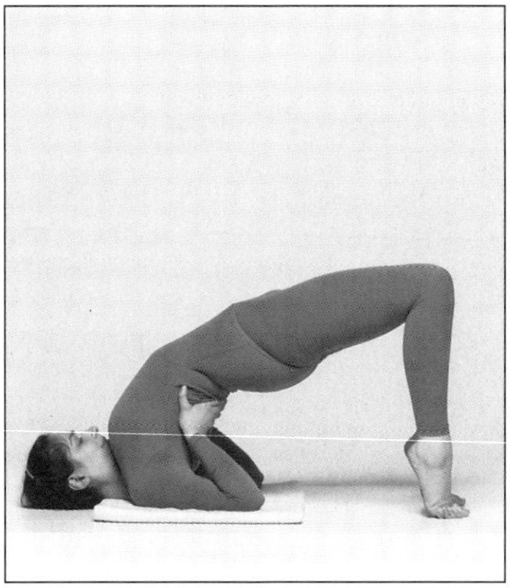

1 Be in Sarvāṅgāsana (p. 108). Press the hands into the rib cage to bring the chest and hips forward. Move the sacrum in. Bend the legs back.

WAYS OF PRACTICING

Lie down, knees bent and a little apart. Raise the trunk, bend the arms, and place the hands under the rib cage.

2 Curve the trunk to the maximum. Exhale and drop the feet to the ground. For a moment, be on the toes, raise the heels, and stretch the hips and lumbar up. Tighten the buttocks. Readjust the elbows and hands. Move the spine and back ribs firmly in. Open the chest. Then bring the heels down. Stay for 15 to 20 seconds, breathing evenly.

● *If the back feels strained, do not continue to the next step.*

3 Straighten the legs one at a time. Maintain the lift of the chest and the extension of the whole body.

Bend the legs and walk the feet in. Inhale and jump up into Sarvāṅgāsana. Then come down.

VARIATION

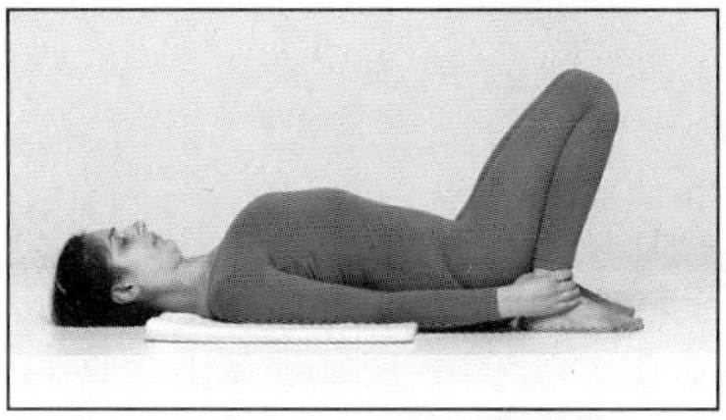

1 Lie on the floor, legs bent and a hip's-width apart. Keep the shoulders down. Catch the ankles.

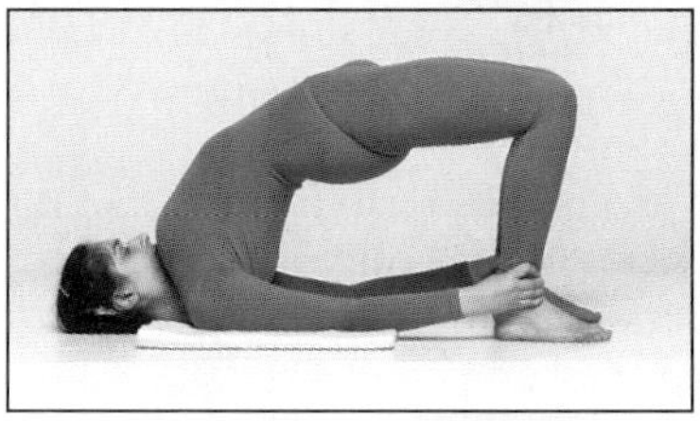

2 Inhale and raise the trunk; lift and curve it.♦♦

WORK IN THE
POSTURE

Be light on the hands.

Raise both the back and the front of the body to increase the arch. Press the shoulders and forearms down to lift the trunk. Press the heels down to stretch the legs.

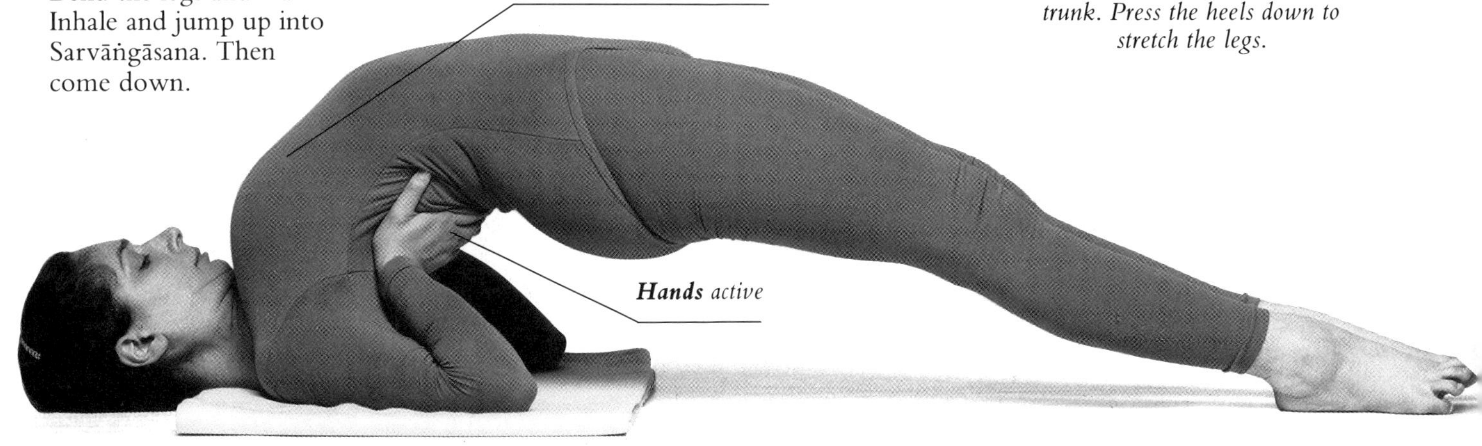

एकपाद सालम्ब सर्वांगासन

Eka Pāda Setu Bandha Sarvāṅgāsana

EKA PĀDA = one leg; *SETU BANDHA* = construction of a bridge;
SARVĀṄGĀSANA = neck-balance

FROM THE arch of the pose the lifted leg elongates upward.♦♦♦

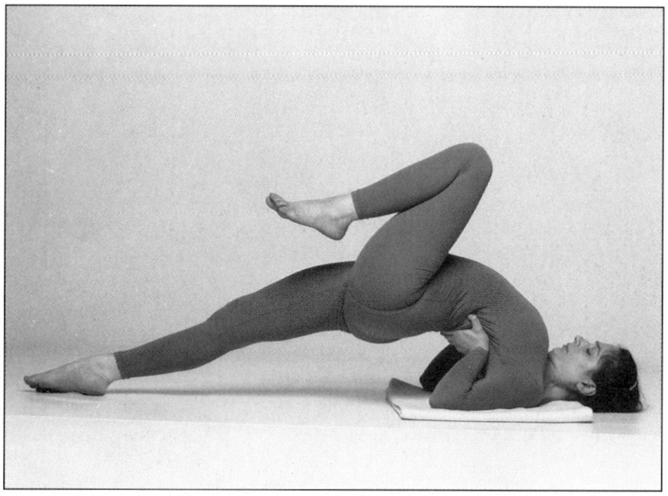

1 Be in Setu Bandha Sarvāṅgāsana (opposite). Keep the back of the body firmly lifted. ▷Bend the left leg over the abdomen, keeping the knee in line.

WAYS OF PRACTICING

Keep the right leg bent when stretching the left leg up.

Drop back into the pose from Eka Pāda Sarvāṅgāsana (p. 111).

2 Exhale and straighten the left leg vertically up. Tuck in the kneecap and extend the heel and the toes up. Lift the left hip. Do not let the legs turn outward. Stay for 10 to 15 seconds, breathing evenly.

Exhale and bend the left leg over the abdomen; then take it down.◁

Repeat from ▷to◁ with the right leg up.

Jump up into Sarvāṅgāsana, or come down.

Focus *Combining effort and understanding*

Vigorous effort coupled with fine understanding is required to master the postures. Maximum effort, to extend further and to use muscles with more strength, needs to be directed and analyzed. To build up stamina and strength, do less than the maximum, pause to reflect and become steady, then increase the effort until the maximum is reached. Or, exert to the utmost without force, then relax, and repeat. This leads to further understanding.

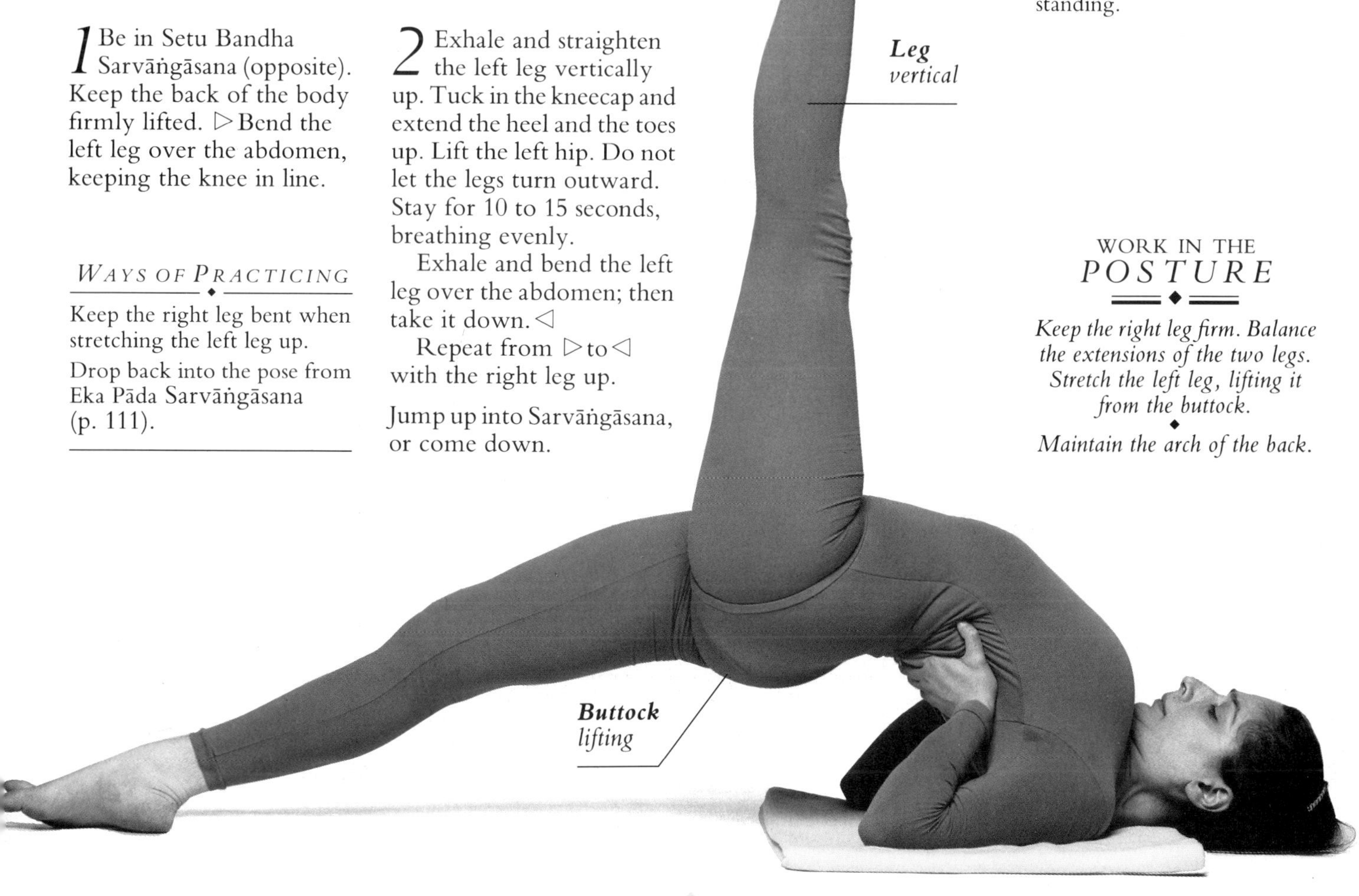

WORK IN THE
POSTURE

Keep the right leg firm. Balance the extensions of the two legs. Stretch the left leg, lifting it from the buttock.
♦
Maintain the arch of the back.

सालम्ब सर्वांगासन

Sālamba Sarvāṅgāsana (on chair)

SĀLAMBA = with support; *SARVĀṄGĀSANA* = neck-balance

THE BACK is supported and arched, allowing the chest to open and the internal organs to stretch. This pose calms the emotions.♦♦

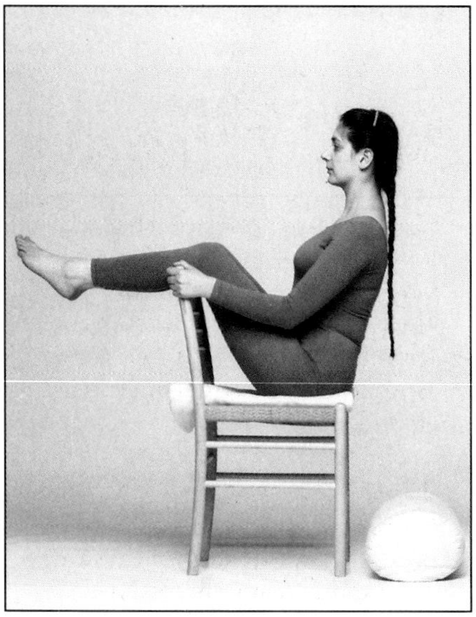

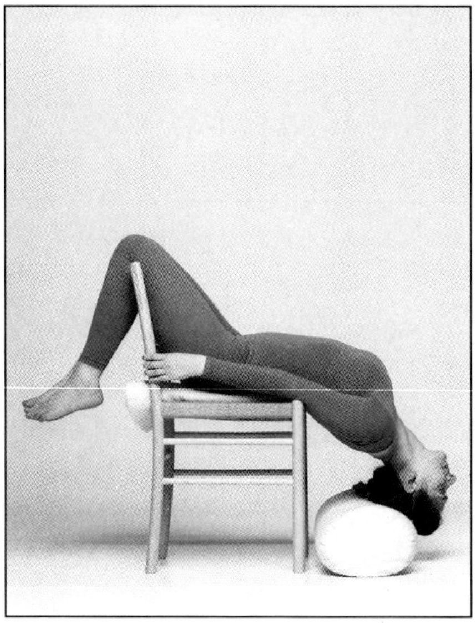

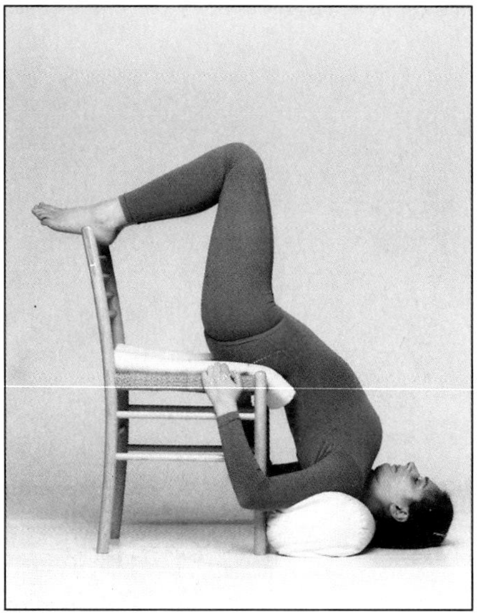

1 Place a chair on a nonslip surface. Put a blanket over the front edge of the seat. Place a bolster or a pile of blankets in front of the chair. Sit astride the chair, facing the back. Move closer to the back. Hold the chair.

Raise the legs one at a time over the back of the chair, keeping them bent. Sit evenly.

Ways of Practicing

Place the chair about 18 in away from a wall to support the feet.

Place a blanket over the back of the chair for comfort.

Place a folded blanket under the head if it feels strained.

Place a bolster behind the legs to lessen the arch of the back.

Tie the thighs together with a belt to relax the legs.

Follow this posture with Ardha Halāsana (p. 110). Place a stool near the head beforehand.

2 Lean back. Still holding the chair, move the buttocks 2 to 3 in toward the front edge of the chair. Lower the back carefully, curving the waist over the front edge of the chair until the head reaches the bolster. Do not constrict the neck.

Focus *Choosing the right equipment*
Any chair, stool, or bench used for Yoga practice should be strong and stable. It should be of a suitable height and width, and should not tip up or collapse when the body weight is placed at one end. Test this by sitting on the extreme edge (which should be straight, not shaped).

3 Slide further down until the head is on the floor, the shoulders on the blankets and the sacrum rests on the seat of the chair. Rest the feet on the back of the chair. Hold the sides of the seat. Do not let go of the chair. Adjust the back of the chair if necessary, by moving the sacrum away from the waist.

Reflection
Emotions sway the mind from moment to moment, disturbing steadiness and peace. In Yoga it is considered that the emotional heart lies at the center, below the physical heart. This center becomes opened and stabilized by the āsanas, making the mind strong, able to withstand emotional strains.

सालम्ब सर्वांगासन

4 Without disturbing the trunk, take the hands one at a time in between the chair legs to hold the back legs, or the sides of the seat. Straighten your legs and stretch the trunk and the legs up. Gripping firmly with the hands, press the back ribs in and open the chest.

Stay, breathing evenly, for 5 to 10 minutes or longer.

Coming out of the posture

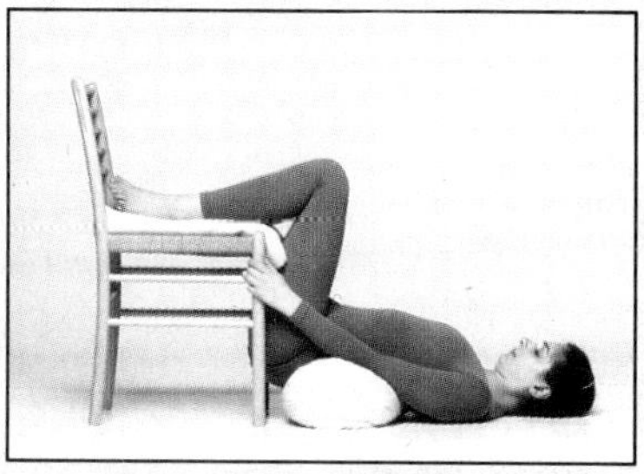

Come down carefully as the lower back may hurt after being pressed down on the chair. Bend the legs and rest the feet on the back of the chair. Bring the arms from under the chair and hold the seat.

Gradually ease the body off the chair, bringing the feet on to the seat. Push the chair away until the hips lie on the bolster.

Come down completely, bending the legs and turning to the side.

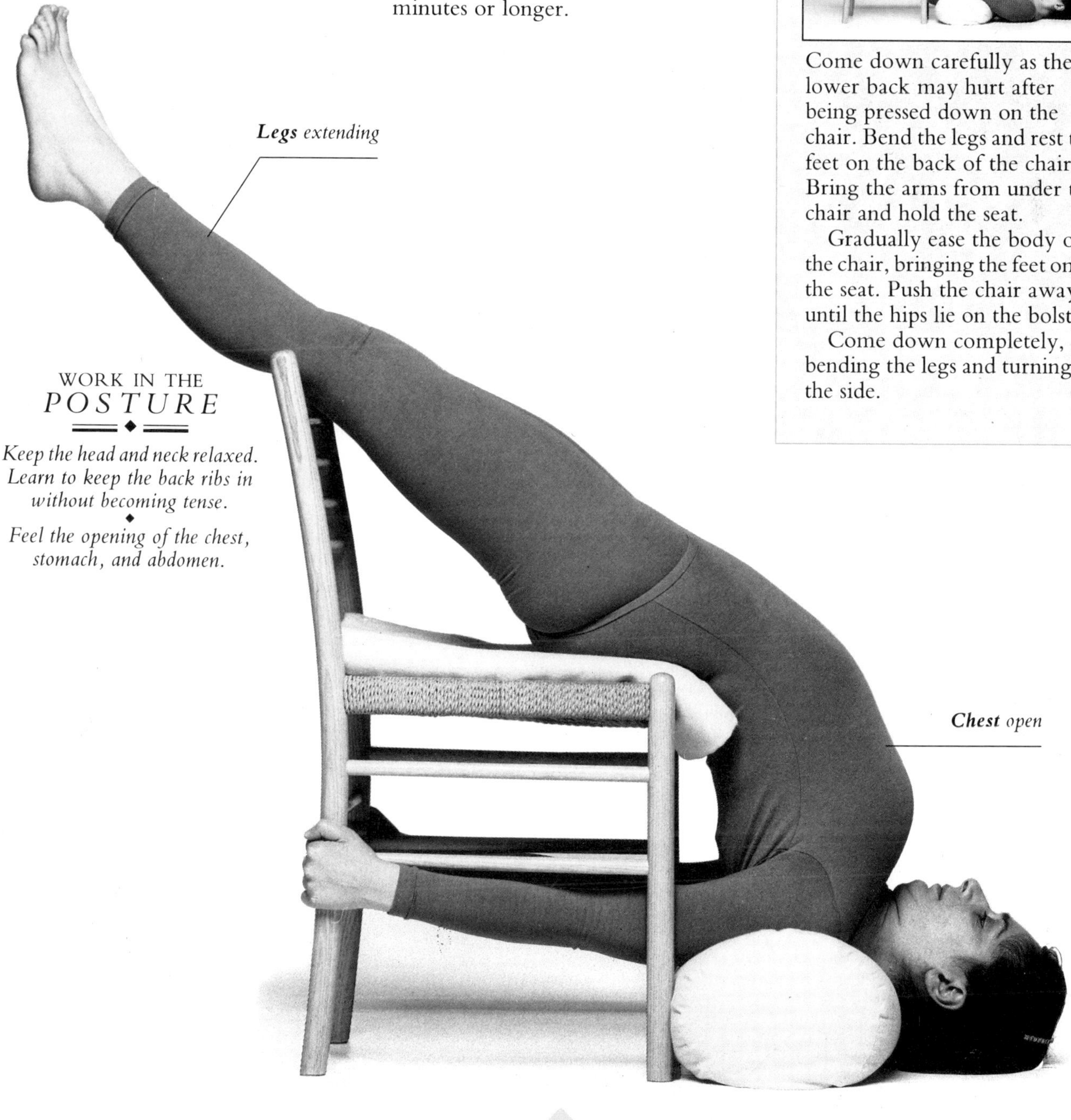

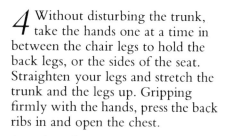

WORK IN THE
POSTURE

Keep the head and neck relaxed. Learn to keep the back ribs in without becoming tense.

◆

Feel the opening of the chest, stomach, and abdomen.

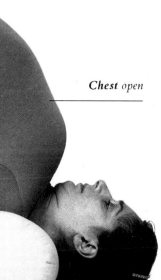

सेतुबन्ध सर्वांगासन

Setu Bandha Sarvāṅgāsana (on bench)

SETU BANDHA = construction of a bridge; *SARVĀṄGĀSANA* = neck-balance

THIS IS a recuperative posture as the lungs open while the body is at rest.♦♦

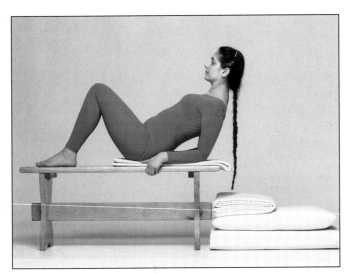

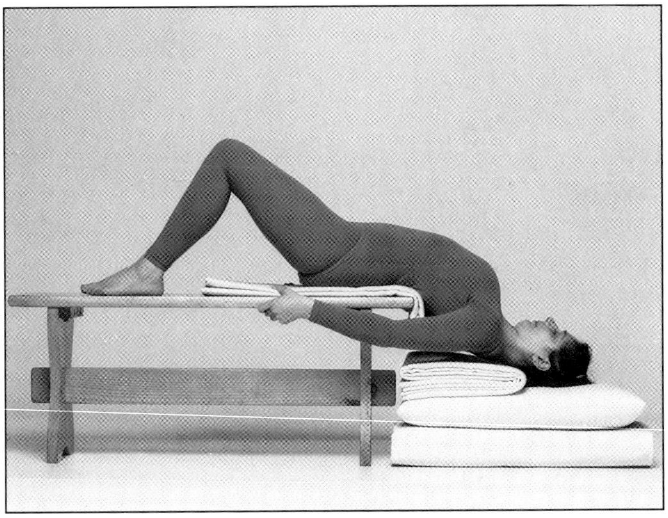

1 Place a thick folded blanket over one edge of a bench or coffee table. On the floor in front of this place 1 or 2 firm bolsters or several blankets, long enough to take the shoulders, head, and upper arms. Place a small pillow or blanket halfway across, to support the shoulders. Sit with the feet on the bench, legs bent, about 2ft away from the edge and facing away from it. Holding the bench, lean back onto the elbows. Check that the trunk and legs are in line.

2 Exhale and carefully lie back, curving the waist over the edge of the bench until the shoulders rest on the top blanket and the head is on the bolsters. Keep the sacrum on the bench. Move the sacrum and the flesh of the buttocks away from the waist.

WAYS OF PRACTICING

Adjust the height of the bolsters according to the flexibility of the spine.

To relax further, tie a belt around the mid-thighs. If there is a helper to undo the belts, tie the legs just above the ankles, below and above the knees, and at the tops of the thighs.

Raise the feet onto a bolster if the back aches.

3 Straighten the legs away from the trunk, then relax them. Lift the rib cage so that the upper chest opens and breathing becomes deeper. Take the arms over the head and relax.

Stay, breathing evenly, for 5 to 10 minutes or longer.

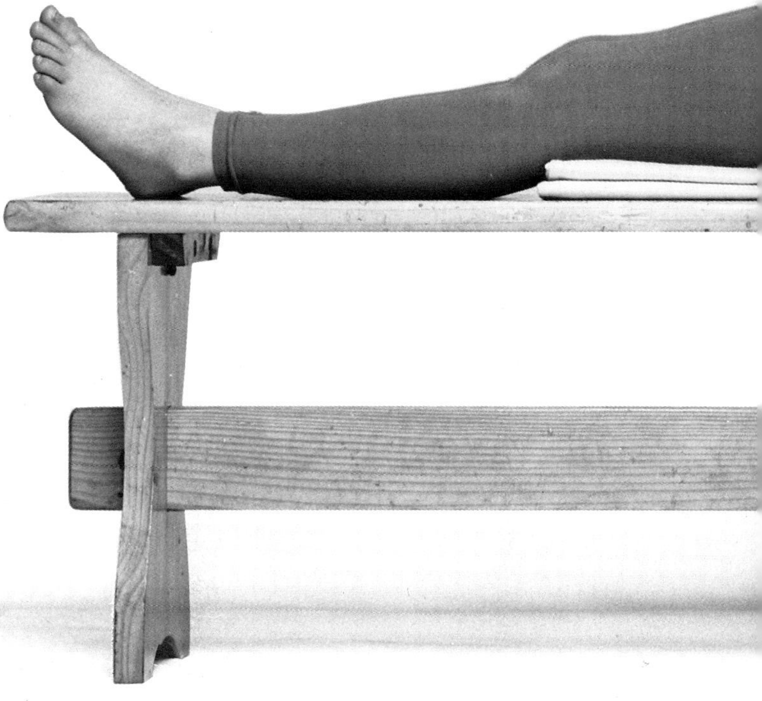

सेतुबन्ध सर्वांगासन

Coming out of the posture

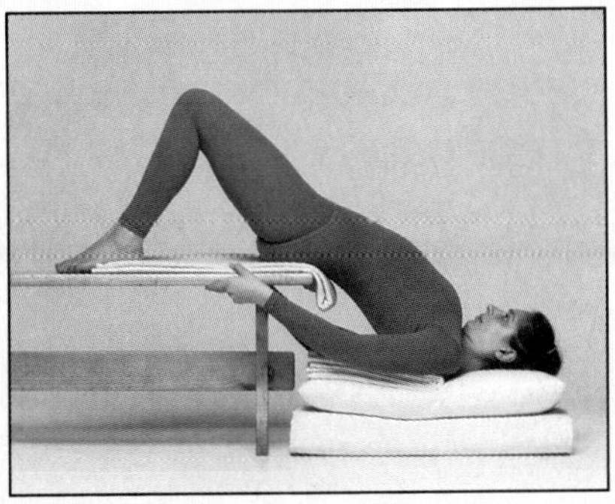

1 Hold the bench and bend the legs, keeping the feet on the bench. Carefully slide back in the direction of the head. When the coccyx reaches the edge, pause so as not to come down with a bump.

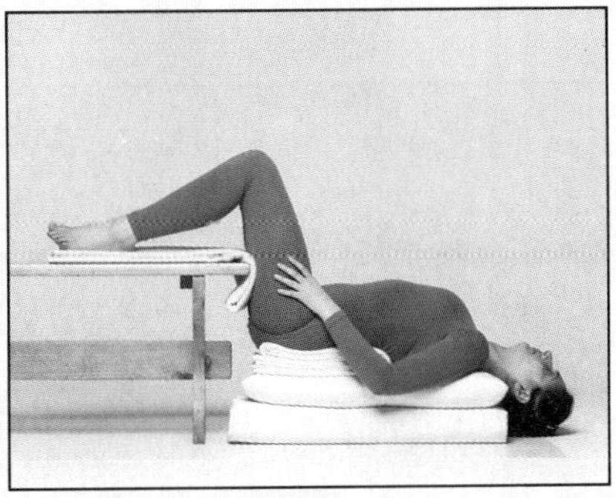

2 Move the hips down and rest the lower back on the bolsters. Come down completely, turn to the side, and get up.

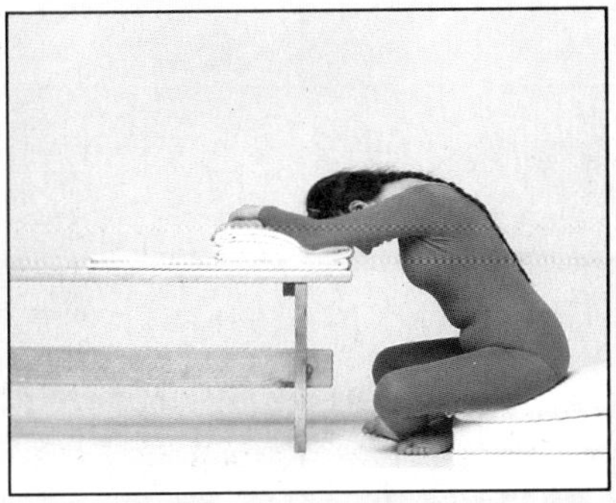

3 Sit with the legs simply crossed in front of the bench and rest the head on it, until the back returns to normal.

WORK IN THE
POSTURE

Stretch the abdomen toward the chest, the chest away from the abdomen.

◆

Let the edge of the bench press into the bottom of the rib cage to arch the back more. Keep the head and neck relaxed and press the shoulders down.

◆

Learn to let go. Enjoy the relaxation.

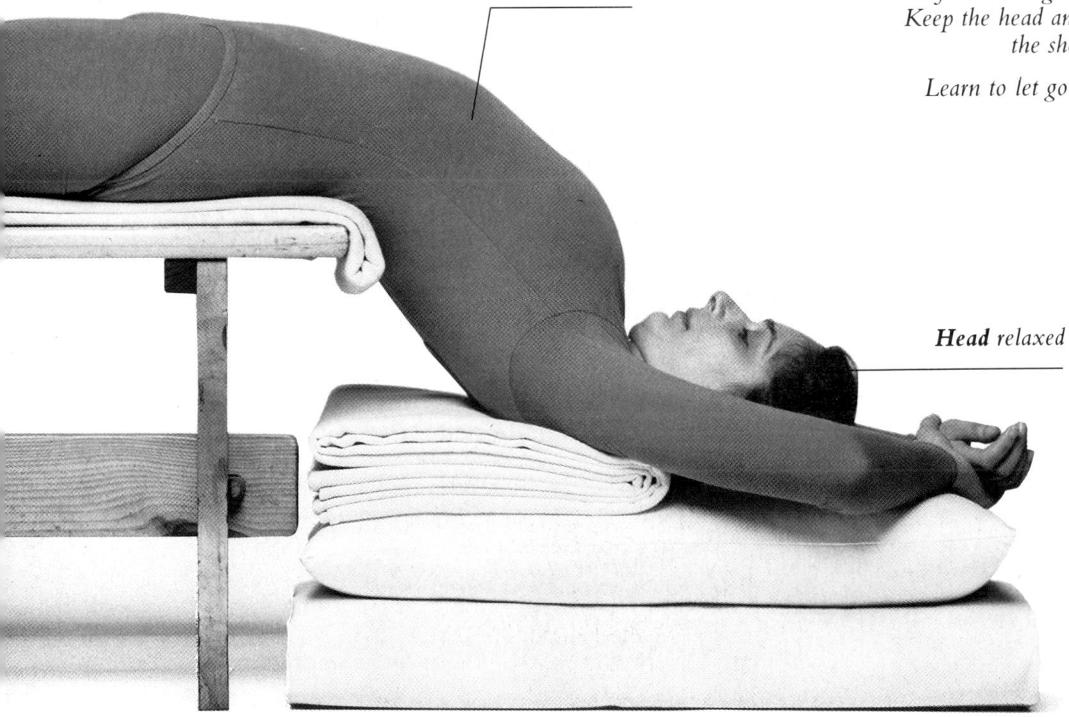

विपरीत करणि

Viparīta Karaṇi

VIPARĪTA = inverted; KARAṆI = a particular type of practice

THIS IS a restful practice, where the body is inverted without effort.♦

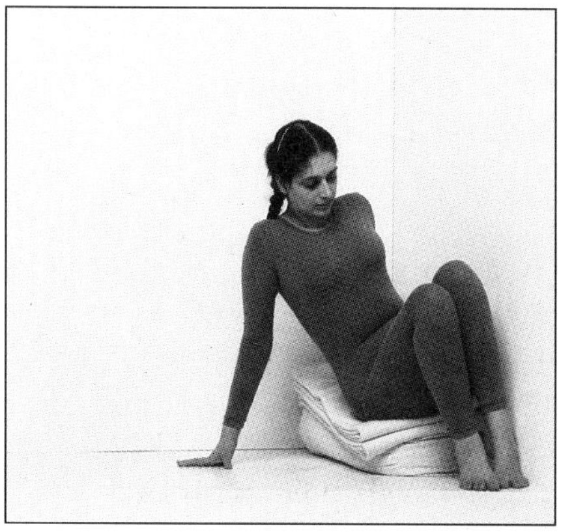

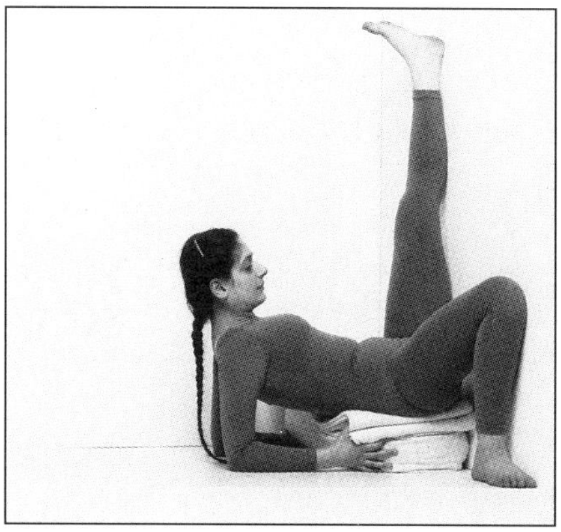

1 Place a pile of blankets or a bolster against a wall. The width of the support depends on the length of the trunk. A taller person will need a higher and wider support.

Sit sideways on the edge of the bolster, with one hip touching the wall. Bend the legs. Keep the hands on the floor.

2 Prepare to slide 90° around, with the help of the hands. One at a time, raise the legs onto the wall and take them sideways to a vertical position. At the same time swivel the trunk around in the opposite direction until it is in line with the legs. Keep both buttocks touching the wall.

3 Keeping the hips down, curve the trunk, and lie back over the blankets, head on the floor. Press the shoulders down and extend the chest. Place a blanket under the head if necessary.

Turn the upper arms out and take them over the head.

Stay, breathing evenly, for 5 to 10 minutes.

Slide back to rest the hips on the floor. Bend the legs, turn to the side, and get up.

WORK IN THE POSTURE

Keep the groin down. Do not slide away from the wall.

♦

Feel the opening of the abdomen and the chest. Rest completely.

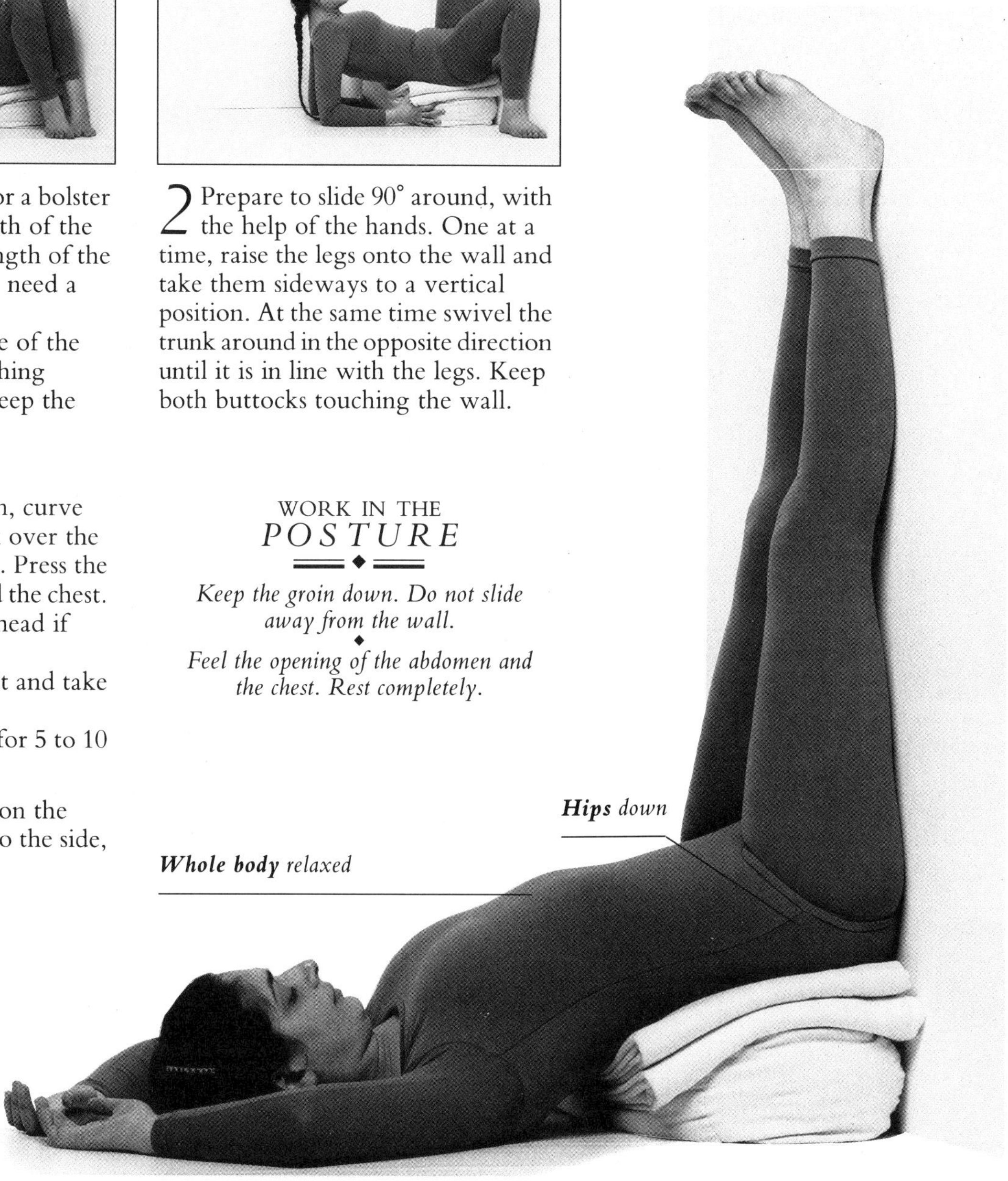

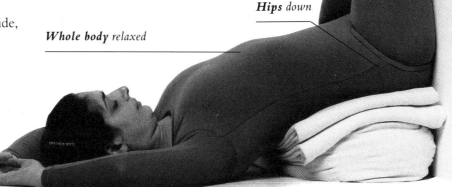

BALANCINGS

You must hold the balance by the intelligence of the body – by instinct or the sense of equilibrium – and not by strength. When you keep the balance by strength, it is physical action; when you keep it by the intelligence of the body, it is relaxation in action.

B. K. S. IYENGAR[1]

The balancing poses develop lightness, strength, and agility. Tremendous control is achieved over the body. Muscle tone is developed. Coordination and concentration increase.

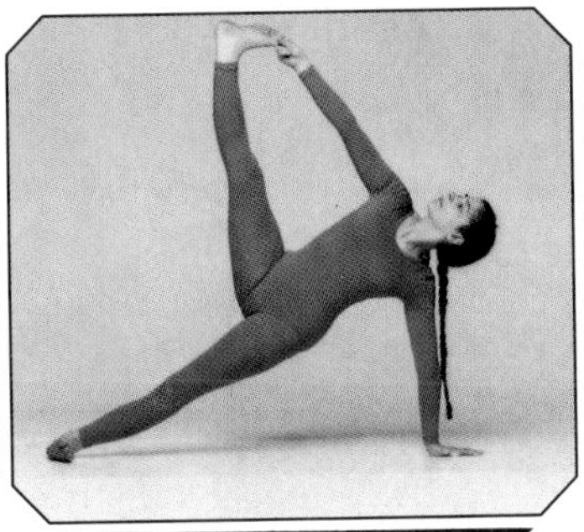

GUIDELINES FOR PRACTICE

Although the balancings strengthen the arms, they also require strong wrists. These are developed by the practice of Adho Mukha Śvānāsana (p. 90), Ūrdhva Mukhā Śvānāsana (p. 91) and Adho Mukha Vṛkṣāsana (p. 96). Sometimes it is helpful to tie a bandage around each wrist for more support.

In the beginning it is advisable to keep a cushion on the floor in front of the head, or at the back of it, when practicing, to break a possible fall.

If the wrists become tired, rest in Uttānāsana with the fingers pointing back and the palms facing up.

The neck has a tendency to compress when balancings are done from Śīrṣāsana II (p. 107). The back and neck need to be strong and well trained through practice of the other *āsanas*. Ūrdhva Dhanurāsana practiced afterward relieves the compression of the neck.

CAUTIONS: Do not do balancings for 12–18 months after an abdominal operation. Do not do them during menstruation or pregnancy.

Be careful if the wrists are weak or injured.

लोलासन

Lolāsana

LOLA = swinging to and fro; pendant earring

THE BODY swings backward and forward between the arms, developing lightness.♦♦♦

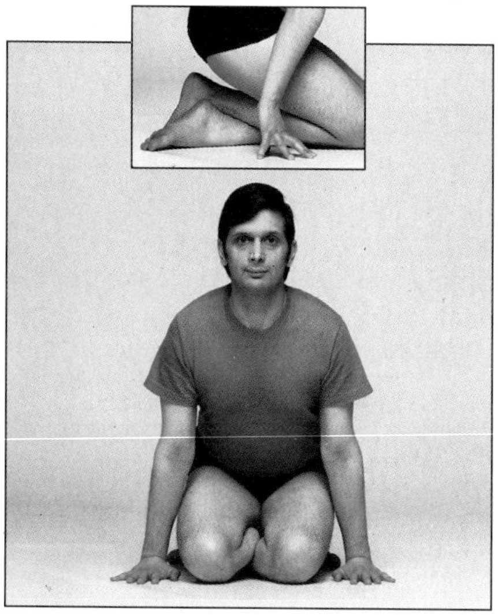

1 Kneel with the palms down beside the knees, pointing forward and with the fingers spread. ▷Raise the buttocks, place the right ankle over the left, then sit again. Lean forward.

Ways of Practicing

Place the hands on bricks.

WORK IN THE POSTURE

Keep the weight equal on both hands.
Stretch the upper arms strongly up.

Draw the thighs up toward the trunk and the shins up toward the thighs.
Stretch the toes back.

Focus *Placing the hands*
Keep the hands facing forward and in line. Extend the palms and fingers and press them down. Press down the heels of the hands, especially the thumb side. Stretch the forearms away from the wrists.

For a stronger, lighter balance, bend the knuckles.

2 Straighten the elbows, press the palms into the floor; exhale and lift the trunk and legs off the floor, with the crossed feet close to the perineum. Draw the legs up and balance on the hands. Swing backward and forward two or three times.

Exhale and come down. Stretch out the legs.◁

Repeat from ▷to◁, changing the legs.

Reflection
Yoga enhances all the faculties of the body and maintains them at their peak. The postures increase vigor, pliability, stamina, and resilience. They also develop firmness and lightness. These qualities are transferred to the mind. Thus a finely tuned body is considered necessary for spiritual growth.

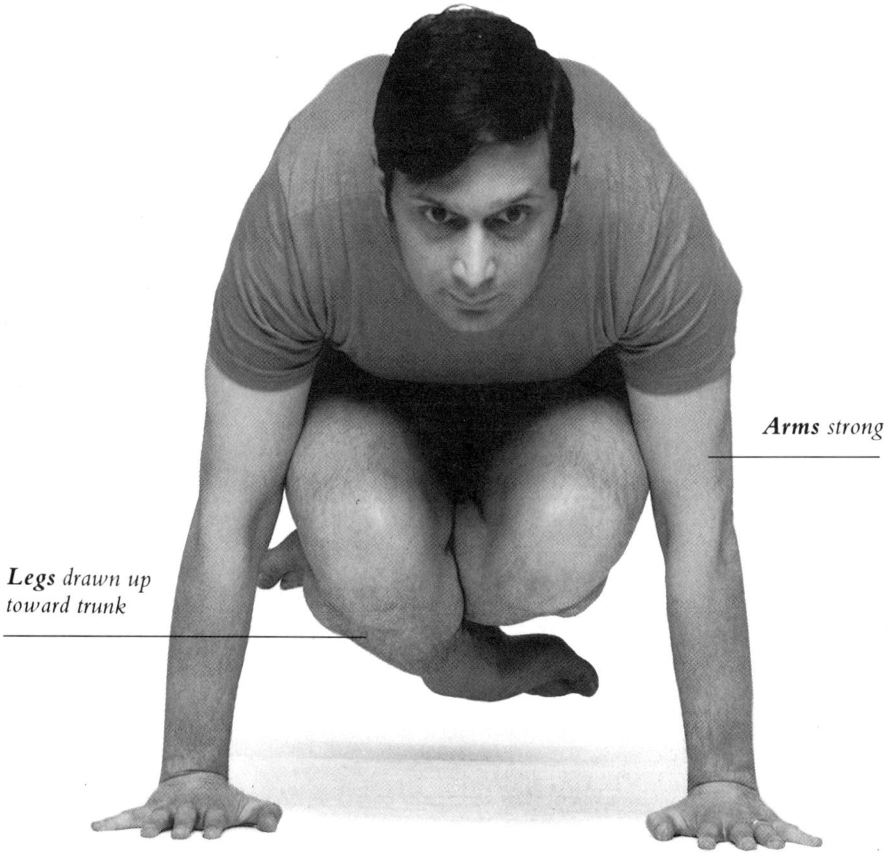
Arms *strong*
Legs *drawn up toward trunk*

एक हस्त भुजासन

Eka Hasta Bhujāsana

EKA = one; *HASTA* = hand; *BHUJA* = arm, trunk of an elephant

THE ARMS lift the heavy weight of the legs.♦♦♦

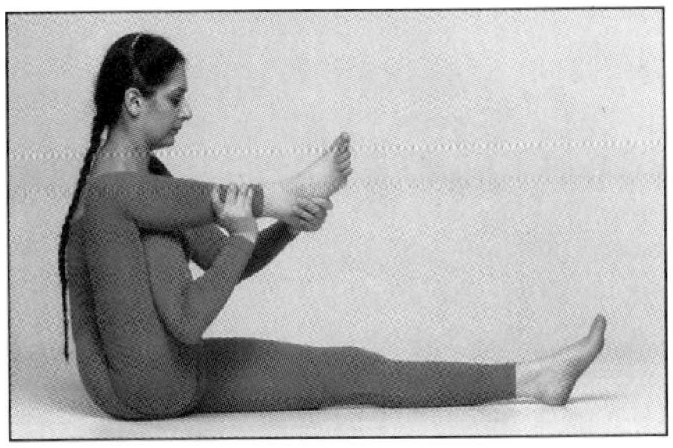

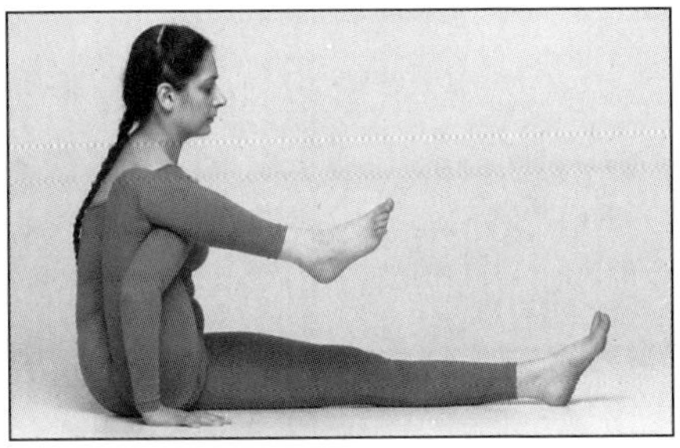

1 Sit in Daṇḍāsana (p. 52). ▷Keep the left leg straight. Bend the right leg and raise it over the right upper arm. Hold the foot with both hands, pull the leg back, and take it as high as possible up the arm.

2 Place the hands beside the hips, with the left arm straight and the right arm slightly bent. Press the right outer thigh toward the trunk so that the leg does not slip. Stretch the foot forward.

3 Press the palms down; exhale and raise the trunk and the left leg above the floor. Keep the leg straight, the kneecap locked, and the foot stretching.

Balance for 5 to 10 seconds, breathing evenly.

Exhale and come down. Take the right leg down.◁

Repeat from ▷to◁ on the left.

WAYS OF PRACTICING

Place the hands on bricks.

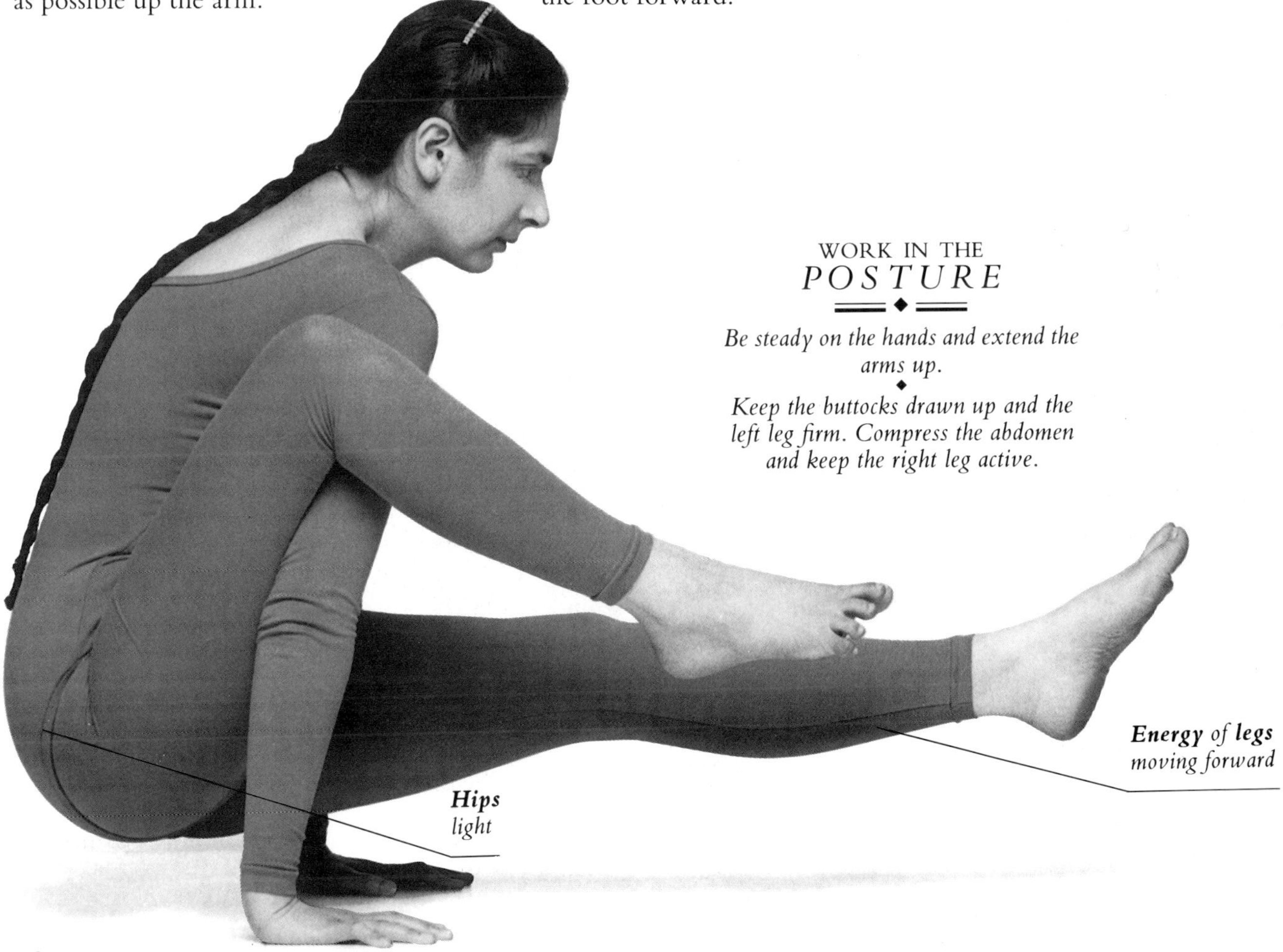
Hips *light*
Energy *of* **legs** *moving forward*

WORK IN THE
POSTURE

Be steady on the hands and extend the arms up.

Keep the buttocks drawn up and the left leg firm. Compress the abdomen and keep the right leg active.

वसिष्ठासन

Vasiṣṭhāsana

VASIṢṬHA = name of a sage

BALANCING on one hand and one leg requires strength and concentration.♦♦♦♦

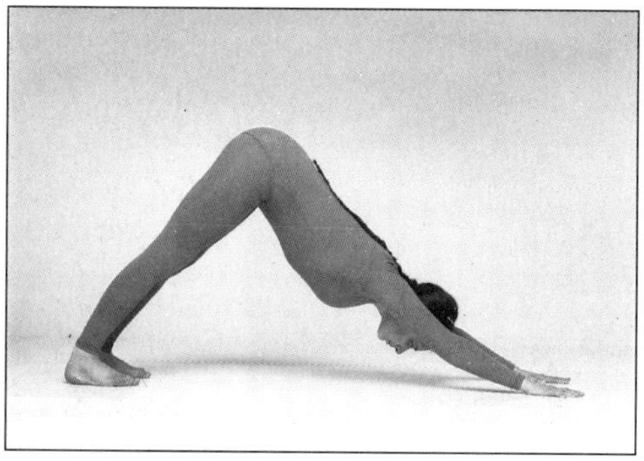

1 Be in Adho Mukha Śvānāsana (p. 90). ▷Put more weight on the left hand, making the right side light.

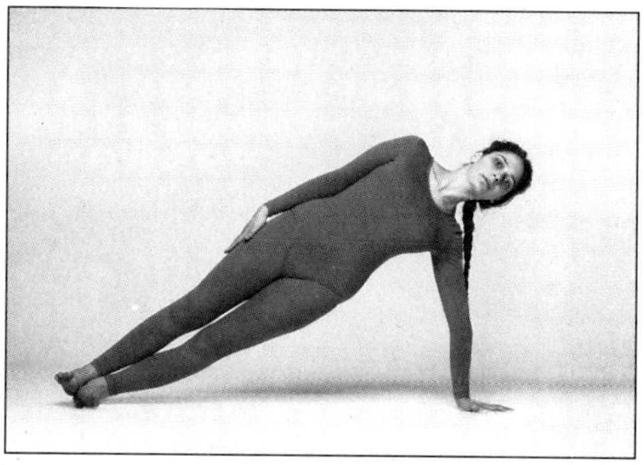

2 Turn the feet and trunk 90° to the right; place the right leg over the left, with the feet together. Keep the right side over the left, head in line with the sternum and slightly back. Rest the right arm along the right side.

Be firm on the left hand and stretch the arm up. Extend the trunk and lift the left hip. Straighten the knees.

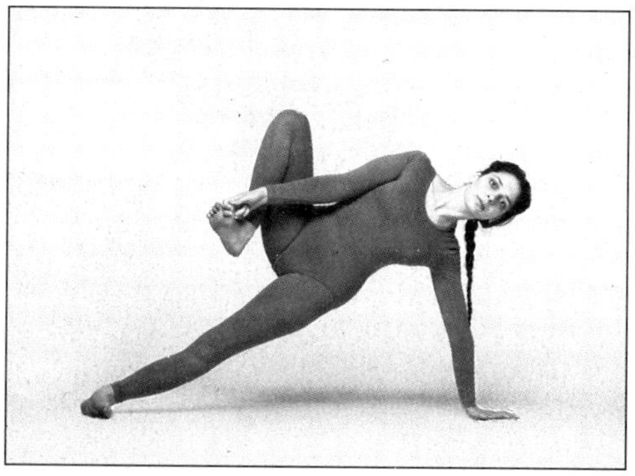

3 Bend the right leg, turning it outward in its socket, with the knee pointing up. Catch the big toe with the thumb, index, and middle fingers.

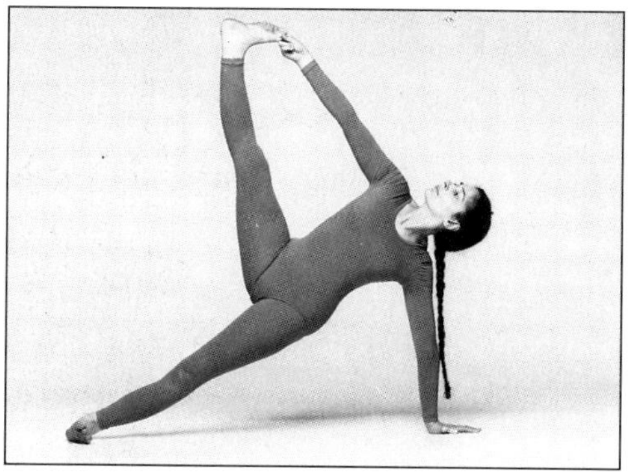

4 Straighten the right arm and leg and stretch them up. Turn the head and look up.

Balance for 10 to 15 seconds, breathing evenly.

Exhale, bring the right arm and leg down. Turn into Adho Mukha Śvānāsana.◁

Repeat from ▷to◁ on the other side. Then come down.

वसिष्ठासन

WORK IN THE
POSTURE

Keep the trunk and left leg in line. Do not let them drop downward.

Bring the hips, waist, and chest slightly forward.

Revolve the left arm outward and tuck in the shoulder blades.

Lift the right leg strongly from the buttock.

Ways of Practicing

Support the left foot against a wall.

Learn to balance in step 2, stretching the right arm vertically up.

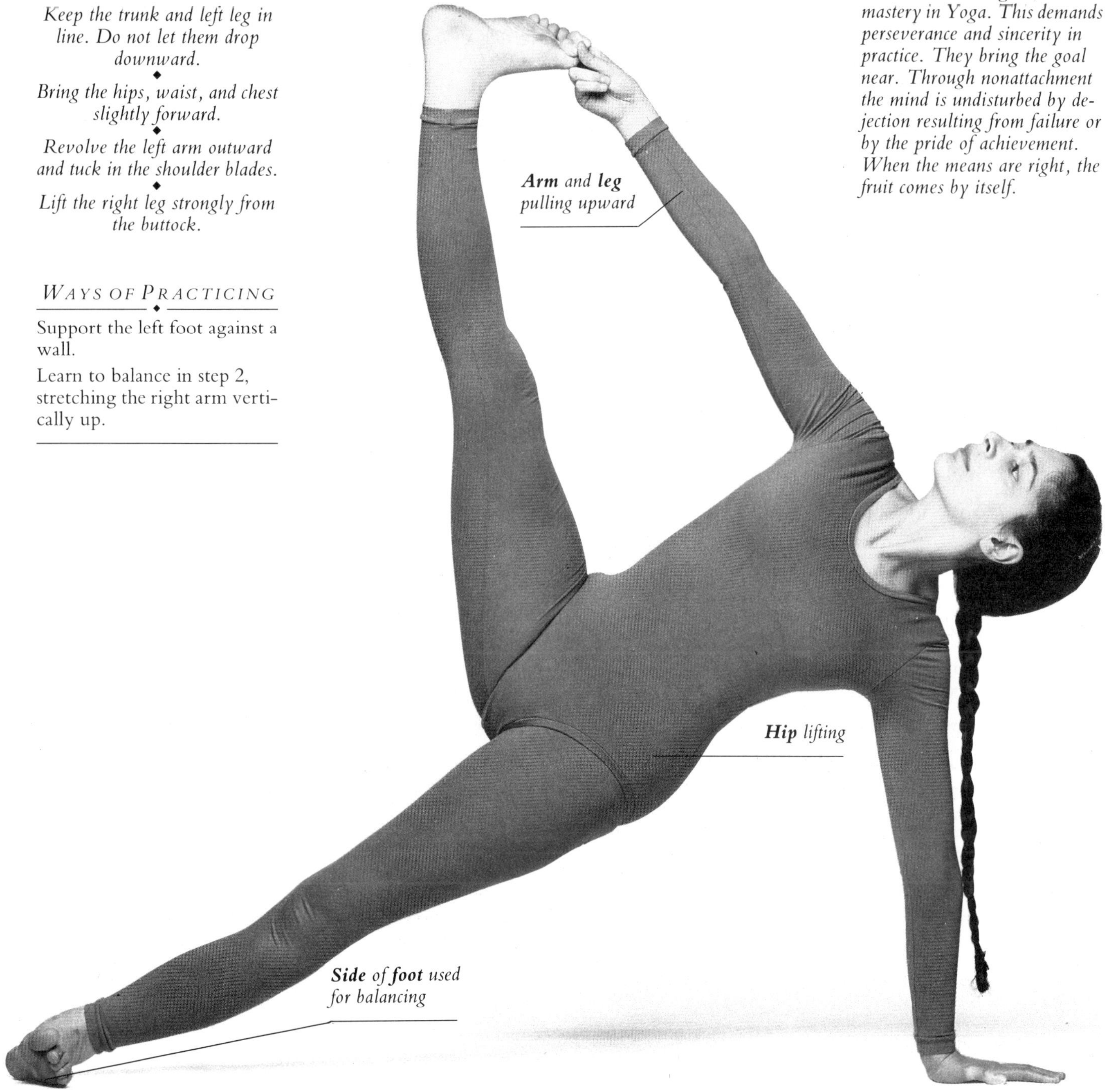
Arm *and* ***leg*** *pulling upward*
Hip *lifting*
Side *of* ***foot*** *used for balancing*

Reflection
Correct effort, without overattachment to the goal, leads to mastery in Yoga. This demands perseverance and sincerity in practice. They bring the goal near. Through nonattachment the mind is undisturbed by dejection resulting from failure or by the pride of achievement. When the means are right, the fruit comes by itself.

अष्टावक्रासन

Aṣṭāvakrāsana

AṢṬA = eight; *VAKRA* = bend; *AṢṬĀVAKRA* = name of a sage

THE BODY bends in eight places: the wrists, elbows, hips, and ankles.♦♦♦♦

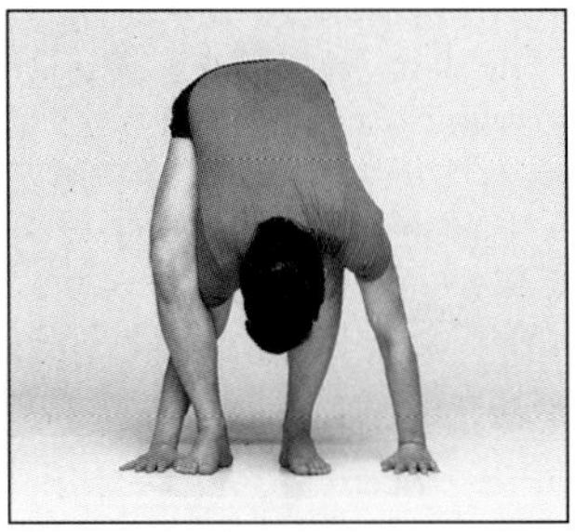

1 Stand in Tāḍāsana (p. 18) with the feet about 1ft apart. ▷ Bend down and place the right palm on the floor a few inches to the inside of the right foot, the left palm to the outside of the left foot. Bend the legs.

Take the right arm behind the right knee and place the hand by the outer edge of the right foot.

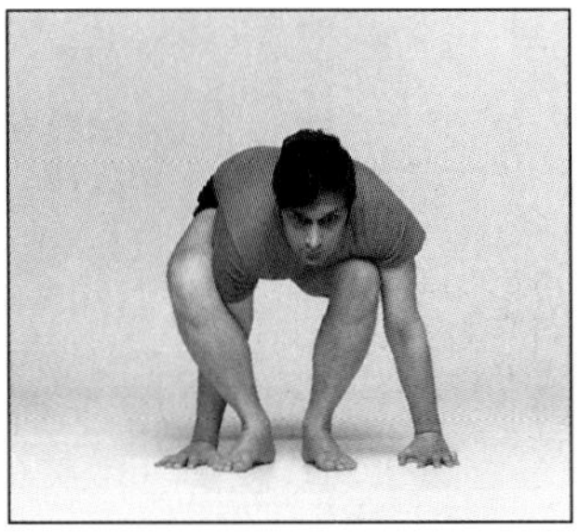

2 Bend the knees more. Take the right thigh as high as possible on the right upper arm. Transfer the body weight onto the hands. Make the feet light.

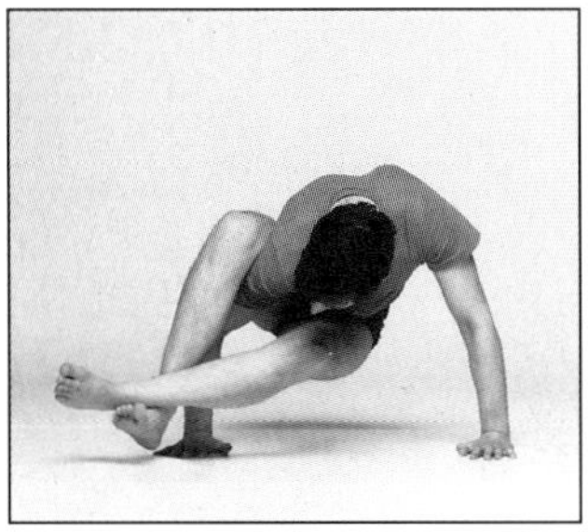

3 Move the feet forward. Cross the left ankle over the right and move the feet to the right. Make the body light.

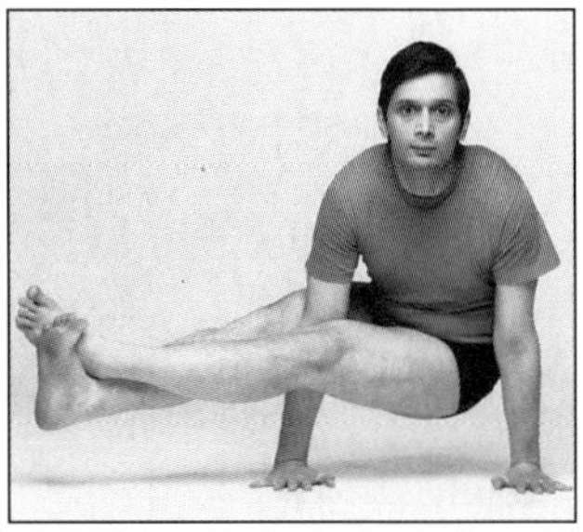

4 Exhale; raise and stretch the legs to the right, straightening the knees. Lift the chest and look up.

Stay for 5 to 10 seconds. Come down or continue to the next step.

WORK IN THE
POSTURE

Make the hands active (see Focus, p. 124). Make the arms strong to keep the body low. Extend the trunk forward. Do not hunch the shoulders or compress the neck.

♦

Stretch the legs strongly. Squeeze the arm with the legs.

5 Bend the arms outward, and take the head and trunk down until they are almost horizontal. Balance for a few seconds, breathing evenly.

Inhale, raise the trunk, and straighten the arms. Uncross the feet, bring them down and stand up. ◁

Repeat from ▷ to ◁ on the left.

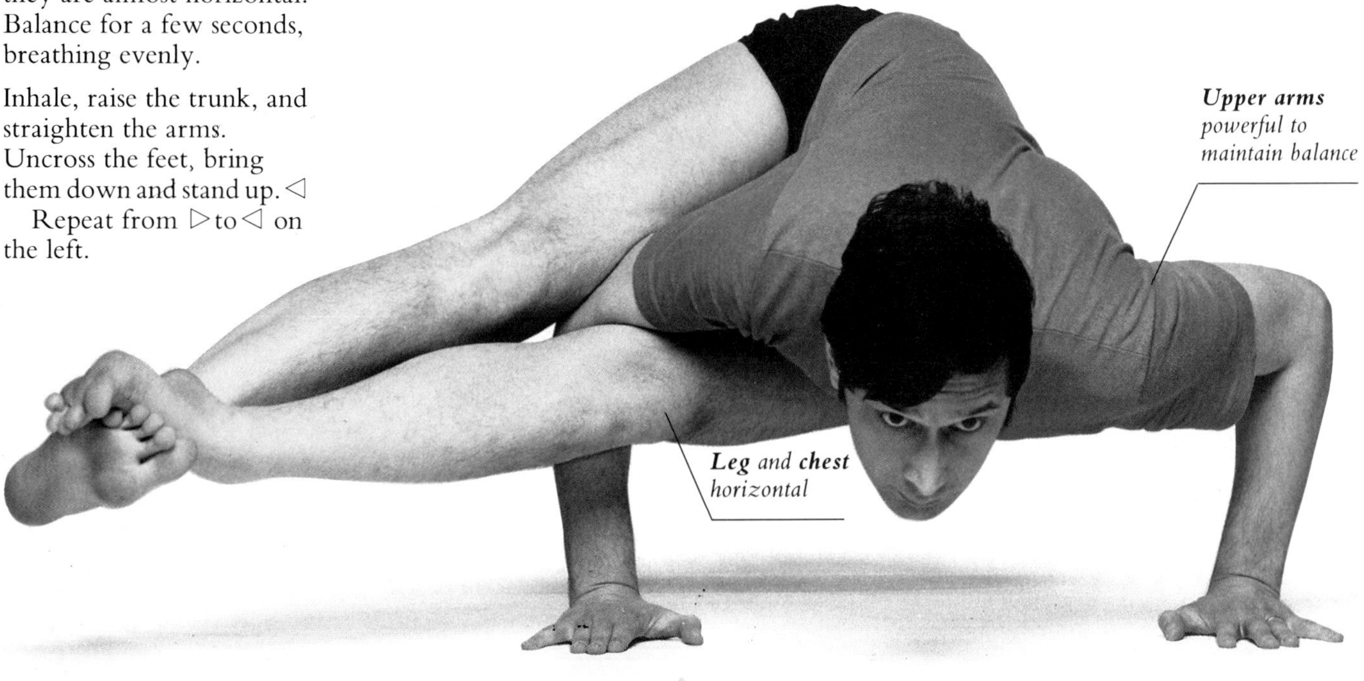
Upper arms *powerful to maintain balance*
Leg *and* **chest** *horizontal*

भुजपीडासन

Bhujapīḍāsana

BHUJA = arm; *PĪḌA* = pressure

THE LEGS press the arms to lift the trunk up. ♦♦♦

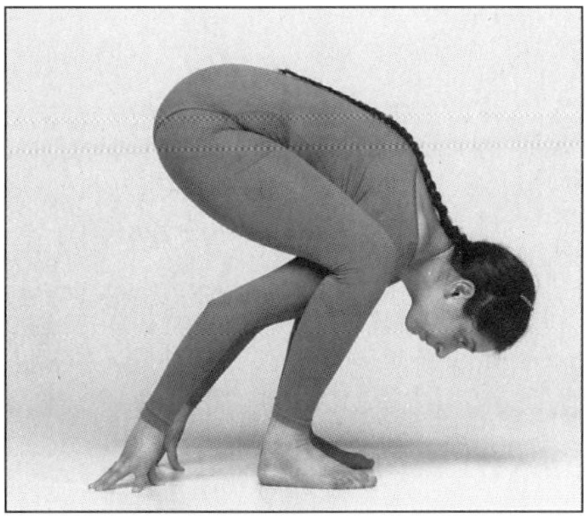

1 Stand in Tāḍāsana (p. 18) with the feet about 1 ft apart. ▷ Bend down and bend the legs. Stretch the arms back between the legs.

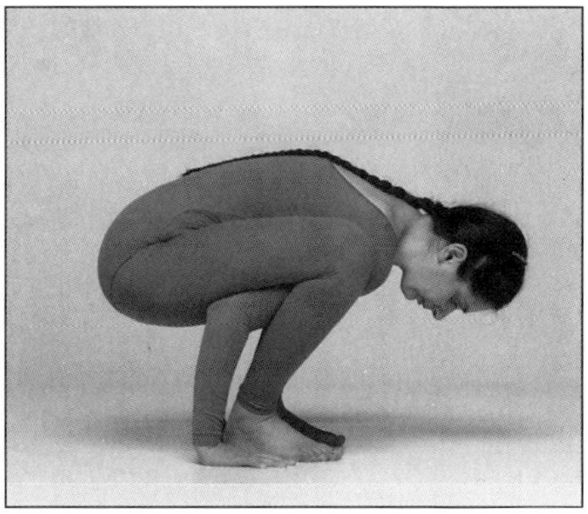

2 Place the palms outside the feet. Rest the backs of the thighs as high as possible on the upper arms. Lean forward; bring the body weight onto the hands and make the feet light.

3 Cross the left foot over the right. Move the feet forward a little. Exhale, press the palms into the floor, and raise the feet. Contract the abdomen and lift the trunk. Straighten the arms. Balance for 5 to 10 seconds and breathe evenly, keeping the chest and head up.

Exhale, uncross the feet, and stand up. ◁

Repeat from ▷ to ◁ with the legs crossed the other way.

WAYS OF PRACTICING

Place the hands on bricks.

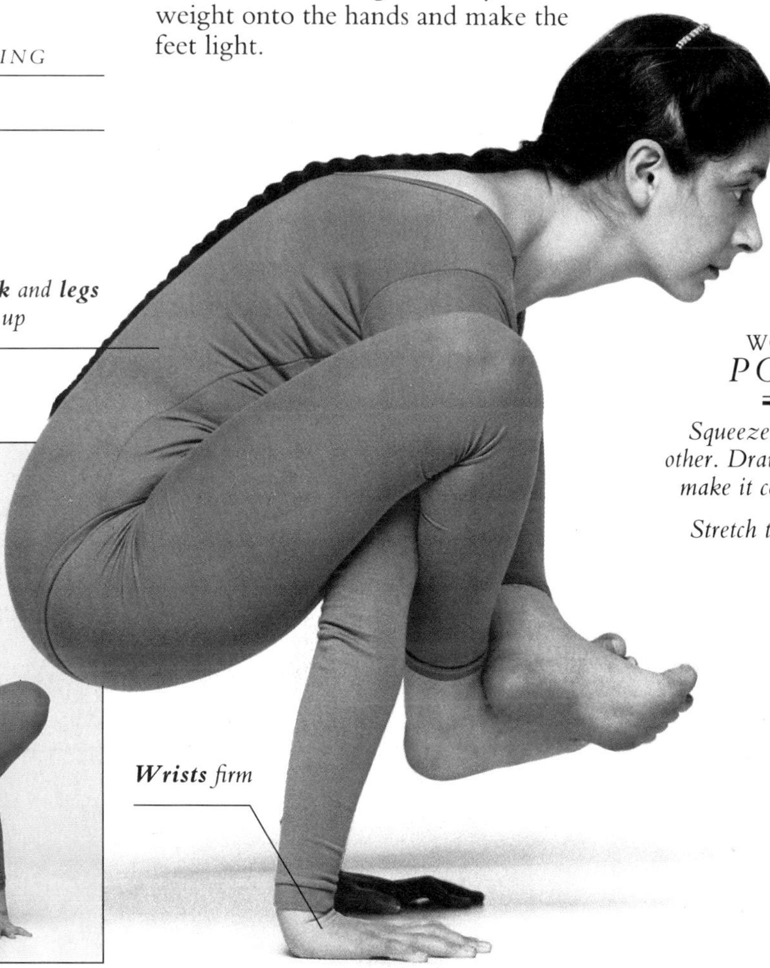

***Trunk** and **legs** rising up*

***Wrists** firm*

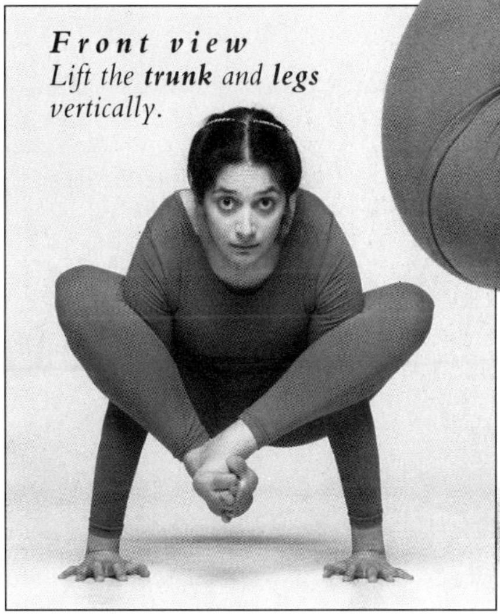

Front view

*Lift the **trunk** and **legs** vertically.*

WORK IN THE POSTURE

Squeeze the legs toward each other. Draw the whole body up to make it compact. Keep it light.

Stretch the arms and lock the elbows.

बकासन

Bakāsana

BAKA = a crane

THIS POSTURE imitates the shape of a bird. The arms become like legs to support the body. ♦♦♦

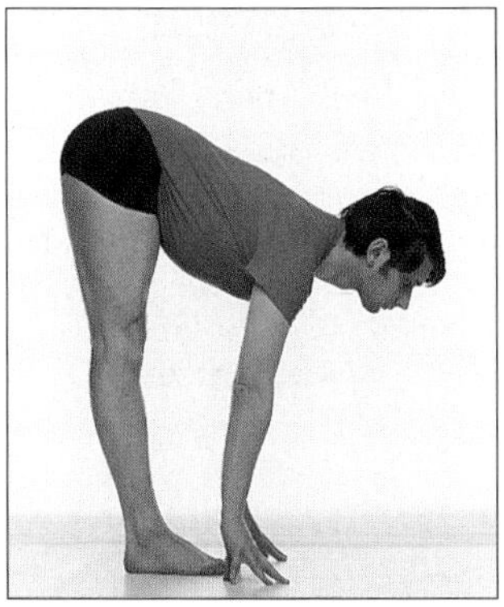

1 Stand in Tāḍāsana (p. 18), feet together. Bend down and place the hands in front of the feet.

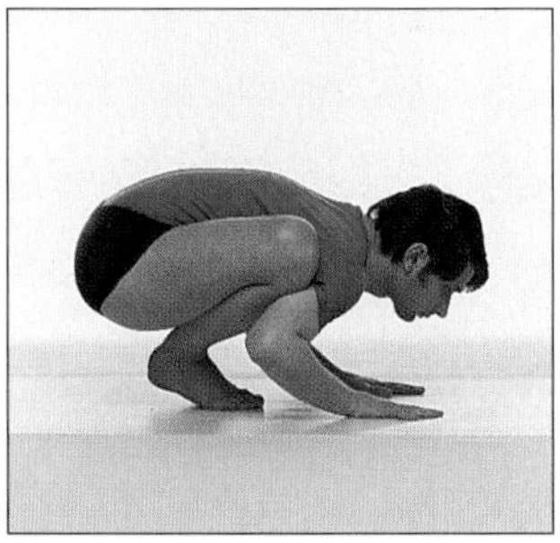

2 Bend the knees and elbows to the sides. Lean forward and take the head and chest down. Place the upper arms under the knees, keeping the palms down. Kneel with the tops of the shins on the upper arms near the armpits, feet together and on tiptoe.

WAYS OF PRACTICING

Place the hands on bricks.

Learn to balance and be light before straightening the arms.

3 Make the feet light and raise them toward the buttocks. If necessary, take them up one at a time. Pause for a moment to steady the balance.

Straighten the arms and raise the trunk and legs as high as possible. Keep the head up. Balance, breathing evenly, for 10 to 15 seconds.

With an exhalation bend the elbows to the sides and come down.

Focus *Raising the legs*
To raise the bent legs, lift the feet, compress the shins toward the thighs and the thighs toward the trunk. Once up, keep the shins and thighs close together, as if they were one limb.

WORK IN THE
POSTURE

Keep the feet lifted. Do not let the legs slip down, but compress them toward the buttocks.

Keep the back rounded and contract the abdominal muscles.

Go on stretching the upper arms.

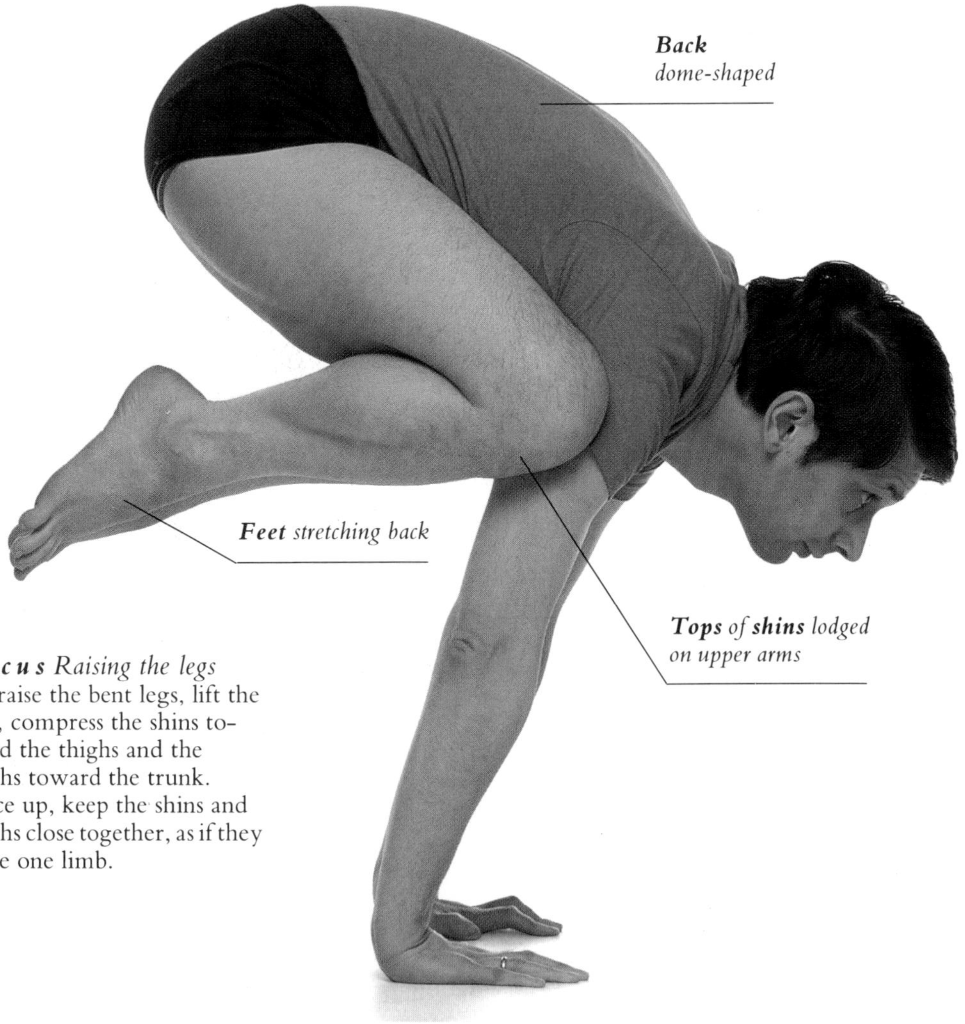
Back *dome-shaped*
Feet *stretching back*
Tops *of* **shins** *lodged on upper arms*

बकासन

Bakāsana from Śīrṣāsana

THE ARMS and shoulders develop strength and mobility.♦♦♦♦

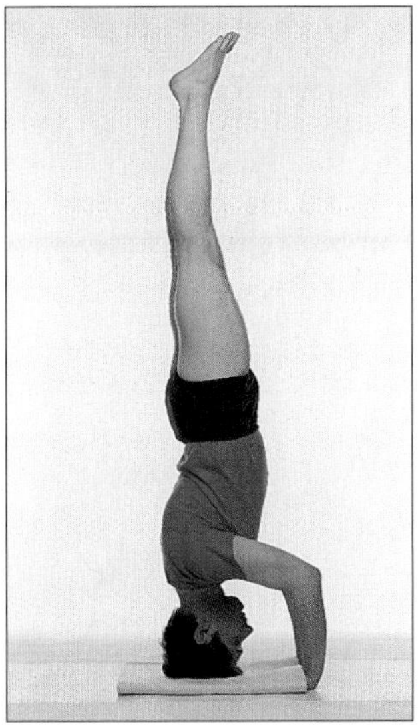

1 Be in Śīrṣāsana II (p. 107).

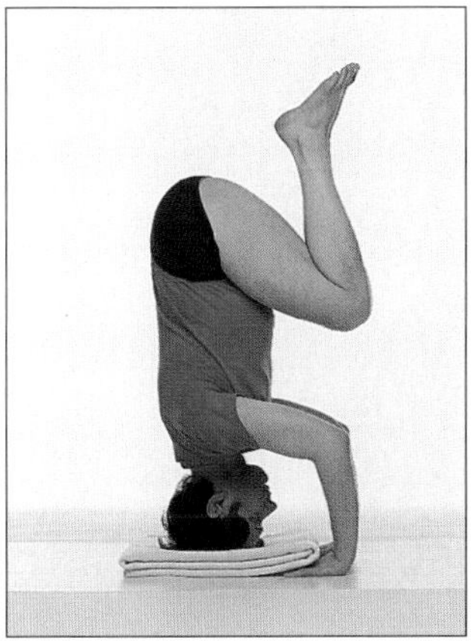

2 Keeping the shoulders lifted and the elbows in, bend the legs toward the abdomen.

WAYS OF PRACTICING

To make it easier to lift, place the head on two or three blankets.

If the neck gets compressed, do Ūrdhva Dhanurāsana (p. 138).

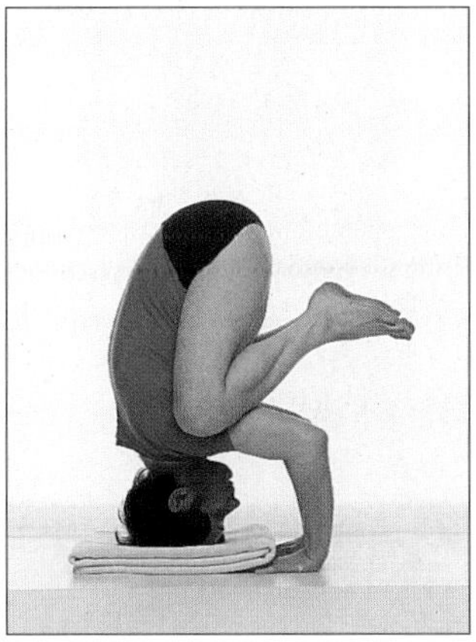

3 Exhale and bring the shins onto the upper arms. Take the knees as high up the arms as possible. Keep the feet lifted. Balance for a moment.

4 Inhale, raise the head and shoulders; start straightening the elbows. Keep the legs pulled up.

Stabilize in this position, so that the legs do not slip down. Bring the outer elbows firmly in and stretch the arms until they are straight, and the trunk is high up.

Exhale, bend the arms, extend the neck down, and place the head on the floor. Raise the legs into Śīrṣāsana II. Come down.

WORK IN THE POSTURE

As for Bakāsana (opposite).

To raise the head, lift the shoulders strongly, and pull the trapezius muscles and shoulder blades toward the waist. Simultaneously stretch the upper arms up.

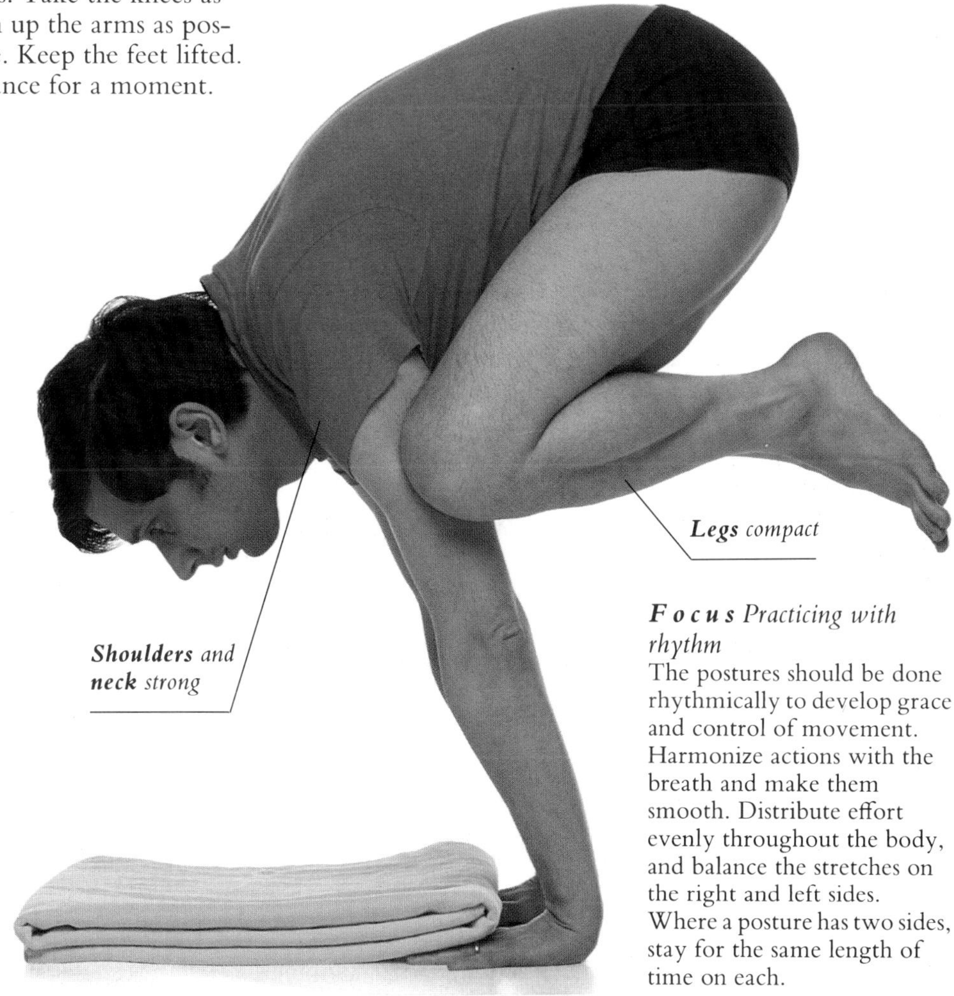
Legs compact
Shoulders and **neck** strong

Focus *Practicing with rhythm*
The postures should be done rhythmically to develop grace and control of movement. Harmonize actions with the breath and make them smooth. Distribute effort evenly throughout the body, and balance the stretches on the right and left sides. Where a posture has two sides, stay for the same length of time on each.

पार्श्व बकासन

Pārśva Bakāsana

PĀRŚVA = sideways; *BAKA* = a crane

THE GRIP on the abdomen keeps the body turned and balanced.♦♦♦♦

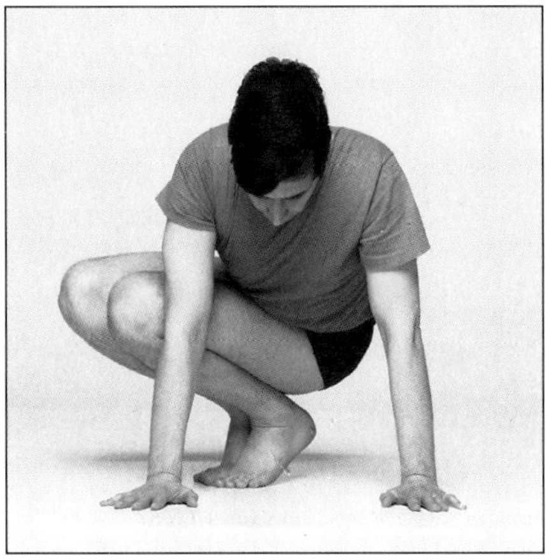

1 Stand in Tāḍāsana (p. 18). ▷Bend down and bend the legs. Place the hands in front of the feet, slightly apart.

Raise the heels and turn the legs and hips almost 90° to the right, with the thighs close to the right upper arm. Keep the head and chest and the hands facing forward.

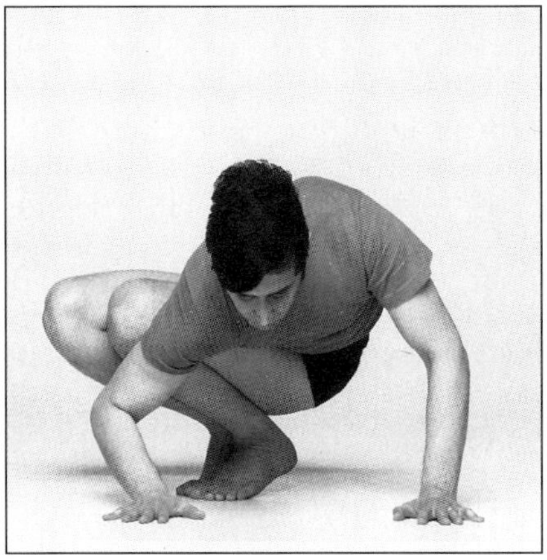

2 Bend the elbows, move the abdomen strongly to the left, and kneel on the right upper arm with both legs. Take the legs as high as possible toward the shoulder. Bring the weight onto the hands.

3 Exhale and lift the feet off the floor, compressing the bent legs. Raise the hips and the trunk. Stretch the arms from the wrists up. The right arm remains slightly bent to support the legs. Balance for 5 to 10 seconds, breathing evenly.

Exhale, release the legs, and turn to the front. Stand up.◁

Repeat from ▷to◁ on the left.

WAYS OF PRACTICING

This posture can also be done from Śīrṣāsana II (p. 107), like the preceding one.

WORK IN THE POSTURE

Keep the left arm strong as a counterbalance to the weight on the right arm.

Turn the trunk more. Contract the abdomen and squeeze it further to the left, while taking the legs to the right.

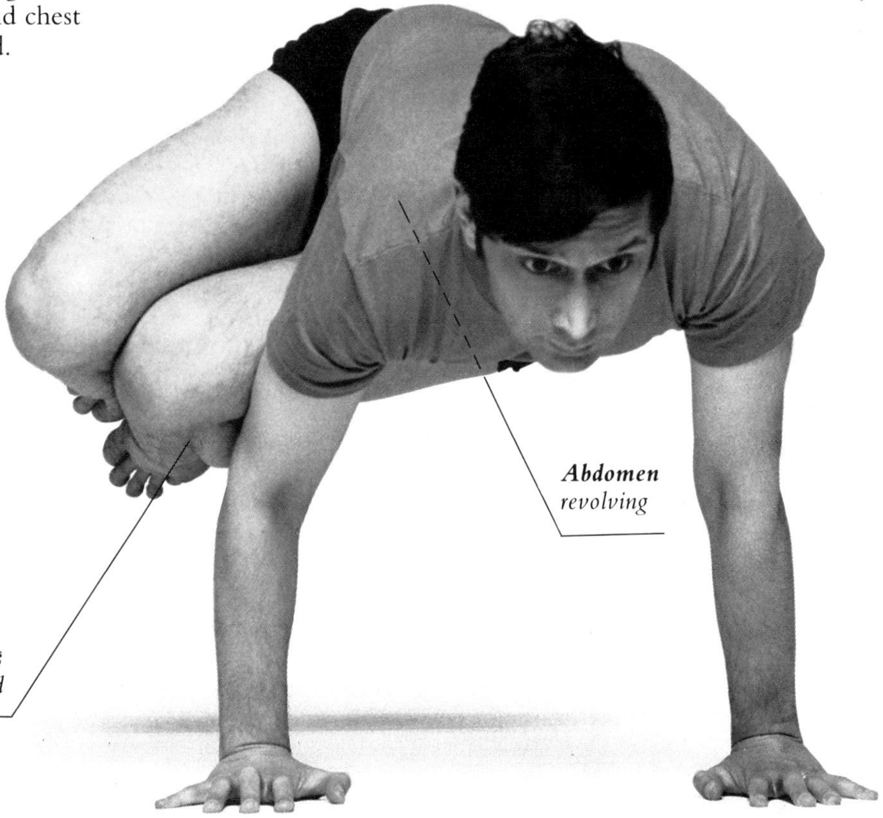
Abdomen *revolving*
Feet *and* **legs** *tucked upward*

BACKBENDS

When the āsana is correct there is a lightness, a freedom. Freedom comes when every part of the body is active. Let us be free in whatever posture we are doing. Let us be full in whatever we do.

B. K. S. IYENGAR

Backbends are rejuvenating. They give energy and courage, and combat depression. They open the chest and make the spine flexible. The arms and shoulders become strong. The mind and body become alert.

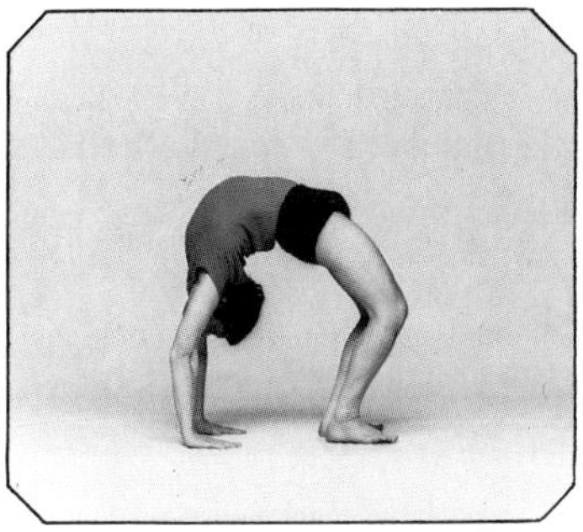

GUIDELINES FOR PRACTICE

It is best to work on a non-slip surface.

Backbends are strenuous and should be started gradually. The instructions given are for the final postures. Beginners and those who are stiff should not force themselves beyond their capacity but should work on Uṣṭrāsana (p. 134) and Viparīta Daṇḍāsana on a chair (pp. 136–7). The body should be toned by practicing these backbends before any of the others are attempted.

Ūrdhva Dhanurāsana (p. 138) is an important posture. The more advanced backbends should be attempted only when this has been completely mastered.

For maximum effect the postures should be repeated at least two or three times. This will ease the back, enabling it to bend more, and will improve the postures generally.

Those who are supple should be careful to develop an even extension along the front and back of the body. Overbending in one part, e.g. the lumbar, will cause injury. Both sides of the trunk must curve evenly.

A feeling of nausea may possibly occur during backbend practice. This is caused by the liver being extended, but it is not dangerous. Headaches can occur if the breath is held inadvertently. Dizziness caused by going up and down is eased by bending forward afterward.

The back should not be strained. If it is sore after backbends, care should be taken to avoid pinching in the lumbar. When practicing, the sacrum and coccyx should move away from the lumbar (see Focus, p. 93).

After backbends the spine should be carefully released. This may be done by twists, especially Marīcyāsana III (p. 73) and Ardha Matsyendrāsana (pp. 74–5), or nonstrenuous forward bends, particularly Janu Śīrṣāsana (p. 59). Here the spine should be released gradually and not stretched by force.

CAUTIONS: Do not do backbends if suffering from heart trouble, high blood pressure, or other serious illnesses, nor during menstruation or in pregnancy.

If suffering from a bad back or injured knees, do backbends only under supervision.

उष्ट्रासन

Uṣṭrāsana

UṢṬRA = camel

THIS SIMPLE backbend makes the shoulders mobile and opens the chest.♦♦

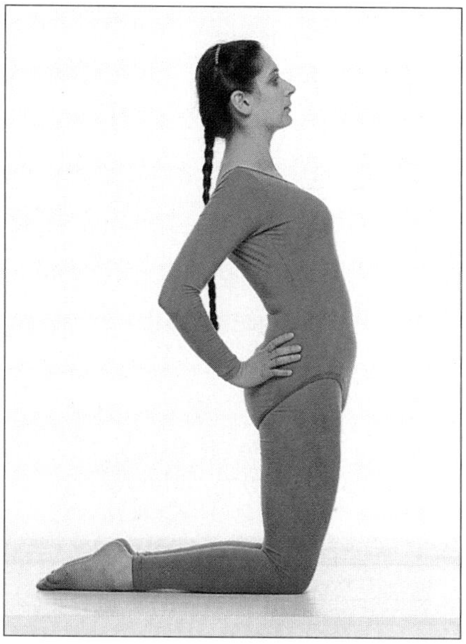

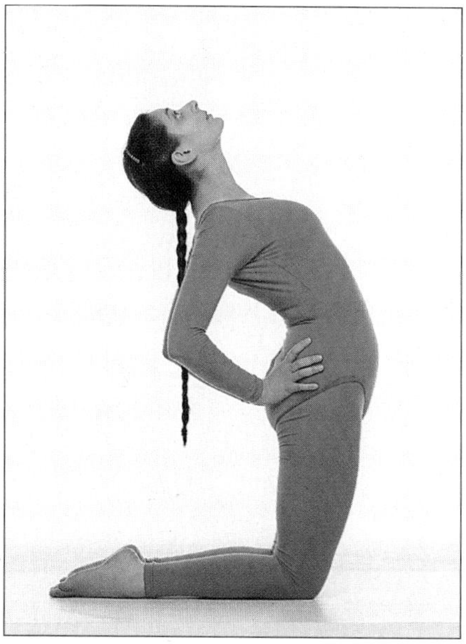

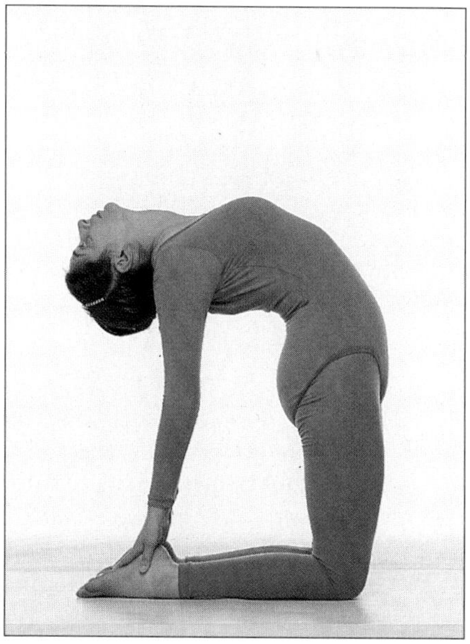

1 Kneel with the thighs perpendicular, knees and feet together, and trunk upright. Keep the knees in line, both sides of the body parallel. Place the hands on the hips. Contract the buttocks and stretch the hips and the trunk up.

Reflection
Knowing the line and detail of the postures is necessary for practicing. It means understanding precisely in what direction and to what degree to move, turn, or stretch, and which part of the body to keep stable. It also means recognizing whether an action is correct or incorrect, and whether or not there is strain. Proper understanding leads to progress in Yoga.

2 Move the tops of the thighs and the hips forward. Exhale and arch back: bring the coccyx, sacrum, and lumbar forward, curve the thoracic spine and take the shoulder blades in, keeping the shoulders back. Stretch the abdomen toward the rib cage and take the sternum and collarbones back. Extend the neck, without straining it.

3 Release the hands, stretch the arms down, and hold the heels, with the palms on the soles and the fingers pointing to the toes. Take the head back and look back.

Stay, increasing the curve of the trunk, for 15 to 20 seconds. Do not hold the breath.

Inhale, release the hands, and come up, using the buttock muscles to lift the pelvis.

उष्ट्रासन

Focus *Beginning backbends*
In backbends the muscles of the back should be soft and the spine should be trained gradually to bend. To do this, be fully aware of the body in the postures and follow all movements mentally. Pay more attention to stiff areas in order not to overwork the supple parts. Do not hold the muscles hard as this prevents movement and may cause injury. Learn to develop a sense of even extension.

WORK IN THE POSTURE

Press the shins down and stretch the feet back.

Turn the arms outward in their sockets and lock the elbows.

Press the lower back firmly forward and the back ribs up. Extend the front of the body over the arch of the back.

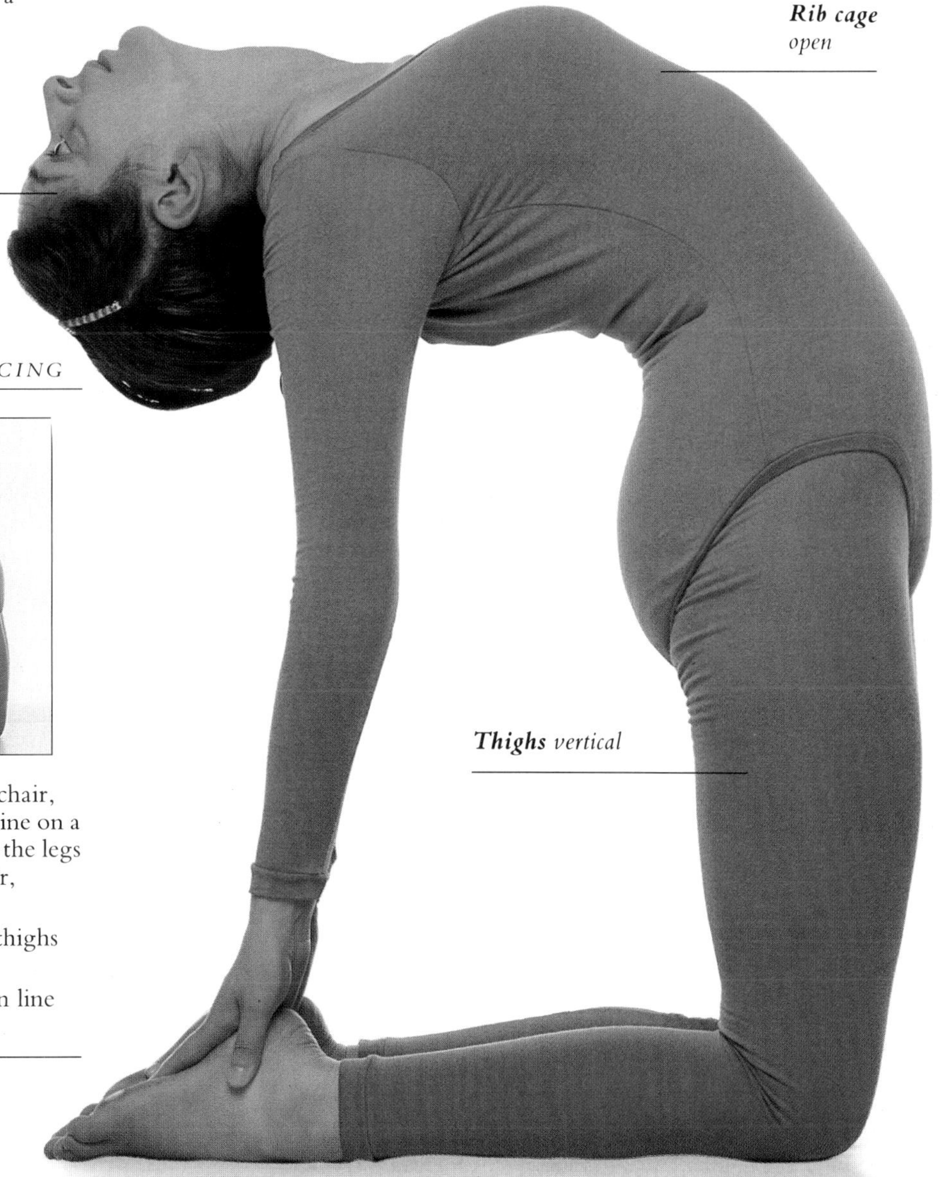
Rib cage *open*
Head *and* **neck** *curving back*
Thighs *vertical*

Ways of Practicing

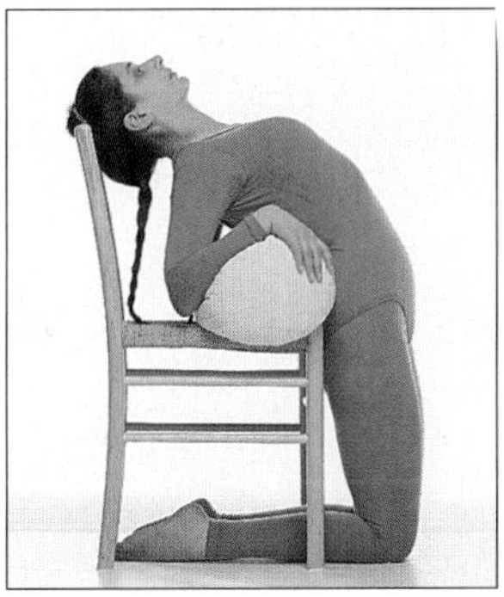

Curve backward onto a chair, supporting the lumbar spine on a bolster or blankets. Place the legs inside or outside the chair, according to its width.

Use a wall, pressing the thighs and pubis toward it.

Keep the legs 1ft apart, in line with the hips.

विपरीत दंडासन

Viparīta Daṇḍāsana (on chair)

VIPARĪTA = inverted; *DAṆḌA* = staff, stick

THE BACK can relax as it arches over a chair. ♦♦

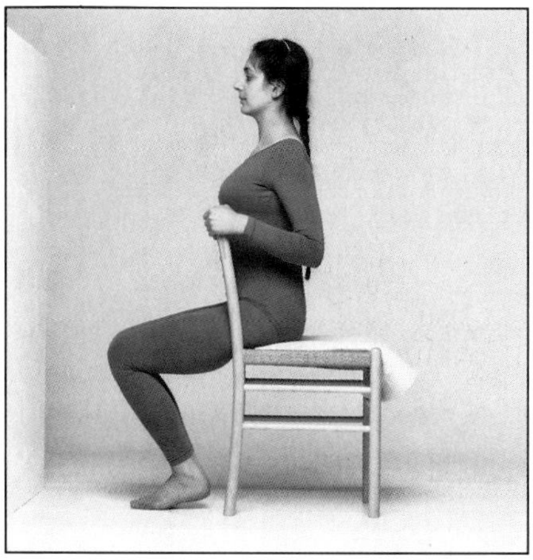

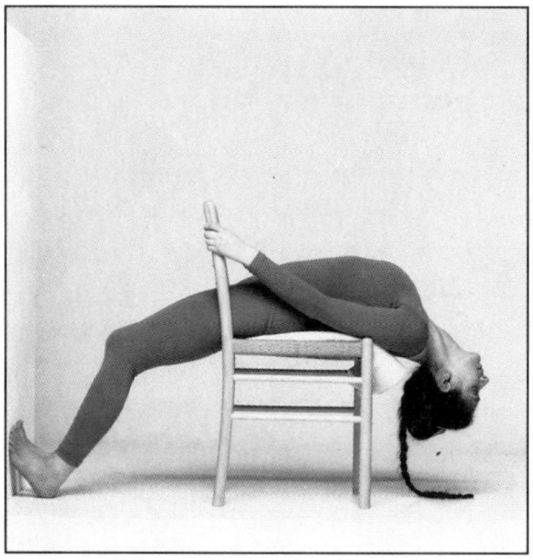

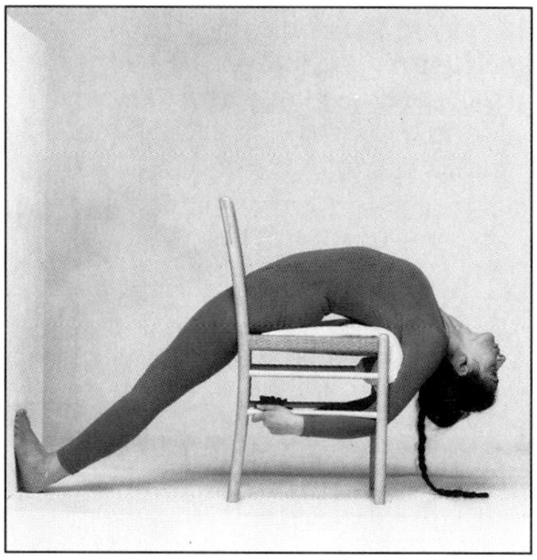

1 Place a sturdy chair (see Focus, p. 118) 2 to $2\frac{1}{2}$ft away from a wall, backing onto it. Put a folded blanket over the front edge of the seat.

Take the legs one at a time through the back of the chair and bring the hips forward so that the bottom of the sacrum rests on the back edge of the chair. Hold the sides of the chairback.

Reflection

Supported āsanas are restful and tone the body with minimum effort. They should not be underestimated as they have a powerful physiological effect. They nourish the nervous system and increase the efficiency of the glandular system, which is essential for physical and mental health. The inner organs stay for some time in positions where they are extended or massaged. Hidden parts of the body and cells are activated. No one can afford to neglect these tremendously beneficial postures.

2 Making the back concave, exhale, lean back, and go down until the back ribs curve over the seat of the chair, just below the shoulder blades. Place the toes 3 to 4in up the wall, the heels on the floor. Keep the legs slightly bent.

WAYS OF PRACTICING

If there is pain in the lumbar spine, place a rolled or folded blanket under it.

If the neck compresses, support the head on a bolster or blankets. This is relaxing.

3 Take the arms between the legs of the chair and hold the back legs or side bars. Straighten the legs by pressing the knees down. Extend the trunk from the groin to the shoulders. Take the head back, extending the chin toward the floor. Gaze back evenly.

Stay for 30 to 60 seconds, breathing evenly, or continue to the next step. Do not strain the back or the neck.

***Legs** firm*

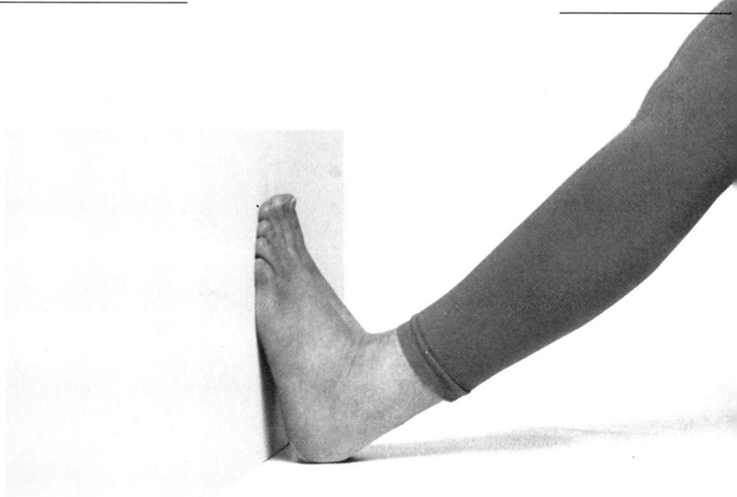

विपरीत दंडासन

4 Keeping the legs firm, take the arms over the head. Stretch them down toward the floor. Do not slide off the chair. Stay for 30 to 60 seconds.

Coming out of the posture
Hold the back of the chair and bend the legs. Carefully come up, lifting the chest. For a few moments lean over the back of the chair. (This will remove any strain in the back.) Come out of the chair.

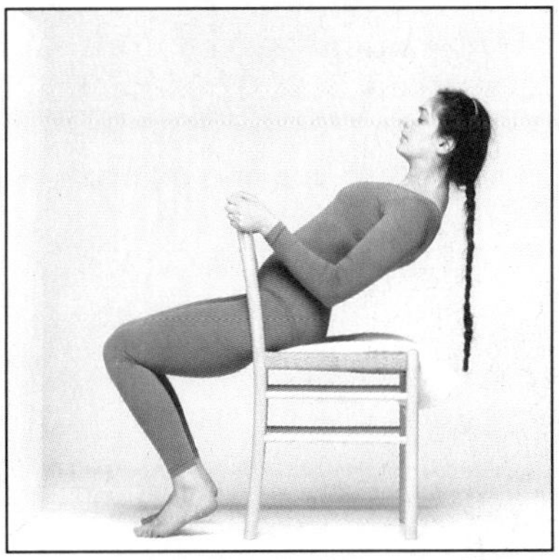

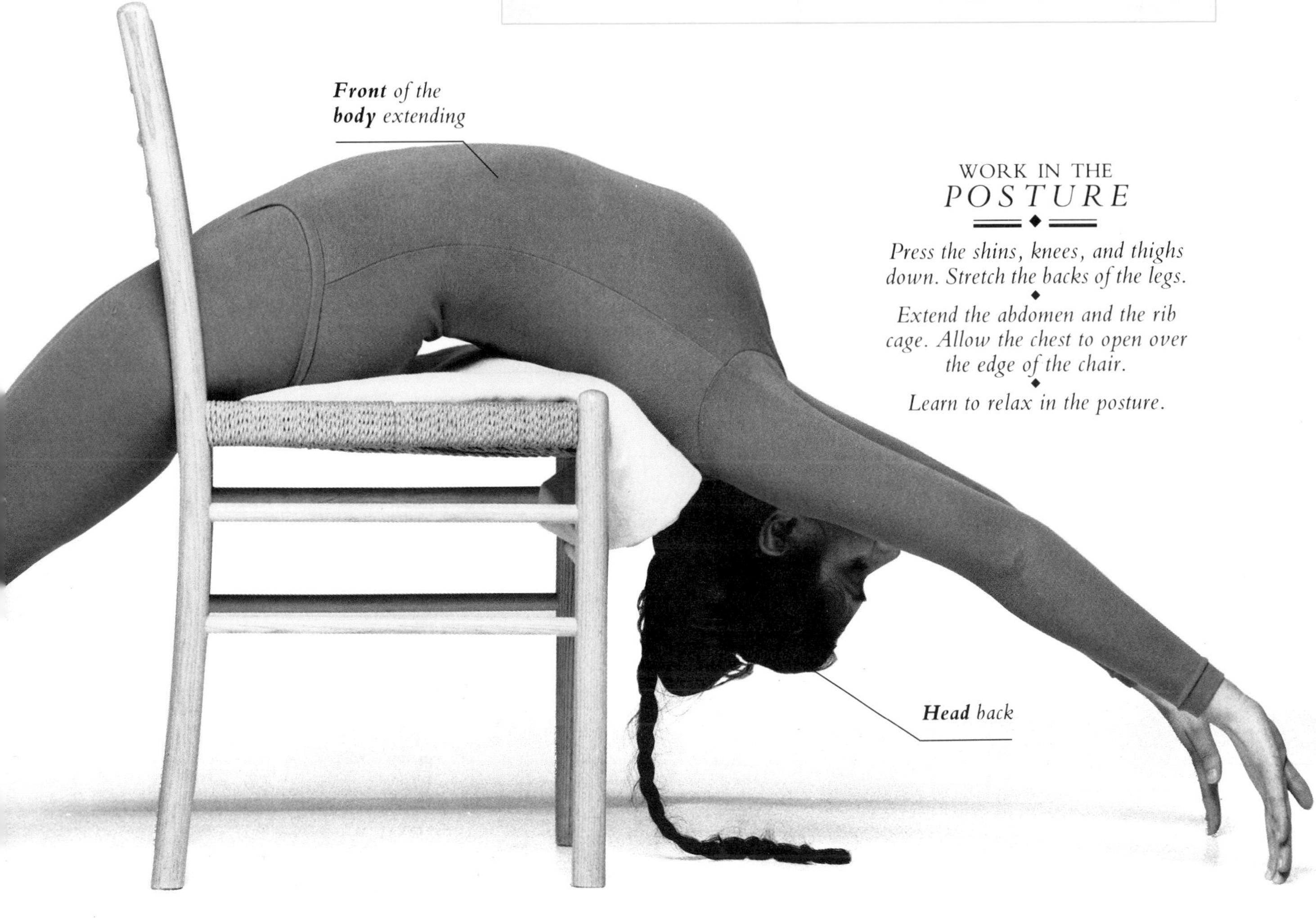

WORK IN THE
POSTURE

Press the shins, knees, and thighs down. Stretch the backs of the legs.

Extend the abdomen and the rib cage. Allow the chest to open over the edge of the chair.

Learn to relax in the posture.

ऊर्ध्व धनुरासन

Ūrdhva Dhanurāsana

ŪRDHVA = upward; *DHANURA* = a bow

THE ARCH of the body rises against the resistance of the arms and legs.♦♦

1 Lie on the floor in a straight line. Bend the elbows and take the arms over the head. Place the hands under the shoulders, fingers spread and pointing toward the feet. Bend the legs and place the feet close to the buttocks, a hip's-width apart.

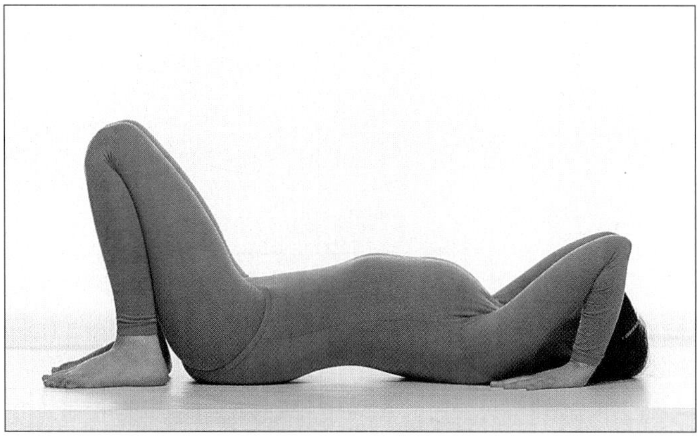

2 With an exhalation raise the chest and hips, take the head back, and place the crown of the head on the floor. Check that the hands are in line. Lift the shoulders and sacrum.

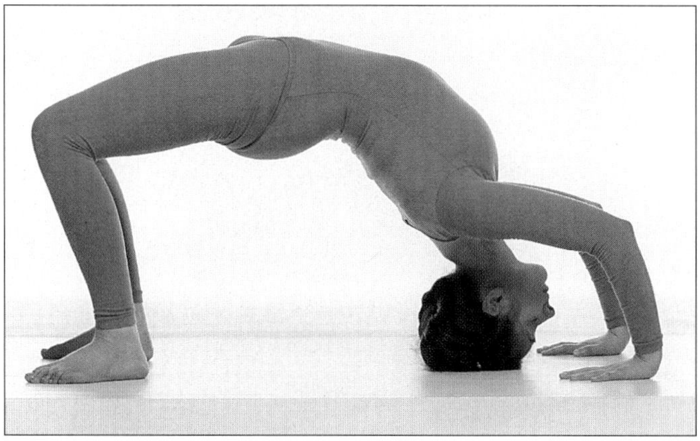

3 Press the hands and feet into the floor and raise the head and trunk. Straighten the arms and stretch the legs up.

Raise the heels and walk the feet in. Bring the chest and upper arms forward. Lift the hips and buttocks. Raise the coccyx, sacrum, and lumbar and move them away from the waist. Pull up the thigh muscles.

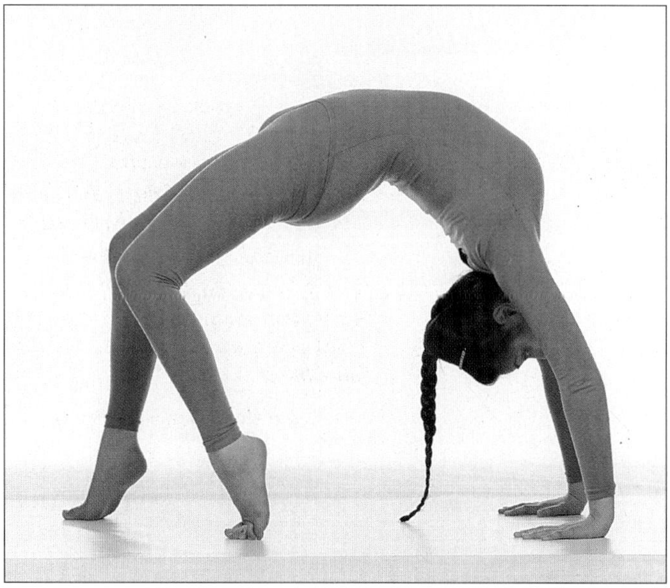

ऊर्ध्व धनुरासन

4 Keeping the height of the coccyx and sacrum, take the heels down. In going down, roll the outer thighs in (see Focus). Move the shoulder blades and back ribs in. Stretch the arms and legs to the maximum. Take the head back, keeping the throat relaxed.

Stay for 10 to 15 seconds or longer, breathing evenly.

Exhale and carefully come down.

Focus *Centering the legs*
In backbends the legs tend to turn outward. This narrows the sacroiliac joint, causing pain. To avoid this, revolve the thighs, knees, and shins inward. Gradually, when freedom of movement comes, center the feet.

Ways of Practicing

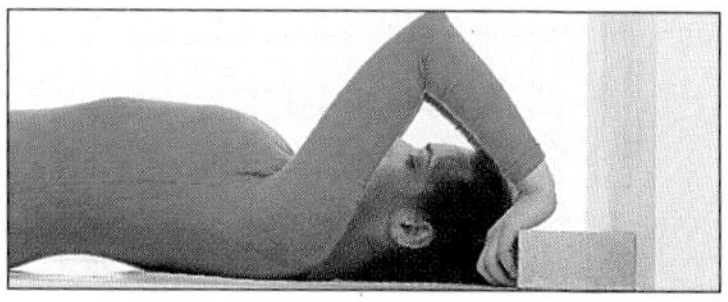

Place the hands on bricks as shown.

To support the arms and keep them in place, tie the upper arms together with a belt, just above the elbows.

To help the lower trunk to lift more, place the feet on two bricks or on a low stool.

Reflection
In normal life the spine degenerates with age. The body becomes shorter and lacks vitality. Bending backward counteracts this process. The spine remains long and pliable and the inner organs open and stretch. The brain is energized through being inverted. The mind remains alert and cheerful.

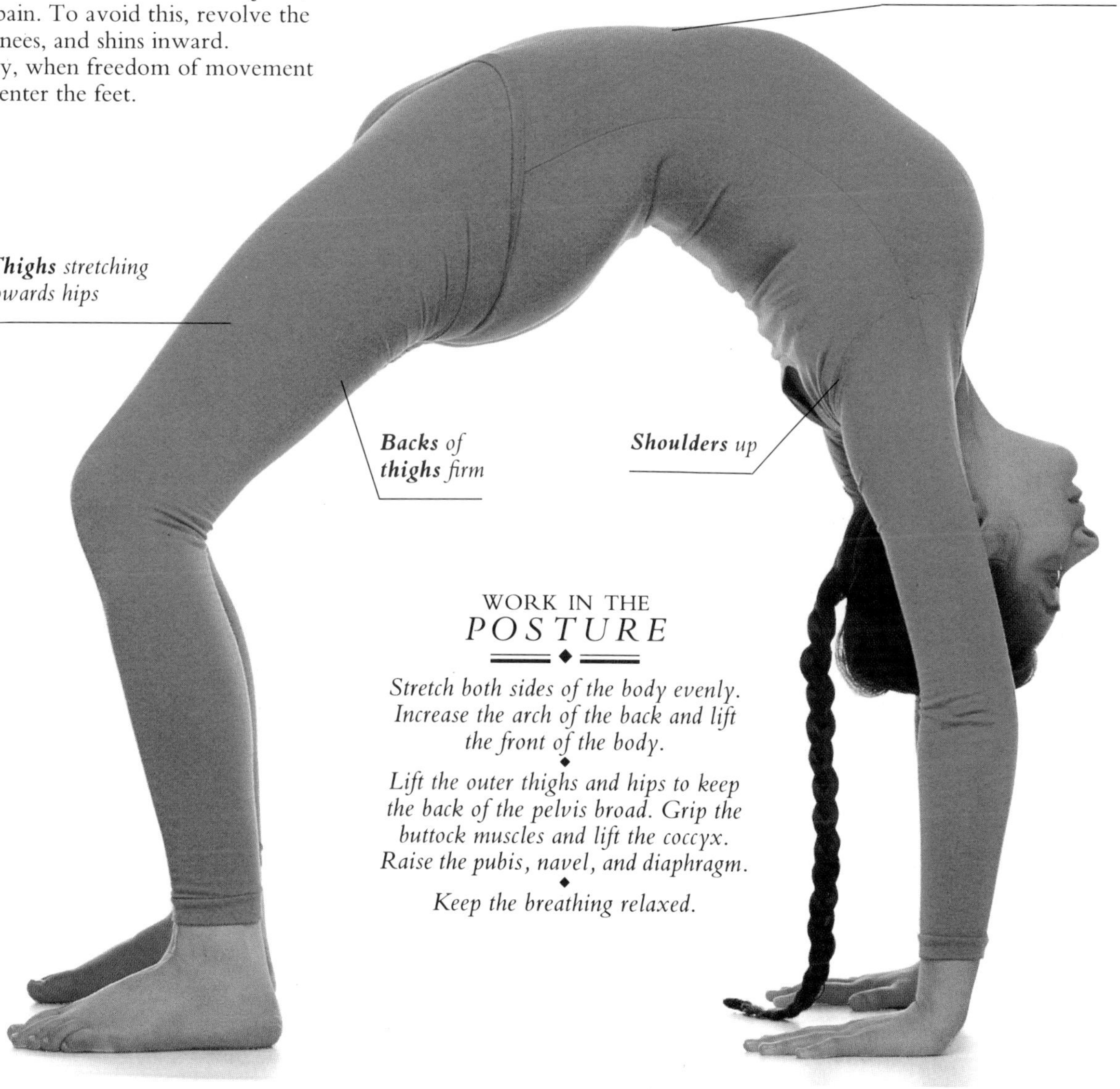
Navel *lifting*
Thighs *stretching towards hips*
Backs *of* **thighs** *firm*
Shoulders *up*

WORK IN THE POSTURE

Stretch both sides of the body evenly. Increase the arch of the back and lift the front of the body.

Lift the outer thighs and hips to keep the back of the pelvis broad. Grip the buttock muscles and lift the coccyx. Raise the pubis, navel, and diaphragm.

Keep the breathing relaxed.

ऊर्ध्व धनुरासन

Ūrdhva Dhanurāsana from Śīrṣāsana

ŪRDHVA = upward; DHANURA = a bow

Dropping back from above makes the back-arch lighter. Both Śīrṣāsana and Ūrdhva Dhanurāsana should be mastered first. ♦♦♦

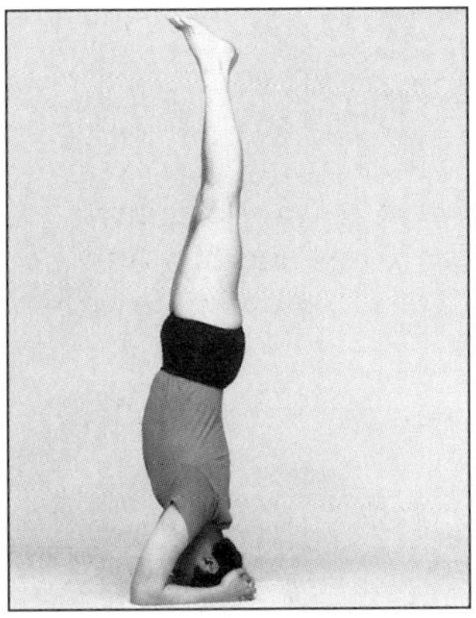

1 Be in Śīrṣāsana (p. 98). Stretch up well.

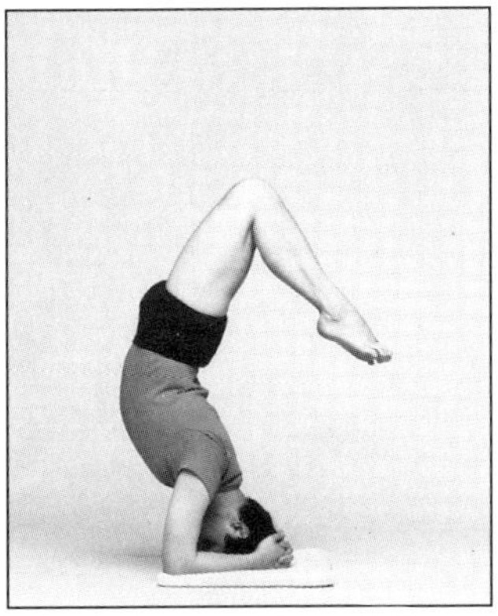

2 Lift the shoulders strongly. Bring the chest forward, making the back concave. Stretch the hips up and bend the legs back.

Arch the trunk, bringing the chest, abdomen, and hips further forward and taking the knees back. Pause to stabilize the position, then arch more and take the feet further down.

Pressing the forearms firmly down, roll more onto the forehead, without compressing the neck.

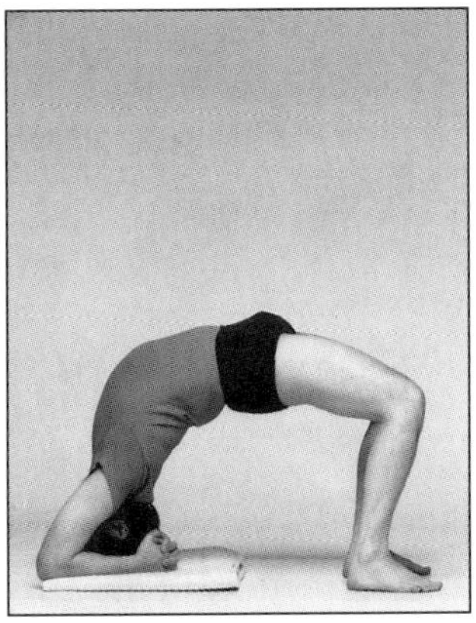

3 Exhale and drop the legs to the ground. Keep the hips lifted.

4 Unclasp the hands and place them under the shoulders. Press them into the ground and raise the shoulders and head. Then straighten the arms, walk the feet in, and arch the back.

Stay, breathing evenly, for 10 to 15 seconds.

Exhale and come down.

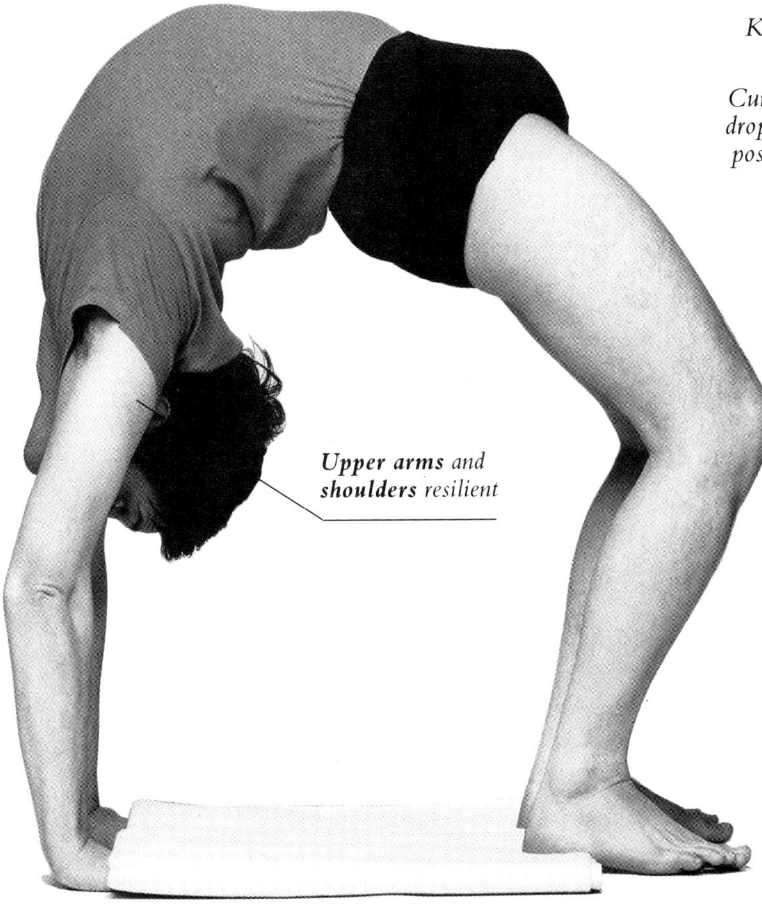

Ways of Practicing

Place a bolster or firm cushion behind the head, in case of a fall.

Place a low stool against a wall; drop the feet onto the stool. Gradually decrease the height.

If the back and neck are strong, repeat the posture 2 or 3 more times.

WORK IN THE POSTURE

Work in the posture as in Ūrdhva Dhanurāsana (p. 138).

♦

Keep the upper arms and shoulders strong.

♦

Curve the back evenly when dropping back. Drop into the posture lightly, not heavily.

ऊर्ध्व धनुरासन

Ūrdhva Dhanurāsana from Tāḍāsana

ŪRDHVA = upward; *DHANURA* = a bow

WHILE CURVING into the back-arch, strength and flexibility are controlled.♦♦♦♦

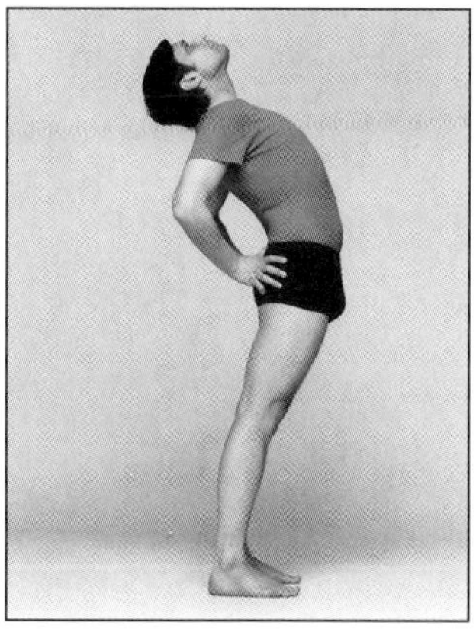

1 Stand in Tāḍāsana (p. 18) with the feet 1ft apart. Place the hands on the hips. Keeping the knees straight and the heels down, bring the thighs and hips forward and start arching the back.

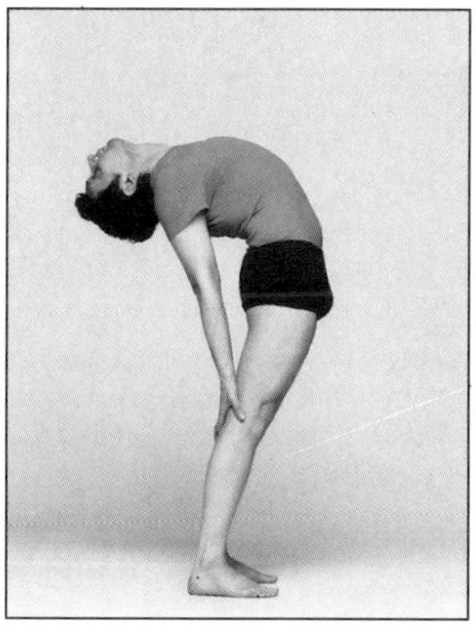

2 Increase the arch: press the sacrum forward, stretch the lumbar spine up, and curve the thoracic spine. At the same time take the hands further down the backs of the legs and look back.

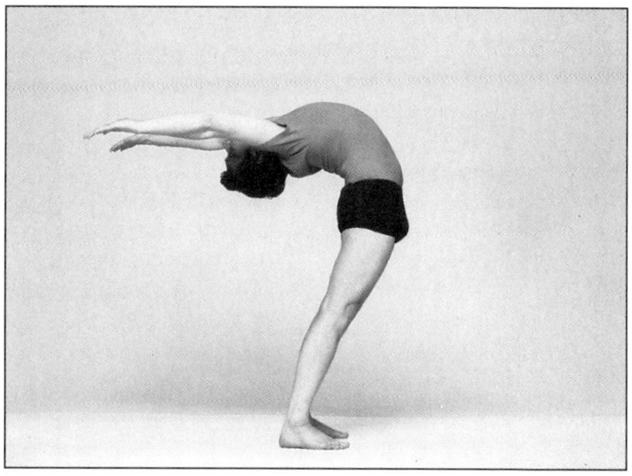

3 Release the hands and raise the arms over the head. Stretch them back and then down, curving the trunk to the maximum.

4 Bend the knees very slightly, resisting the bend with the shins. Drop back onto the hands and immediately, with a springy action, stretch the arms up and straighten them. Walk the feet and hands in.

Stay for 10 to 15 seconds, breathing evenly.

Exhale and come down carefully.

WAYS OF PRACTICING

Stand about 2 ft away from a wall. Curve back, taking the hands onto the wall; crawl the hands down. Come up the same way.

Drop back onto a bed or pile of firm cushions.

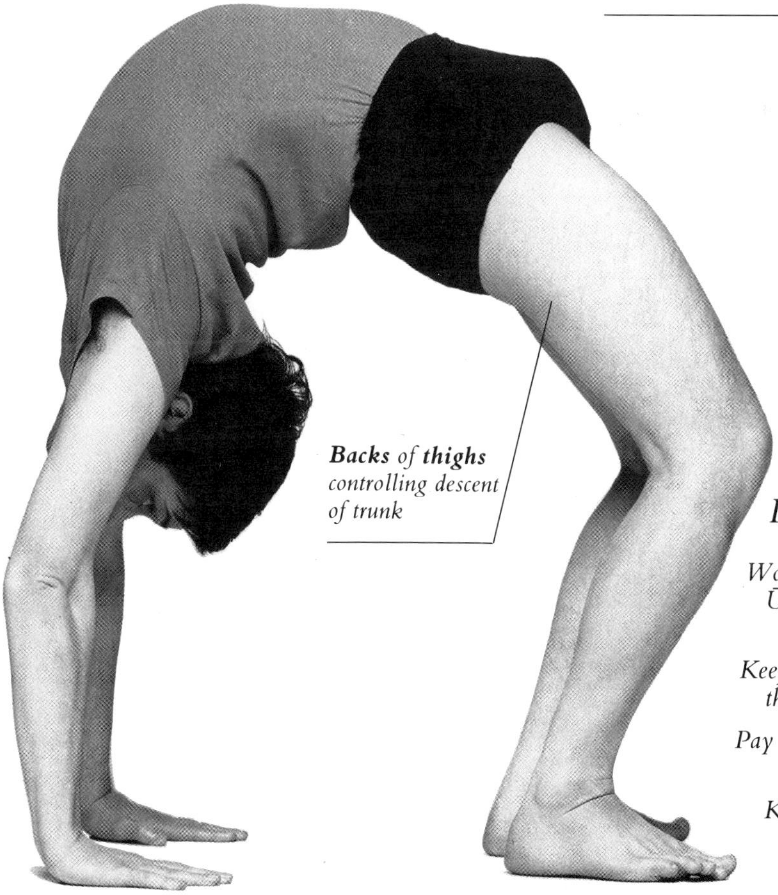
Backs *of* **thighs**
controlling descent of trunk

WORK IN THE
POSTURE

Work in the posture as in Ūrdhva Dhanurāsana (p. 138).

Keep the legs straight until the very last moment.

Pay attention to curving the trunk evenly.

Keep the arms strong.

द्वि पाद विपरीत दंडासन

Dvi Pāda Viparīta Daṇḍāsana

DVI PĀDA = two legs; *VIPARĪTA* = inverted; *DAṆḌA* = stick, staff

THE SHOULDER BLADES must grip the ribs for the chest to open and the hips to lift.♦♦♦

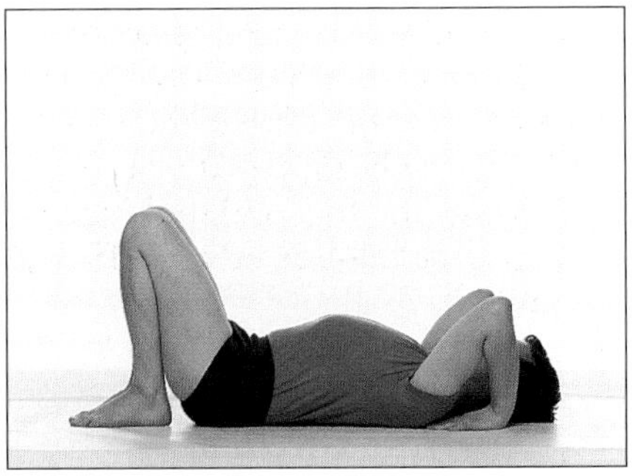

1 Lie on the floor. Bend the knees and place the feet near the buttocks, keeping them together. Bend the elbows and place the palms under the shoulders, fingers pointing toward the feet.

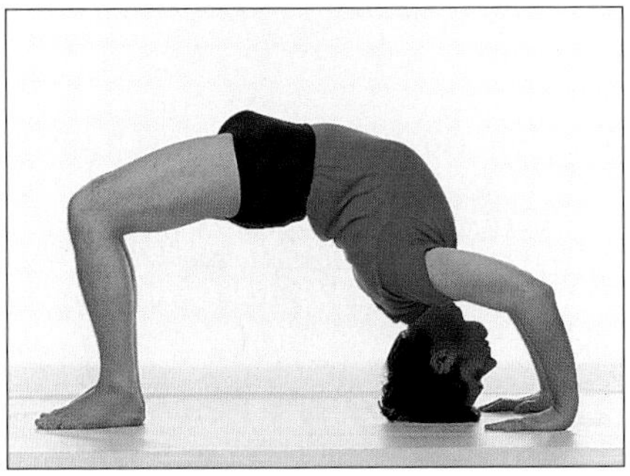

2 Exhale, lift the shoulders and hips, and go onto the crown of the head.

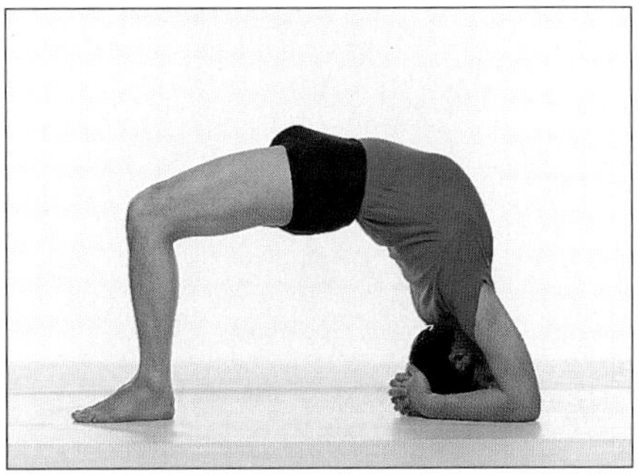

3 Clasp the hands behind the head. Take the elbows in. Stretch the neck and shoulders up and press the back ribs in. Lift the coccyx, sacrum, and thighs. Open the chest. Stay for 10 to 15 seconds, breathing evenly. Exhale and come down or continue to the next step.

4 Keeping the chest and hips up, straighten the legs one at a time. Stay without straining the back, for 10 to 15 seconds, or longer.
Bend the legs and come down.

WAYS OF PRACTICING

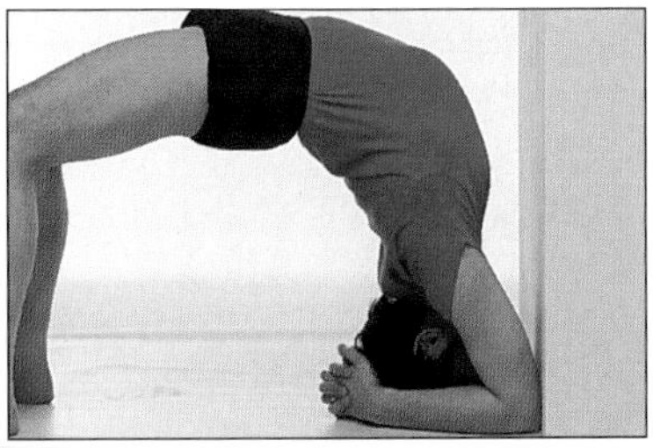

Lie with the head near a wall. In Step 3, place the elbows against the wall and raise the chest.

Raise the feet onto a stool placed against the wall.

Alternative method
Drop back into the posture from Śīrṣāsana (see p. 140).

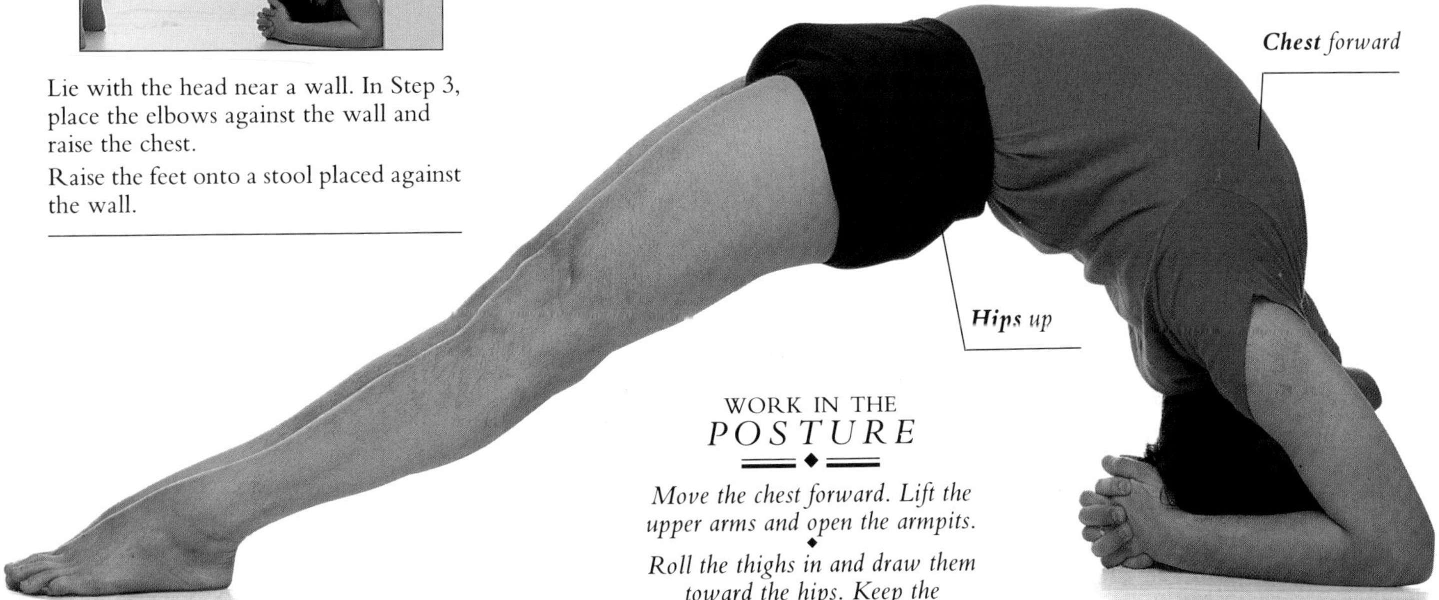

WORK IN THE POSTURE

Move the chest forward. Lift the upper arms and open the armpits.

Roll the thighs in and draw them toward the hips. Keep the buttocks firm.

एक पाद राजकपोतासन

Eka Pāda Rājakapotāsana

EKA PĀDA = one leg; *RĀJA KAPOTA* = king pigeon

THE INDEPENDENT actions of the limbs and trunk unite to create this graceful pose.♦♦♦♦

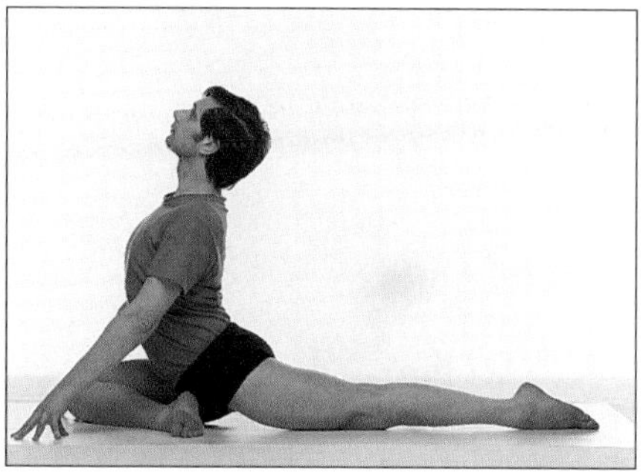

1 Kneel, bend forward, and place the hands on the floor. ▷Bring the right leg forward and bend it, with the knee slightly to the side and the foot in front of the left side of the groin. Keep the thigh down. Stretch the left leg directly back with the front of the leg on the floor. Stretch the hips and trunk up.

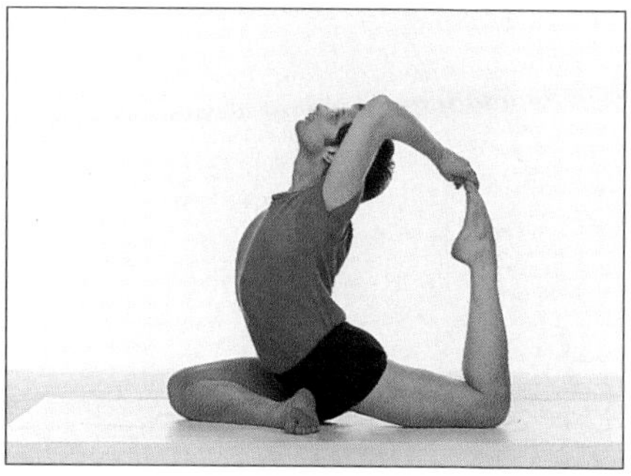

2 Bend the left leg up. Extend the thigh away from the buttock. Press the sacrum and buttocks down. Extend the trunk up, puff the chest out, and curve the upper trunk back toward the left foot. Stretch the left arm back, catch the left toes, and turn the arm up, with the elbow facing the ceiling. Make the body stable.

3 Take the right arm up and back, and catch the foot. Secure the grip of the hands. Bring the foot closer to the head; rest the head on the sole of the foot and look up.

Stay, breathing evenly, for 15 to 20 seconds.

Exhale, release the foot.◁

Change the legs and repeat from ▷to◁.

WAYS OF PRACTICING

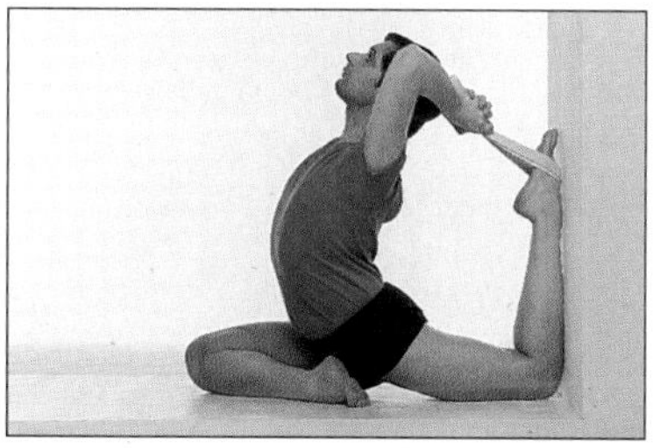

Bend the left leg up against a wall. Put a belt around the foot and pull it toward the head.

WORK IN THE POSTURE

Maintain a steady balance while curving backward. Center the left leg. Keep the left outer buttock down and the sacrum broad. Press the lower back down and extend upward away from it.

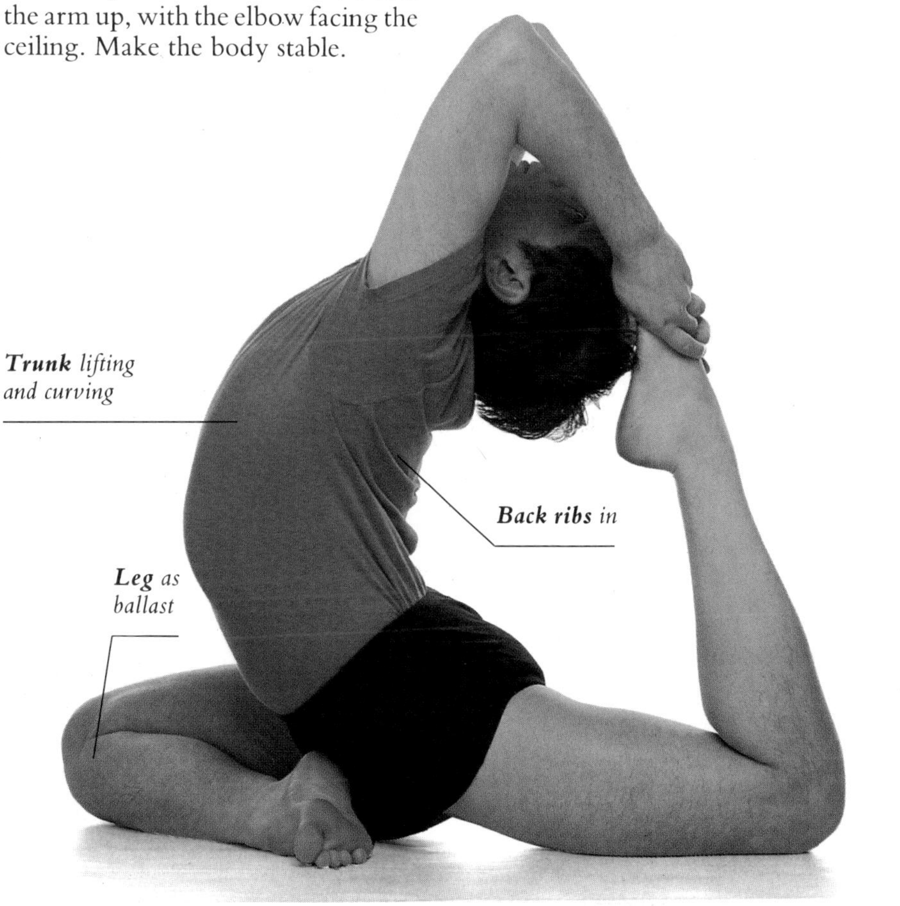
Trunk *lifting and curving*
Back ribs *in*
Leg *as ballast*

कपोतासन

Kapotāsana

KAPOTA = a pigeon

THIS POSE imitates the shape of a pigeon.♦♦♦♦

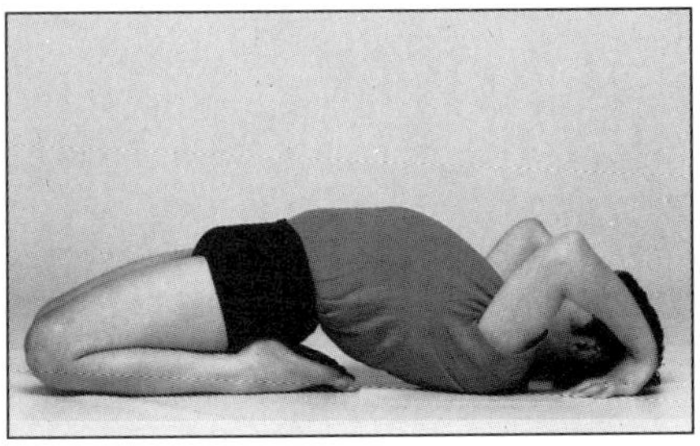

1 Lie in Supta Vīrāsana (p. 82). Bend the arms and place the hands beside the head.

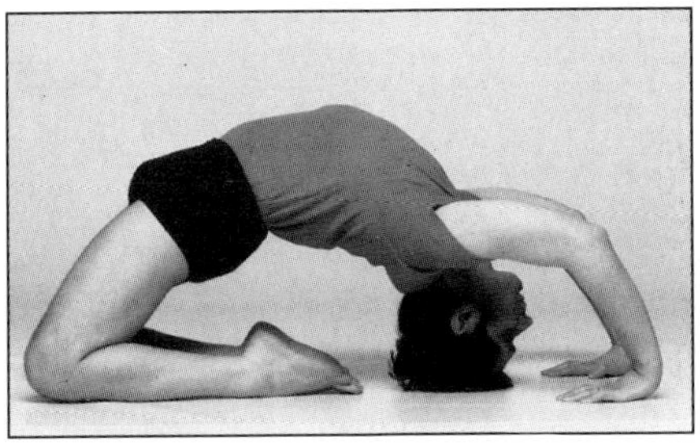

2 Press the hands into the floor, exhale, and raise the hips and trunk. Take the head back and place the crown on the floor.

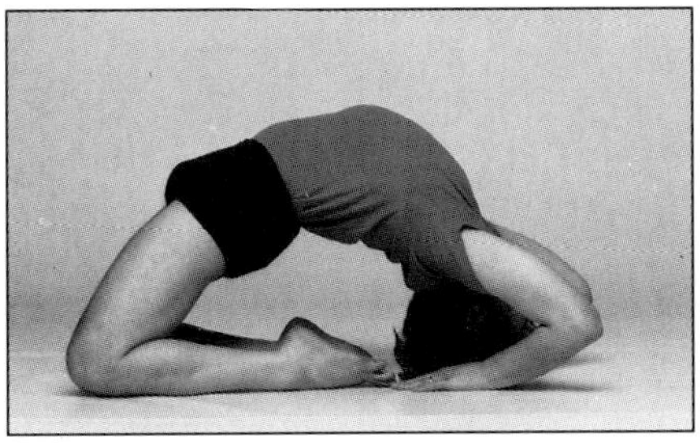

3 Raise the trunk higher and walk the hands toward the feet.

Reach the hands one by one toward the feet.

4 Hold the feet. Take the head back and rest it on the soles. Look back.

Stay, breathing evenly, for 10 to 15 seconds.

Exhale, release the hands, walk them away from the head, and come up.

WORK IN THE POSTURE

Keep the hips and buttocks firm.

Keep the shoulders lifted. Press the shoulder blades into the back ribs and puff the chest.

WAYS OF PRACTICING

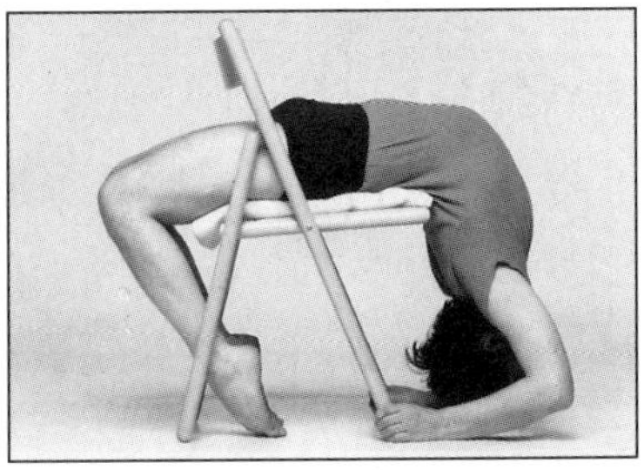

Keep the knees against a wall to stop them slipping.

Use a chair with a bar between the back legs. Go into it as in Viparīta Daṇḍāsana (p. 136). Take the feet under the seat; rest the shins on the bar. Holding firmly, curve over the seat. Take the hands over the head. Catch the front legs of the chair.

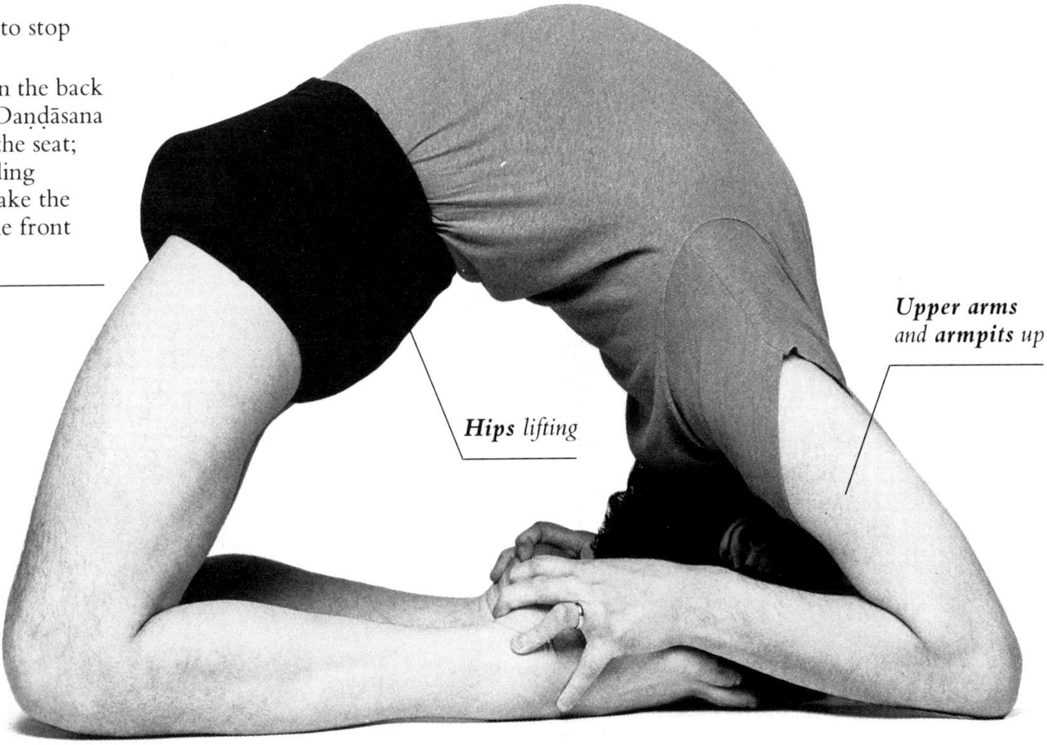

JUMPINGS

Rhythm has to be observed in Yoga more than staying.
B. K. S. IYENGAR

Jumpings are exhilarating and enjoyable. They develop speed, alertness, and stamina. There are two basic kinds. The first is the Sūrya Namaskār, where blood is diffused in the solar plexus. It stimulates the abdominal organs and gives energy. The second is a neck balance and forward bend sequence where blood is supplied to the brain, dispersing depression and lethargy.

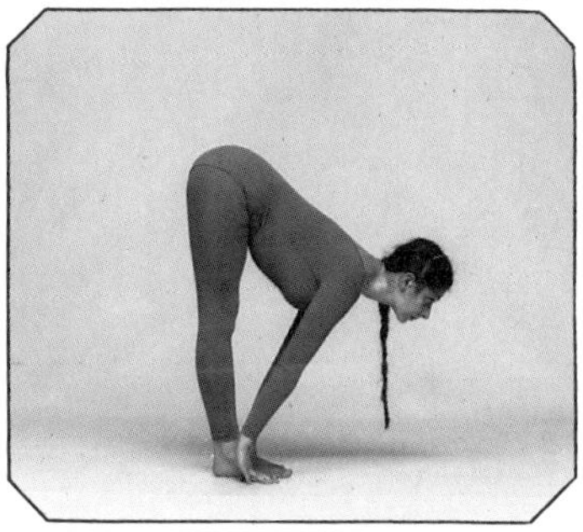

GUIDELINES FOR PRACTICE

The postures are done in quick succession, the sequences being repeated several times and accelerated, according to stamina. As facility is gained, speed will naturally increase.

To jump, both feet are taken off the floor simultaneously.

The sequences should flow smoothly. Care should be taken to move rhythmically from one pose to the next. It is necessary to know the order of a sequence to anticipate each following pose and to prepare for it.

Each posture, though done quickly, should be completed with precision, and with minimal time spent in intermediate positions. The movement of the arms, legs, and trunk should be coordinated to reach the pose at the same time.

The basic sequence should be mastered before other postures are added to it.

Jumpings need to be practiced only occasionally. Sūrya Namaskār (p. 146) may be done at the beginning of a practice session. The neck balance/forward bend sequence (p. 148) may be done at the end.

CAUTIONS: Do not do jumpings if suffering from a bad back or knee injuries or any other medical condition.

Do not do jumpings during menstruation or pregnancy.

सूर्य नमस्कार

Sūrya Namaskār

SŪRYA = sun; *NAMASKĀR* = greeting, salute

THIS IS an ancient Indian practice. Traditionally it is done before sunrise. ♦♦♦

Synchronize all movements with the inhalations and exhalations. Take one or two normal breaths during each posture before jumping to the next.

Stand in Tāḍāsana. Inhale, swing the arms up into Ūrdhva Hastāsana. Exhale, bend down into Uttānāsana. Inhale, raise the head. Exhale, jump back into Adho Mukha Śvānāsana. Inhale, jump lightly onto the tops of the feet into Ūrdhva Mukha Śvānāsana. Exhale, bend the arms, flick the toes under and dip down into Caturaṅga Daṇḍāsana.

Continue, reversing the sequence as follows:
Inhale, jump lightly onto the tops of the feet and straighten the arms into Ūrdhva Mukha Śvānāsana. Exhale, jump into Adho Mukha Śvānāsana. Inhale, jump forward and place the hands by the feet for Uttānāsana, head up. Exhale, take the head down. Inhale, stand up, raising the arms into Ūrdhva Hastāsana. Exhale, bring the arms down into Tāḍāsana.

Repeat the sequence from the beginning two or three times, without a break. At the end, rest in Uttānāsana.

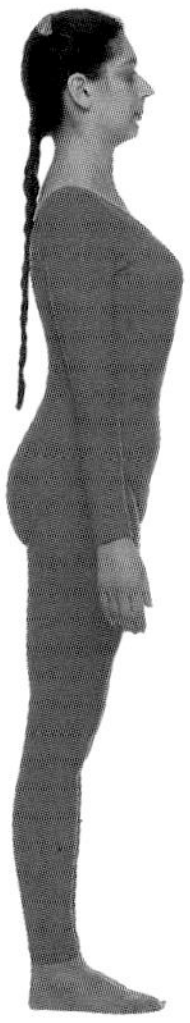
Tāḍāsana

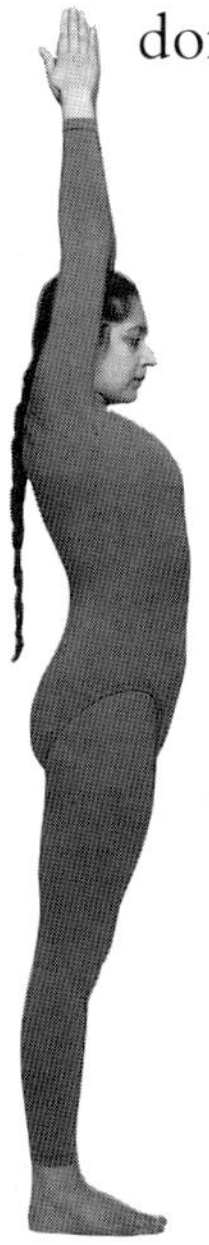
Ūrdhva Hastāsana

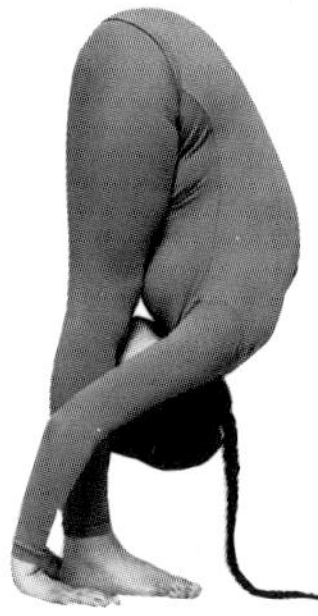
Uttānāsana

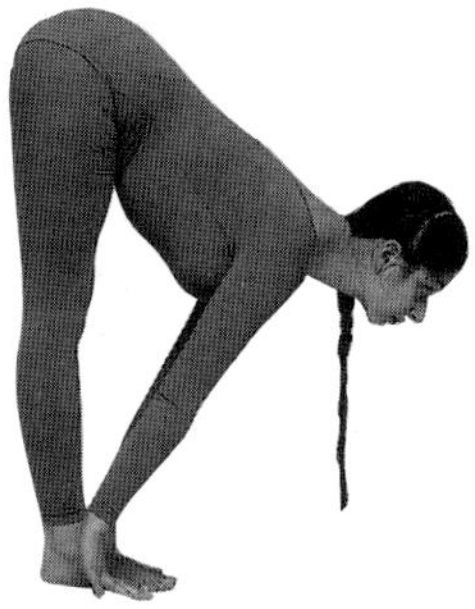
Uttānāsana head up

VARIATION

Tāḍāsana, Ūrdhva Hastāsana, Uttānāsana as above. Then from Adho Mukha Śvānāsana, jump forward via Lolāsana into Jānu Śīrṣāsana, with the right leg bent. Change the legs. Jump back into Adho Mukha Śvānāsana. Repeat from Adho Mukha Śvānāsana in the reverse sequence.

Repeat from the beginning, inserting Ardha Baddha Padma Paścimottānāsana, Triaṅg Mukhaikapāda Paścimottānāsana, Marīcyāsana I and Paścimottānāsana into the sequence in turn.♦♦♦♦

WAYS OF PRACTICING

Vary or extend this sequence by including Nāvāsana, Ardha Nāvāsana, twists, balancings, or standing poses.

Separate the two sides of a pose by Lolāsana and Adho Mukha Śvānāsana.

If Lolāsana is difficult, cross the legs simply and propel the body quickly from Adho Mukha Śvānāsana to the forward bends and back.

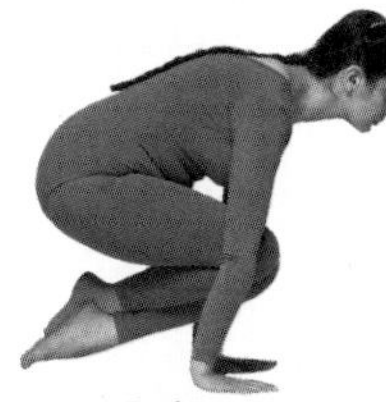
Lolāsana

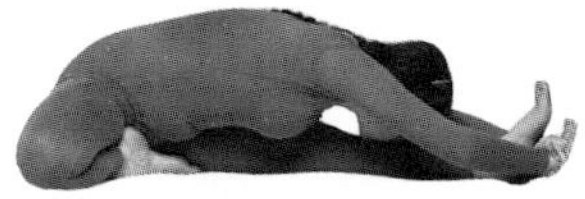
Jānu Śīrṣāsana

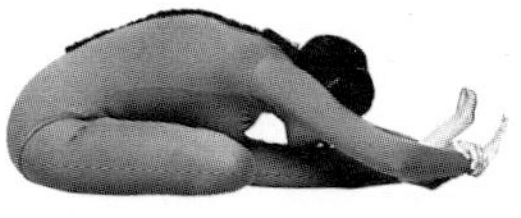
Ardha Baddha Padma Paścimottānāsana

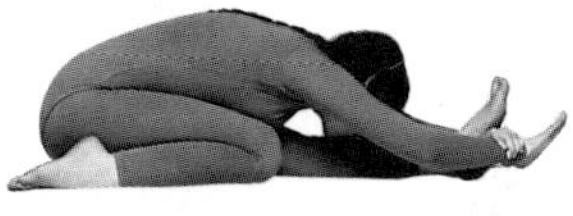
Triaṅg Mukhaikapāda Paścimottānāsana

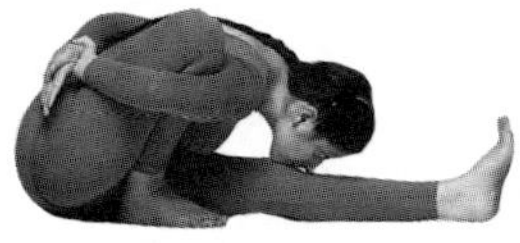
Marīcyāsana I

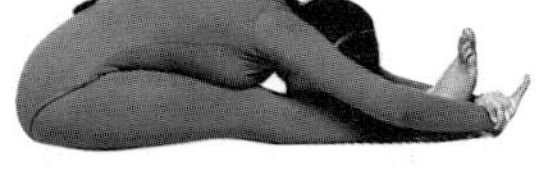
Paścimottānāsana

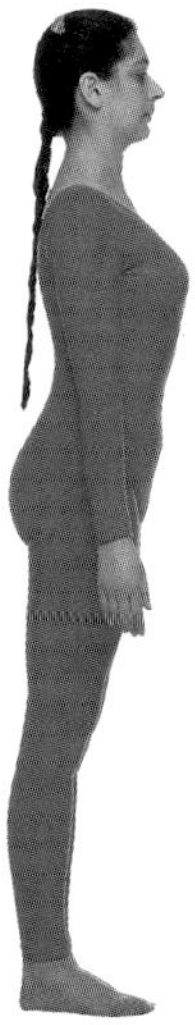
Tāḍāsana

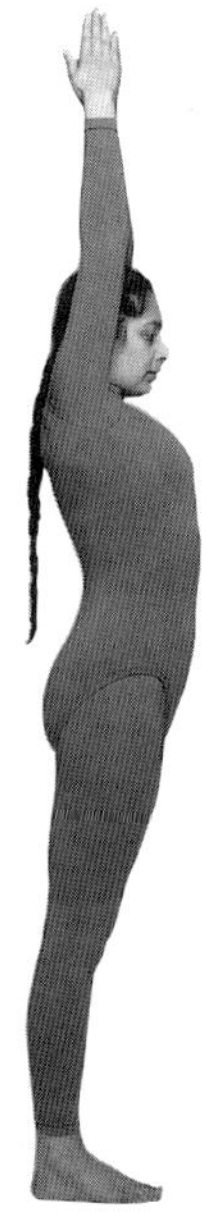
Ūrdhva Hastāsana

Ways of Practicing

Practice jumping from Uttānāsana to Adho Mukha Śvānāsana and back several times. Then add Ūrdhva Mukha Śvānāsana, and finally Caturaṅga Daṇḍāsana (see Simple Jumping Sequence, p. 91).

Omit Caturaṅga Daṇḍāsana from the main sequence.

Vary the order of the last three poses (Adho Mukha Śvānāsana, Ūrdhva Mukha Śvānāsana and Caturaṅga Daṇḍāsana).

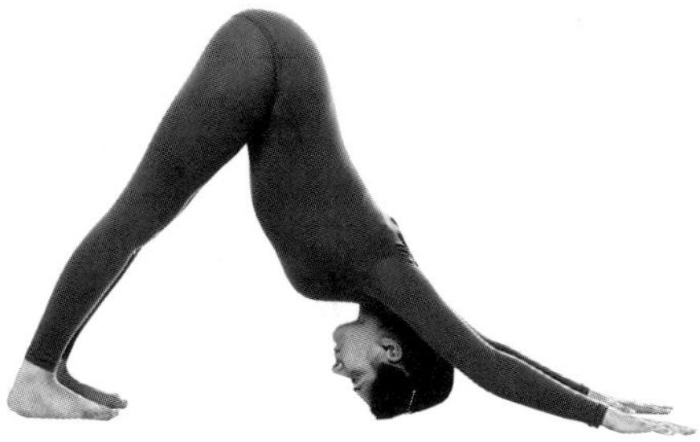

Adho Mukha Śvānāsana

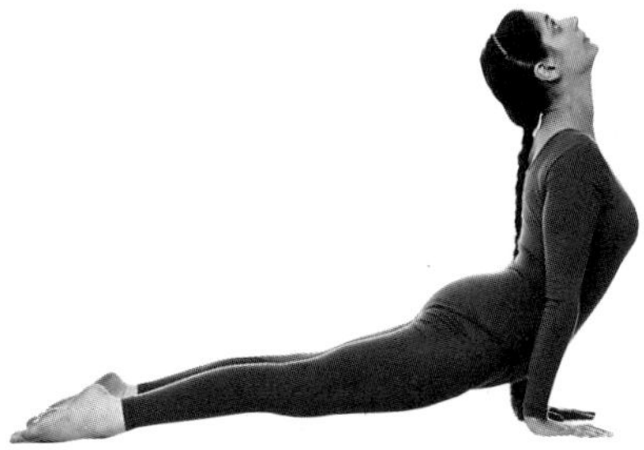

Ūrdhva Mukha Śvānāsana

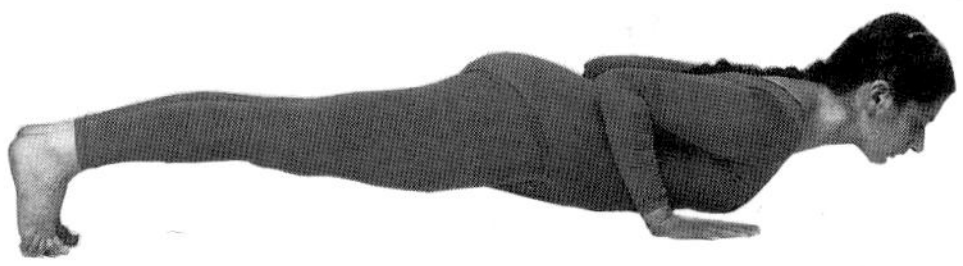

Caturaṅga Daṇḍāsana

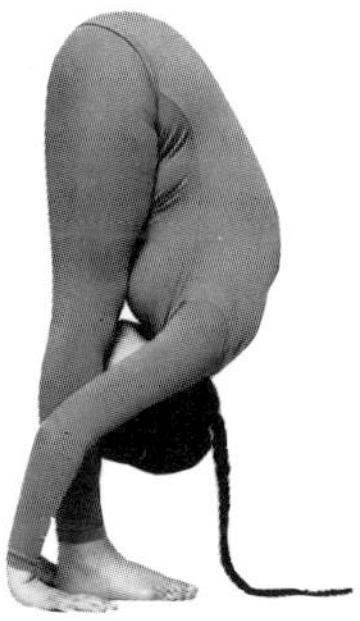

Uttānāsana

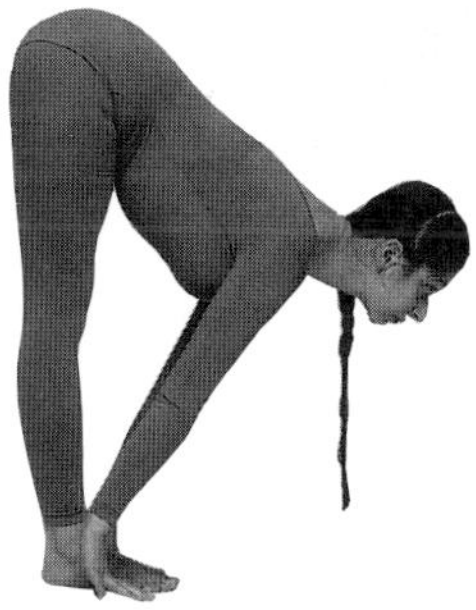

Uttānāsana head up

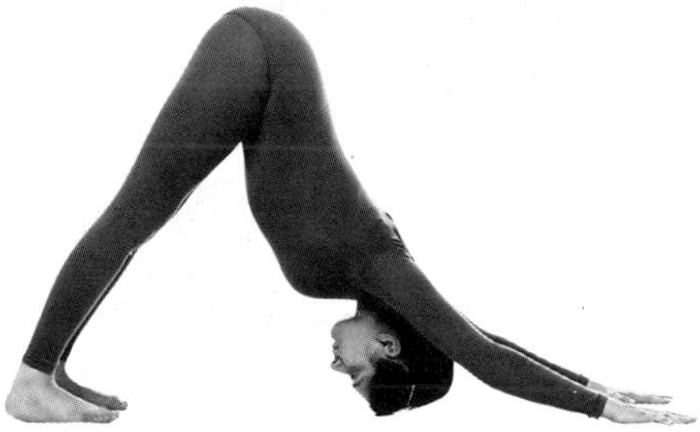

Adho Mukha Śvānāsana

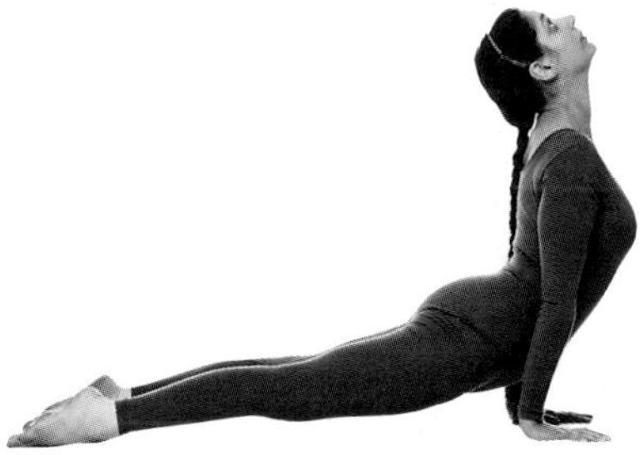

Ūrdhva Mukha Śvānāsana

Sarvāṅgāsana & Forward Bends

THIS HAS a refreshing effect on the brain.♦♦♦

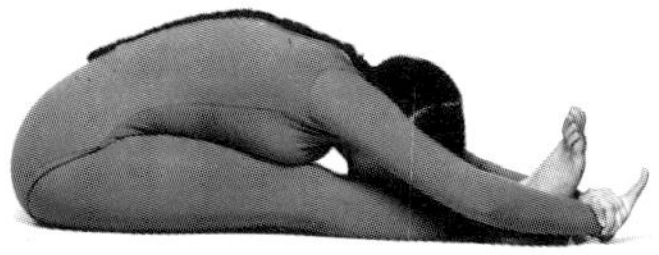

Paścimottānāsana

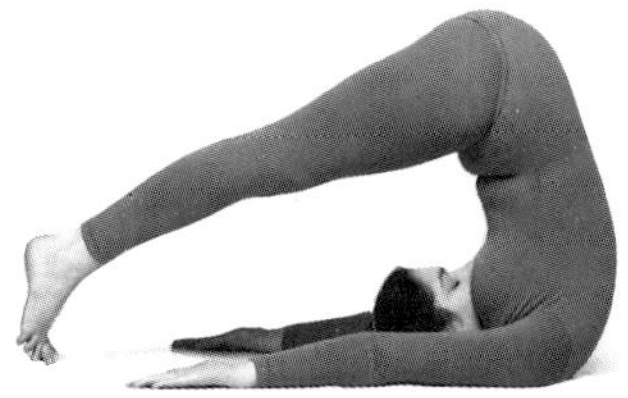

Halāsana

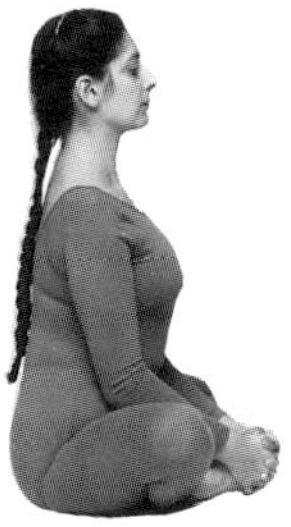

Baddha Konāsana

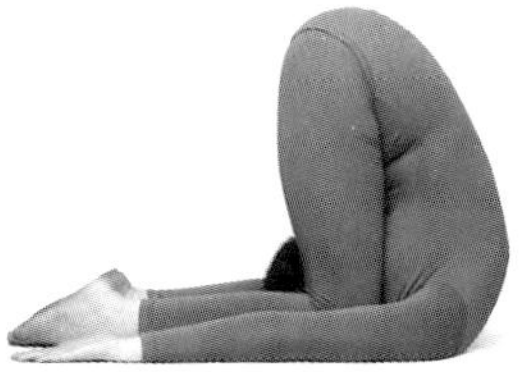

Karṇapīdāsana

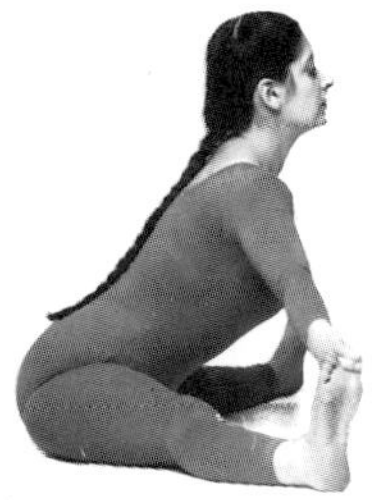

Upaviṣṭa Koṇāsana

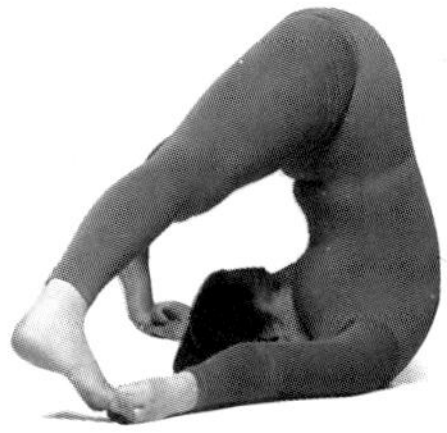

Supta Koṇāsana

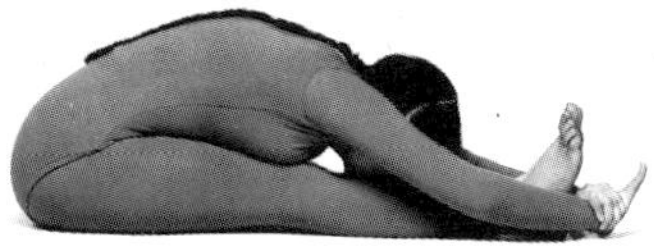

Paścimottānāsana

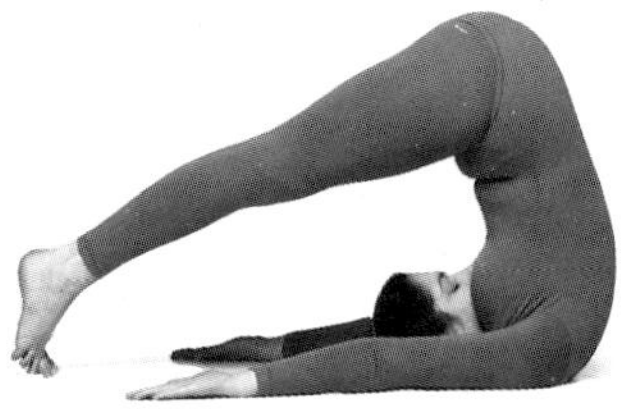

Halāsana

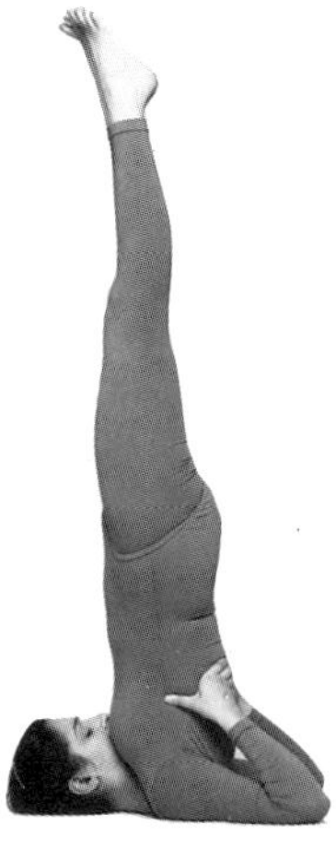

Sarvāṅgāsana

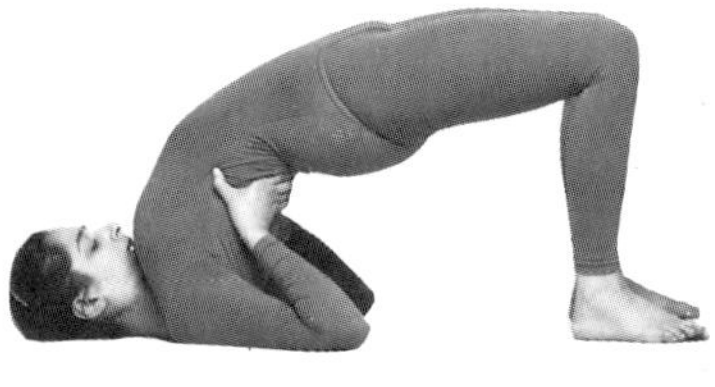

Setu Bandha Sarvāṅgāsana

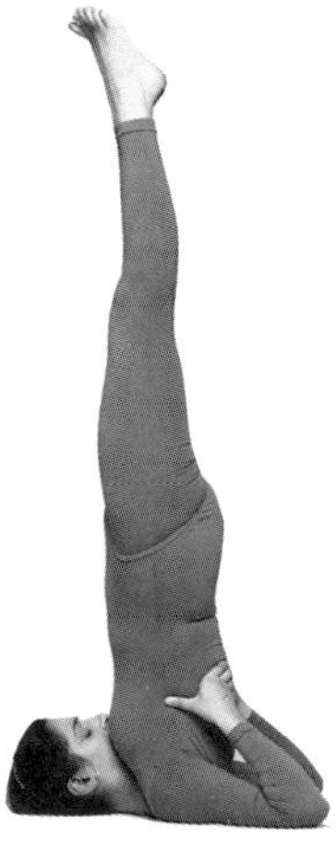

Sarvāṅgāsana

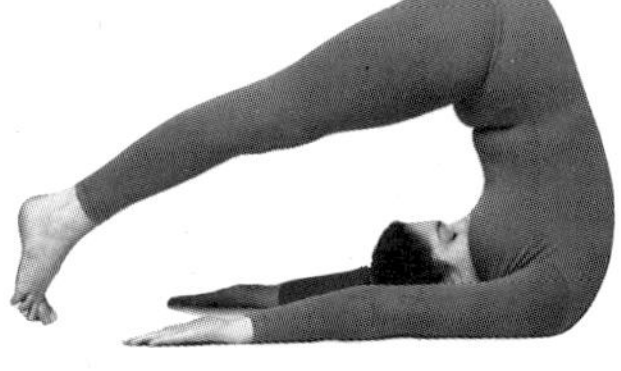

Halāsana

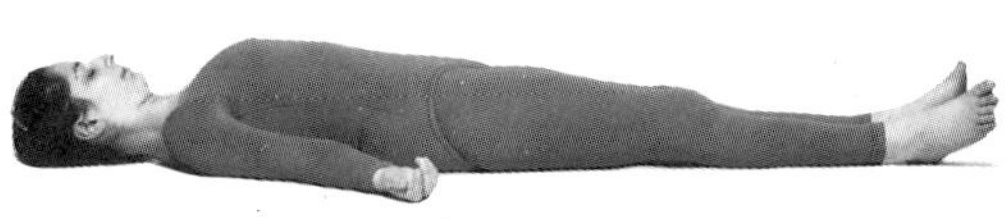

Śavāsana

Do all movements on an exhalation. Take one or two normal breaths during each posture.

Exhale, bend forward into Paścimottānāsana. Exhale, take the arms and legs over the head into Halāsana. Exhale, sit in Baddha Koṇāsana, clasping the feet. Exhale, swing back into Karṇapīḍāsana, arms back. Exhale, swing forward into Upaviṣṭa Koṇāsana, catching the feet. Exhale, swing back into Supta Koṇāsana, holding the toes. Exhale, bend forward into Paścimottānāsana. Exhale, swing back into Halāsana. Exhale, raise the legs into Sarvāṅgāsana, supporting the back. Exhale, bend the legs back, and drop back into Setu Bandha Sarvāṅgāsana. Exhale, jump up into Sarvāṅgāsana. Exhale, go into Halāsana. Exhale, slide down into Śavāsana.

Ways of Practicing

Extend or vary the sequence to include all the Sarvāṅgāsana variations and forward bends in pairs.

RELAXATION

Detail and precision of the body lead to mastery of the art of relaxation.
B. K. S. IYENGAR

Relaxation is a blessing. It brings peace to body and mind. The mind is introverted, developing the faculty of self-awareness.

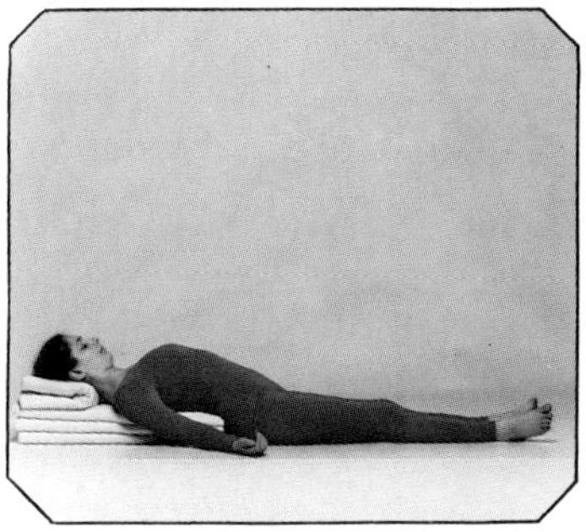

GUIDELINES FOR PRACTICE

It is important to be warm during Śavāsana (p. 150), as the body metabolism slows down. It is better to be covered with a blanket than to wear restrictive clothing. Even socks may constrict the toes.

The disciplined awareness of Śavāsana requires practice and a quiet mind. In the beginning there may be a tendency to fidget or go to sleep, and attention is required to counteract this. The regular practice of *āsanas* greatly aids the ability to relax.

Śavāsana should normally be done after āsana practice, to allow the *āsanas* to take their effect in the body. Occasionally the *āsanas* done are so relaxing that a separate relaxation period is not necessary. Or they may be so invigorating that Śavāsana is impossible and their energy is carried straight into working life.

Those who are tense or suffering from stress should tie a bandage around the forehead and eyes.

Śavāsana may be done both prior to and during Prāṇāyāma practice. It can be used to separate different methods, to rest the back and the lungs, to open the chest, and to make the mind calm. In this case it is helpful to do it with the chest supported.

CAUTIONS: Do not do Śavāsana if suffering from mental illness, depression, or phobias. Do relaxing postures where the chest is supported instead (see Remedial Programs).

If panic occurs during Śavāsana, keep the eyes open but quiet.

If suffering from hyperventilation or epilepsy, seek advice from a specialist teacher.

शवासन १

Śavāsana I

ŚAVA = a corpse

IN RELAXATION the body lies as still as a corpse and the mind is at peace. Once the posture is mastered, quietness can be called upon at will.♦

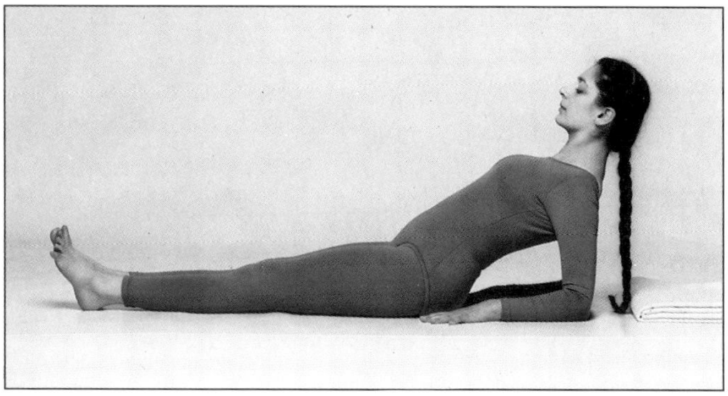

1 Sit in Daṇḍāsana (p. 52). Lean back onto the elbows. Check that the trunk and legs are in line.

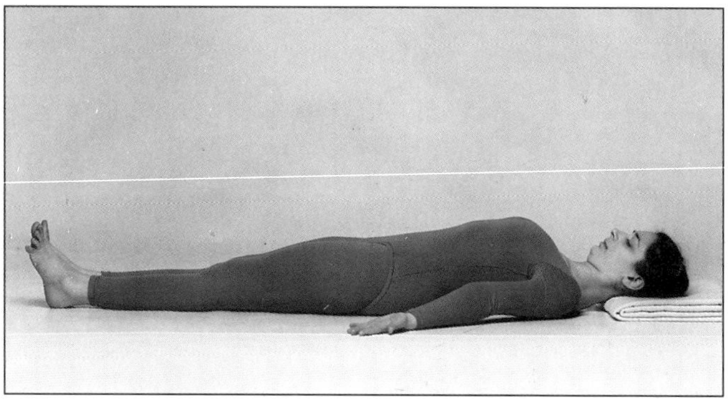

2 Lie down, lowering the back vertebra by vertebra. Place a pillow under the head and neck. Settle the back on the floor. Extend the trunk, arms, and legs prior to relaxing them.

HEAD AND NECK

Keep the head straight and move it away from the trunk. Be on the center of the back of the skull. Let the eyebrows and bridge of the nose face the ceiling. Extend the neck and throat, and relax them. Do not raise the chin. If there is tension in the throat, readjust the position of the upper back and head.

BACK

Move the shoulders away from the head and press them down. Move the shoulder blades and the back ribs in to open the chest.

Bend the legs slightly, raise the hips, and extend the lower back toward the legs. With the help of the hands, broaden the buttocks away from the sacrum. Then place the sacrum down evenly and straighten the legs.

ARMS

Turn the upper arms out, palms up. Extend the arms and hands, then relax them. Keep them slightly away from the trunk, with the corresponding parts of each arm, wrist, and hand on the floor and the fingers curling naturally.

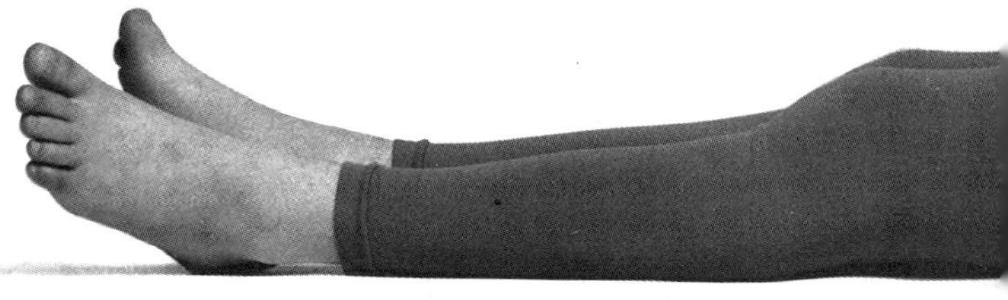

शवासन १

Front of the Body

Widen the collarbones outward and move them toward the head. Open the rib cage; do not let the sternum sink in. Move the chest away from the abdomen. Keep the abdomen relaxed.

Legs

Extend the legs and feet. Then let them drop evenly to the sides, with the corresponding part of each leg and foot touching the floor.

3 Close the eyes. Keep the breath normal. Make it quieter. Do not let the mind wander, but keep the attention on the body. Keep the eyes still and relax the face. Allow the body to sink into the ground.

Stay quietly for 5 to 10 minutes or more.

Then slowly open the eyes. Bend the legs, turn to one side, and stay for a moment; turn to the other side. Then get up from the side.

Ways of Practicing

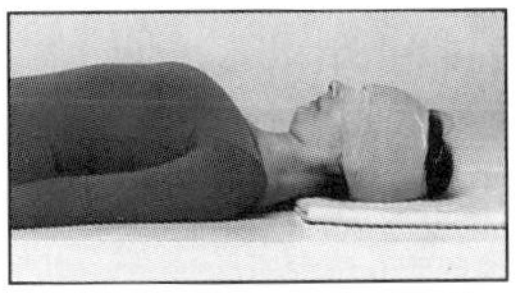

Spread the legs a little further apart to relax the abdomen.

Tie a bandage around the forehead and eyes to ease tension and migraine. Do not use a crêpe bandage. To remove the bandage, unwind it carefully.

If lying flat is uncomfortable, or in case of backache, bend the legs to a right angle and support the calves on a chair.

Focus *Adjusting the body*
Any wrong position of the body hinders relaxation. After lying quietly for a few moments, observe any unevenness. Spend some time adjusting and aligning the posture. Correct it carefully, with minimum disturbance, to center the body and head. Then do not move the body again. If another defect becomes apparent, remember when next practicing not to commit the same mistake.

Reflection
The mind is changeable and subject to moods. It is affected by internal and external circumstances. When the body is still, the state of the mind can be observed. It may be dull and sleepy, or restless and unable to settle. Both lethargy and agitation need to be overcome. Śavāsana disciplines the mind to be quiet and watchful.

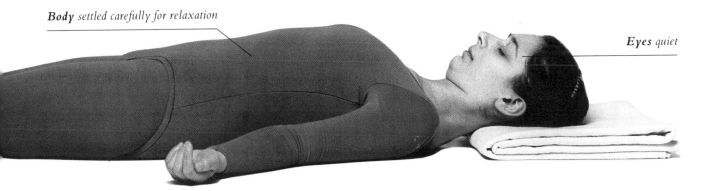

Body *settled carefully for relaxation*

Eyes *quiet*

शवासन १

Śavāsana II

ŚAVA = a corpse

THE MIND is trained to be indrawn, refining the relaxation.♦♦

1 Lie evenly on two or three blankets folded lengthwise under the lumbar, chest, and head (or on a bolster). Hold this against the lumbar while going down. Place another blanket under the head so that the forehead does not drop back.

2 Adjust the body carefully as in Śavāsana I (step 2, page 150).

3 Close the eyes by drawing the upper lids down. Keep them still. Relax the eyeballs and sink them deep into their sockets.

Draw the skin of the forehead away from the center outward, to smoothe out any wrinkles. Then release the skin from the hairline down toward the eyebrows. Relax the temples.

Relax the skin of the face. Release the tension from the corners of the eyes, nose, and lips. Relax the skin of the nose and cheeks.

Do not clench the jaws or teeth. Rest the tongue on the lower palate.

Release the tension around the ears. In listening for external sounds, the auricular passages harden. To relax the ears, draw the hearing inward, as if listening to internal sounds.

Make the skin soft and sensitive, from the head to the fingers and toes. Learn to draw inward away from the skin.

Still all thought processes. Do not let the ego rise or the mind wander.

Draw the gaze of the eyes down, into the rib cage. Begin to observe the breath. Mentally follow the course of the normal inhalations and exhalations. Make the breath softer and quieter. Let the mind merge in the breath.

Stay for 5 to 10 minutes or longer, maintaining the stillness of the body and mind.

Then slowly open the eyes, allowing them to focus gradually. Bend the legs, turn to one side, and stay for a moment; turn to the other side. Then get up from the side.

WAYS OF PRACTICING

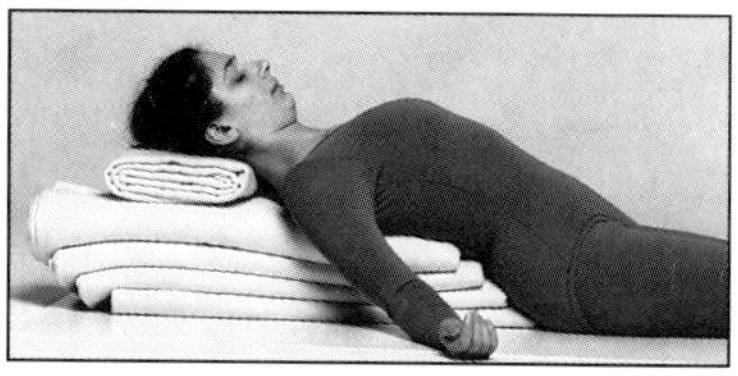

Lie back on a stepped arrangement of blankets. This is good for people with heart and respiratory problems, and in pregnancy.

Reflection
The skin becomes sensitive through the practice of āsanas, moving and stretching in harmony with the body. It is the boundary between the internal and the external world. In Śavāsana it is trained to relax. The more the skin relaxes, the deeper the experience of Śavāsana. Mind and body draw inward away from the skin, penetrating the subtle inner functions and sounds of the body. They become still. This state of peaceful awareness leads to meditation.

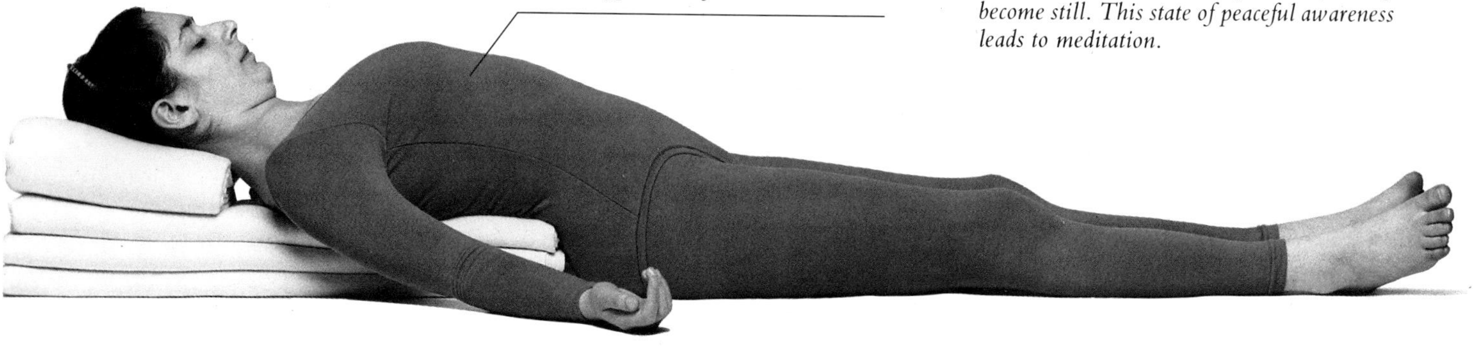

***Trunk** supported to facilitate relaxation*

PART II

THE MIND

PRĀṆĀYĀMA & PHILOSOPHY

Control of the mind is said to be the highest Yoga. It is like the control of an unruly horse, which must be made to obey its rider.

BHAGĀVATA PURĀṆA, XI.20

Study of the Self

The end of analysis is the beginning of discrimination. The end of discrimination is the beginning of knowledge.

B.K.S. IYENGAR

Svādhyāya, the study of the self, is the second cornerstone in the practice of Yoga. It leads to knowledge (*jñāna*) and answers the second need of humanity, satisfaction of the mind.

Acquiring Knowledge

Knowledge is a gift of the mind and marks the human being from the animal. It is both theoretical and practical and has to be acquired by study and experience.

For Yoga students, *svādhyāya* comes through sincere practice. The student has to learn to open mind and heart to all aspects of Yoga. This effort is worthwhile as understanding of oneself brings mental and physical assurance. It also brings an awareness that the principles of philosophy need to be put into practice.

The appeal of *svādhyāya* may not at first be apparent, as the benefits derived from *āsana* practice are immense. However, it adds a further dimension to Yoga and is essential for those who wish to proceed deeper into the subject. The body and mind attain a state of quietness, and the boundary is crossed between physical practice of Yoga and practice with understanding. In this way a spiritual awareness is acquired.

Svādhyāya has several dimensions. On the practical level it involves the development and control of the mind through the mastery and refinement of the breath (*prāṇāyāma*), and through the practice of stilling the senses (*pratyāhāra*). The mind must also be enriched by the study of philosophy.

According to Yoga philosophy, the mind is the instrument of perception and action. The Sanskrit word for mind is *manas*. Mind is one of the primordial principles of nature. It is part of the greater principle of consciousness (*citta*).

Citta has three components: mind, intellect, and ego, and is permeated by three qualities: lightness, which makes the mind clear, intelligent, and peaceful; energy, giving it driving force that can be used for good or bad; and inertia, producing stability as well as dullness. The interplay of these qualities gives rise to mood swings.

Breath and the mind are closely linked. Usually the state of mind affects the breath. It becomes agitated and shallow during moments of excitement. When it is quiet and deep, the mind becomes calm. In *prāṇāyāma,* breath is used to change the mental state. The mind is trained to follow the course of the breath, and, by so doing, its scattered thoughts are channeled inward.

The calming of the mind through *prāṇāyāma* leads to a state of quietude. With practice, this is prolonged and deepened. Different types of *prāṇāyāma* induce different states of awareness. Just as the many types of *āsanas* need to be practiced in order to tone and sensitize the whole body, so also a variety of *prāṇāyāmas* are necessary for a complete experience.

The senses, too, are quietened by *prāṇāyāma* and drawn towards the inner world. By nature, the eyes, ears, nose, tongue, and skin are attracted to their objects, constantly seeking new experiences. Detaching them from their objects and drawing them inward leads to a state that is self-contained, where nothing external is required. This is the "desireless" state (*prātyāhāra*). Once achieved, the distinction between everyday life and spiritual life is known.

Study of the self is furthered by familiarity with Yoga philosophy, which gives guidance on how to achieve equanimity. The study of philosophy exercises and sharpens the mind and puts individual concerns into perspective. It gives a base of understanding so that practice can be structured and ever-developing. By explaining the purpose behind practices and rules, it helps to maintain interest in the subject.

Applied to life, Yoga philosophy provides a yardstick by which to gauge whether thoughts and actions are correct. Thoughts often change and actions can be wrong. Philosophy is the means by which we analyze and build upon experience, avoiding past mistakes.

The following pages describe the techniques for *prāṇāyāma* and *pratyāhāra* and outline the Yoga philosophy.

प्राणायाम

Prāṇāyāma

In the work of Prāṇāyāma, the back is the blackboard, the air comes to write, and the mind holds the chalk.
B.K.S. IYENGAR

Prāṇāyāma calms and strengthens the mind and creates a feeling of internal space. It generates a store of energy in the body. Once the lungs are strong, it increases their capacity.

It consists of three types of control of the breath: inhalation (*pūraka*), exhalation (*recaka*), and retention (*kumbhaka*). In these processes the breath is extended, expanded, and refined.

Guidelines for Practice

Prāṇāyāma is attempted only when the body, nervous system, and lungs have been strengthened by *āsana* practice. This usually takes at least two years. As breath is subtle, even more care has to be taken over it than over the *āsanas*.

Śavāsana is a preparation for prāṇāyāma.

Prāṇāyāma should be started gradually, a little at a time. Even a few minutes are beneficial. With practice, the time spent can be increased.

Prāṇāyāma is best practiced in the early morning or evening, in an airy room. The stomach and bowels should be empty.

It is not advisable to do it immediately before or after strenuous *āsanas,* as these disturb the breath and the lungs. It may be practiced after a quietening *āsana* session consisting of supported inverted poses.

The breathing methods given here are first practiced in Śavāsana with the back supported. This trains the lungs for Prāṇāyāma, without causing strain. The chest opens and breathing becomes easier. When it becomes steady, the same techniques can be done while sitting.

Sitting straight for Prāṇāyāma requires practice. The body should rise upward. The legs should be comfortable, so that they do not disturb the sitting position.

The stages given should be practiced in their appropriate order, to master the different techniques.

Exhale completely before beginning any of the techniques. One cycle consists of one inhalation and one exhalation.

If a cycle becomes disturbed, it should be completed and followed by two or three normal breaths. The reason for the mistake should be analyzed before starting again.

Cautions

Do not continue with Prāṇāyāma if the lungs get tired or if there is fatigue or irritation, as it is then injurious. Instead, lie down and relax. Lie down also if the back aches.

If you panic or choke, make sure the abdomen is not tensing.

If the head becomes hot, this is a sign of overstrain. Lie in Śavāsana to recover.

Do not do deep inhalations if suffering from hypertension or heart problems.

Do not do deep exhalations if suffering from hypotension or depression.

If suffering from tension, cover the eyes with a soft cloth or tie a bandage round the forehead and eyes. (The bandage should be firm on the forehead but light on the eyes.)

Normal Breathing (lying down)

HERE NORMAL breathing is introduced as a breathing practice.♦♦

Lie on one or two blankets folded lengthwise under the lumbar, chest, and head (see Focus, below right, and Śavāsana, p. 152). Place another blanket under the head. Settle down until the mind and body become quiet. Relax the face. Close the eyes. Lie in Śavāsana for three to four minutes.

Direct the gaze downward into the chest. Become aware of the chest. Observe the rise and fall of the chest as normal breathing takes place. Gradually make each breath smooth, soft, and rhythmic, and of similar volume. Feel both sides of the rib cage moving evenly out and in. Feel the mind becoming quieter and more peaceful. The breath will gradually become slower and deeper, penetrating further into the chest cavity. Do not go to sleep.

Stay, breathing evenly, for five to ten minutes.

Continue with the next technique or remove the support from under the back and lie flat, with a blanket under the head only. After a few minutes, bend the legs, turn to the side and come up.

Caution

Prāṇāyāma is a very powerful practice. It deals with the life force. Mistakes made in āsanas *result at worst in a torn muscle. Mistakes made in prāṇāyāma may affect the nervous system and the brain. For this reason it is essential to learn under the guidance of an experienced teacher.*

Refinement of the Technique

- Keep the eyes still and indrawn throughout. Keep the attention on the breath so that the mind and breath act in unison. Still all other thoughts, as these are disturbing and create tension.
- Breathe evenly through both nostrils. Fill and empty the lungs equally on the right and left sides. Keep the flow of breath on the two sides parallel.

Focus *Using blankets for Prāṇāyāma*

Fold a blanket to a length of $2\frac{1}{2}$ to $3\frac{1}{4}$ft and a width of 8 to 10in. Place it under the back from the lumbar to the head. To open the chest more, add two or three more blankets.

Place the blanket horizontally under the rib cage, just below the shoulder blades. Take the upper arms under the ends of the blanket.

Make a stepped arrangement of blankets (see p. 152).

In each case support the head on one or two folded blankets to raise it above the level of the chest. Make sure the forehead does not drop back and the chin does not lift.

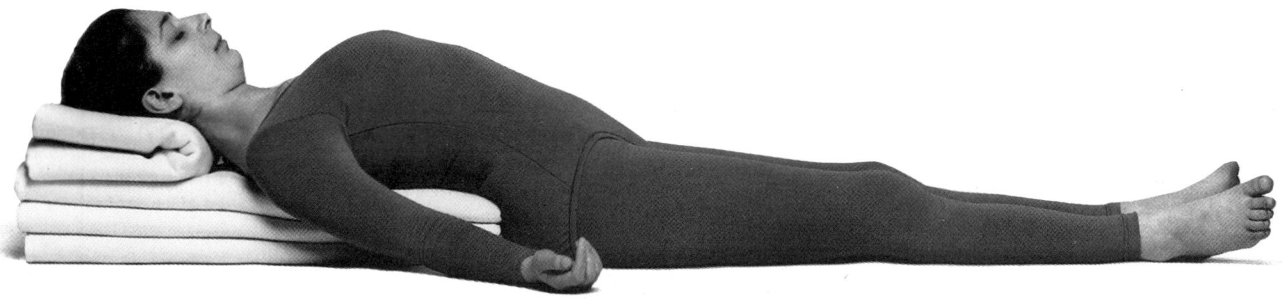

Normal Breathing (sitting)

THIS GIVES training in sitting as well as in normal breathing.♦♦♦

Sit in Sukhāsana (p. 53) on two folded blankets. Place the fingertips beside the hips and stretch the trunk up. Bend the elbows and rest the backs of the hands on the thighs. Relax the upper arms and elbows and take them slightly back. Relax the palms and fingers.

Raise the coccyx, sacrum, and lumbar. Draw the pubis and lower abdomen toward them. Extend the spine up. Stretch the sides of the body and raise the rib cage. Keep the sternum and the collarbones up. Bring the armpits and the chest forward, widen the shoulders and take them back. Pull down the back of the shoulders and the shoulder blades. Move the back ribs in and make the dorsal spine concave.

Keep the head straight, the eyes level, and the crown facing the ceiling. Lift the back of the skull. Keep the ears perpendicular. Close the eyes and draw the eyeballs into their sockets. Draw the gaze of the eyes back and down into the chest.

Sit for a few moments, observing every movement of the body. Counteract the downward trend of the spine and lower back.

Without collapsing the chest, extend the back of the neck toward the skull and lower the head. Do not constrict the throat.

Watch the normal course of the breath. Make it regular. Observe the various movements of the breath in the rib cage. Gradually the upright position of the body will be supported by the breath.

Stay for five to ten minutes. Then relax in Śavāsana.

When practicing: sit against the wall, with a blanket folded behind the waist and rib cage.

Sit in Padmāsana (p. 59), Vīrāsana (p. 50) or Baddha Koṇāsana (p. 57).

To learn to relax the hands, keep them face down on the knees.

If the knees are strained, support them on a blanket.

Refinement of the Technique

- Do not inflate the abdomen, but keep it drawn in and up from below. Keep the anus lightly closed to maintain a lift of the coccyx.
- With every inhalation let the chest rise and the crown of the head go down. Do not collapse the chest while exhaling.

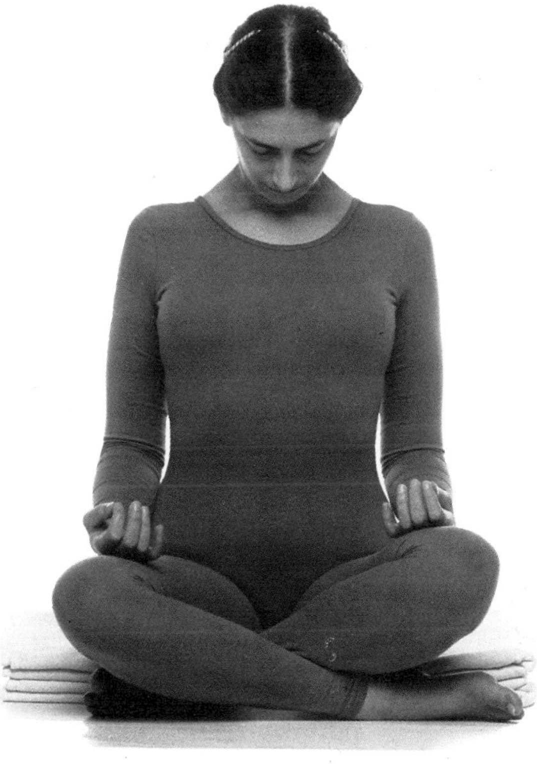

उज्जायी प्राणायाम

Ujjāyī Prāṇāyāma (lying down)

UḌ = extreme; *JĀYI* = conquering, subduing

THROUGH DEEP breathing, energy is diffused in the body.♦♦

1: DEEP INHALATION, NORMAL EXHALATION

Those suffering from lack of energy and low blood pressure should concentrate on this method to increase their oxygen intake.

Lie down for Prāṇāyāma (see p. 156). Relax for three to four minutes. Take a few normal breaths, finishing with an exhalation.

▷Inhale slowly and deeply, lengthening the breath without straining. Draw the breath in at both sides of the septum (nasal bone). While inhaling, feel the lungs and front ribs opening outward and up. Keep the brain passive.

Exhale normally, as if relinquishing the breath with a sigh. Keep the throat and nasal passages relaxed. Do not allow the rib cage to collapse.◁

From ▷to◁ forms one cycle of breath. Repeat six or more cycles, then rest. Finish the practice or continue with the next technique. Later do more cycles at a stretch.

Refinement of the Technique

- Keep the face and the eyes still. Do not strain but go on relaxing. Do not tense the arms or fingers when inhaling.
- Keep the motion of the breath, the lungs, and the ribs parallel. Make the inhalations soft and observe how the chest gradually opens.

2: DEEP EXHALATION, NORMAL INHALATION

The practice of exhalation is calming and helps to reduce high blood pressure. The brain becomes quiet.

Lie down for Prāṇāyāma (see p. 156). After relaxing, take a few normal breaths, finishing with an exhalation.

▷Inhale normally.

Keeping the lift of the top chest, exhale slowly from the back of the nostrils. Do not strain. Control the outflow of breath, keeping it soft and smooth. Do not jerk. Mentally follow the exhalation and experience the increasing sense of calm.◁

Repeat from ▷to◁ for six or more cycles, keeping them of even length. Then rest and finish the practice at this point or continue with the next technique.

Refinement of the Technique

- As the exhalation comes to an end, relax the abdomen further.
- Let the flow of exhalation be even from both lungs and nostrils. Do not let the air gush out. Do not inhale before finishing the exhalation.

3: DEEP INHALATION AND DEEP EXHALATION

Lie down for Prāṇāyāma (see p. 156). Rest for a while. Then take a few normal breaths, finishing with an exhalation.

▷Take a long, slow, deep inhalation, drawing the breath in along the septum. Start by lightly depressing the skin and flesh of the pubis and lower abdomen and drawing them toward the diaphragm. This opens the rib cage more. Inhale until the breath reaches the top outer corners of the chest and the collarbones.

Maintaining the lift of the chest, exhale slowly and deeply, without straining the throat. Control the outflow of breath, so as not to jerk. Do not suddenly collapse the ribs.◁

Repeat from ▷to◁ for six or more cycles. Then rest and finish the practice, or continue with the next technique.

Refinement of the Technique

- Do not inflate the nostrils but keep them passive throughout.
- Keep the inhalations and exhalations steady. Take normal breaths in between to help achieve this.
- Experience how the whole body from the pubis to the collarbones becomes involved in the breathing.

उज्जायी प्राणायाम

Ujjāyī Prāṇāyāma (sitting)

THE BACK of the body supports the breath as it rises and falls. This is practiced in several stages.♦♦♦

1: Deep Inhalation, Normal Exhalation

Sit for Prāṇāyāma (see p. 157). Close the eyes and lower the head. Take a few normal breaths, finishing with an exhalation.

▷Inhale deeply and steadily, drawing the lower trunk up, filling the chest to the collarbones.

Keeping the lift of the chest, exhale normally.◁

Repeat from ▷to◁ for six or more cycles. Raise the head and sit quietly for a few moments. Lie down and rest, or continue with the next technique.

Refinement of the Technique

- Do not let the head lift. Hold the body steady. Keep the lumbar region and the spine ascending and the chest well open.

2: Deep Exhalation, Normal Inhalation

Sit for Prāṇāyāma (see p. 157). Take a few breaths, finishing with an exhalation.

▷Inhale normally.

Exhale slowly and deeply, without allowing the body to shorten.◁

Repeat from ▷to◁ for six or more cycles. Raise the head and sit quietly for a few moments. Lie down and rest, or continue with the next technique.

Refinement of the Technique

- Keep the exhalations smooth. Do not collapse the top of the chest, but allow the bottom ribs to relax gradually.

3: Deep Inhalation, Deep Exhalation

Sit for Prāṇāyāma (see p. 157). Take a few normal breaths, finishing with an exhalation.

▷Take a full deep inhalation, opening the chest well. Exhale slowly and deeply, keeping the trunk drawn up.◁

Repeat from ▷to◁ for six or more cycles, breathing steadily and keeping the transition between inhalation and exhalation smooth.

Raise the head and sit quietly for a few moments. Then lie flat and relax, or continue with the next technique.

Refinement of the Technique

- Keep the chest up and the head down. Do not strain. Relax the eyes and throat.
- Keep the length and volume of the breath even.

***Focus** Deep inhalation and exhalation*

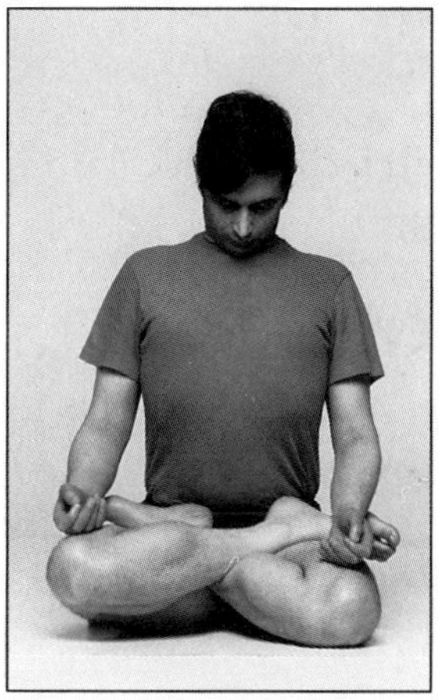

Deep inhalation

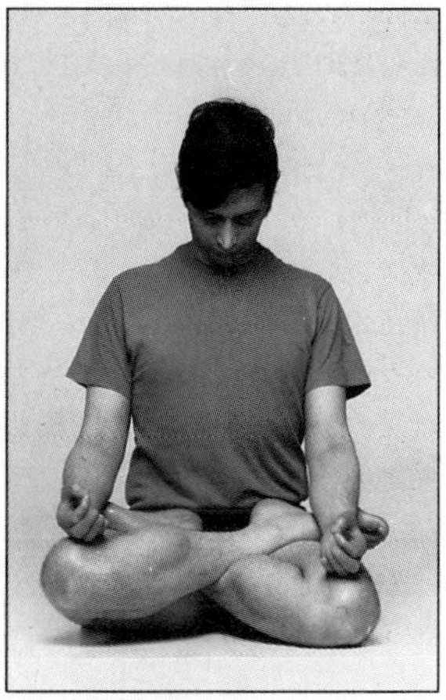

Deep exhalation

Deep inhalation

While drawing the breath in, stretch the spine and trunk up from the base. Draw the abdomen slightly back, lift the floating ribs, and open the chest. Move the lower back ribs in, in an upward direction. At the same time take the shoulders back and move the shoulder blades in, in a downward direction. The upward and downward stretches of the back meet at the seventh dorsal vertebra; press this in to keep the chest lifted.

Deep exhalation

While exhaling, maintain a subtle extension of the trunk. Keep a grip on the top outer corners of the chest and on the back ribs, to control the outflow of breath. Do not allow the mind to sink, the chest to deflate suddenly, or the spine to drop. Let the breath subside gradually.

Caution

The lungs should never feel strained. If fatigue is experienced doing continuous cycles of Prāṇāyāma, take a few normal breaths between each cycle.

कुम्भक

Kumbhaka

KUMBHA = an earthen pot

LIKE A pot, the rib cage must be full or empty. There is an almost imperceptible pause at the end of ordinary inhalation and exhalation. In Prāṇāyāma this is accentuated and prolonged. Breath and its motion are suspended.♦♦♦♦

Antara Kumbhaka

ANTARA = internal

This is retention of breath after inhalation. It distributes energy in the form of breath.

Sit for Prāṇāyāma (see p. 157). Close the eyes and take the head down. Take a few normal breaths, ending with an exhalation.

▷Take a fast, sharp, full inhalation and pause. Lightly draw the lower abdominal area up, without tensing. Keep a light, muscular grip on the top outer corners of the chest and keep the top of the sternum lifted. Spread the breath evenly in the lungs. Do not strain the lungs, face, or throat. Keep the skin soft.

Maintaining the grip on the top of the chest, quietly exhale. Relax the abdomen. Take a few normal breaths to rest the lungs.◁.

Repeat from ▷to◁ for four or more cycles. Raise the head and sit quietly for a few moments. Lie down and rest, or continue with the next technique.

Refinement of the Technique

- Learn to maintain the fullness of the chest without shaking.

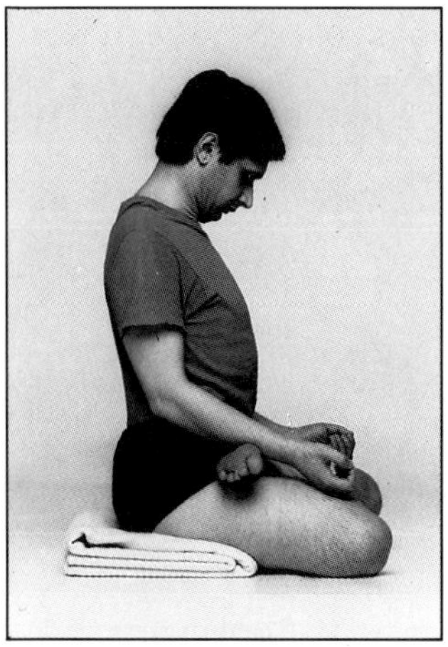

Before retention

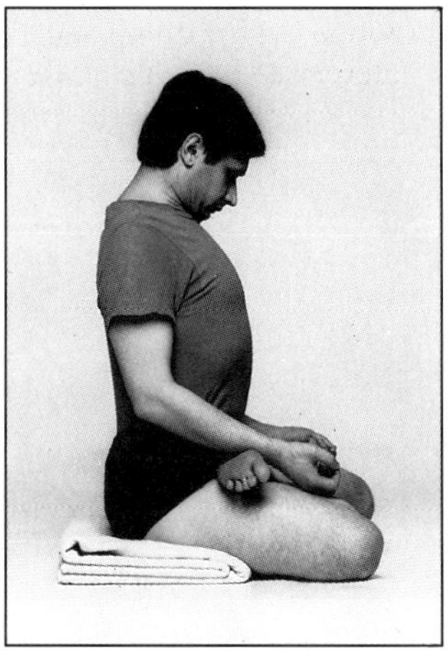

After retention

Bāhya Kumbhaka

BĀHYA = external

This is the pause after exhalation. It is not generally practiced on its own.

In practice this is carried out during Viloma Prāṇāyāma (see p. 161). Use the pause at the end of exhalation to maintain complete quietness of the mind. The pause should be natural, not held by force.

Do not concentrate on Bāhya Kumbhaka until Prāṇāyāma has become natural and Antara Kumbhaka has been learned.

Reflection
Prāṇa is the universal life force pervading the cosmos. It is more subtle than air. During prāṇāyāma, breathing is made more refined; this life energy is distilled from the air, and is distributed and stored within the body. The universal energy unites with the individual soul in the form of breath. In exhalation the mind and ego are subdued as the outgoing breath flows back into the external universe.

Focus *The difference between normal breathing and prāṇāyāma*
Normal breathing is a natural process requiring no thought or understanding. Air enters the lungs and is expelled through the expansion and contraction of the diaphragm. The volume and quality of the breath depend on the physical and emotional state of the individual.

Prāṇāyāma involves the complete mastery of the length, volume, flow, and quality of the breath. The rib cage is made to open completely and the lungs to fill and empty consciously. Control of the diaphragm is fundamental to achieving this.

During inhalation draw the daiphragm to the side and keep it still. Expand the front and side ribs from inside while keeping the back of the body firm. During exhalation release the diaphragm without jerking.

Observing and quieting the diaphragm calms the mind and emotions.

विलोम प्राणायाम

Viloma Prāṇāyāma (lying down)

VILOMA = against the grain or natural order

THE BREATH does not flow naturally but is interrupted by pauses and consciously directed to various parts of the body.♦♦♦

1: *Interrupted Inhalation, Long Exhalation*

Divide the inhalations into three, following the divisions of the body: (1) pubis to pelvic rim; (2) pelvic rim to diaphragm; (3) diaphragm to collarbones.

Lie for Prāṇāyāma (see p. 156). Close the eyes and relax for a few minutes. Take a few normal breaths, finishing with an exhalation.

1 Inhale partially, simultaneously drawing the skin and flesh of the pubis toward the ground and toward the pelvic rim. Pause for a few seconds to distribute the breath in the pelvic area.

2 Inhale partially, simultaneously drawing the skin and flesh of the abdomen from the pelvic rim to the diaphragm. Pause in order to distribute the breath in the abdomen.

3 Inhale completely, simultaneously opening the chest to the collarbones and to the side ribs. Pause to fill the whole rib cage.

Exhale slowly and smoothly. Take two or three normal breaths, until the lungs are rested.◁.

Repeat from ▷to◁ for six or more cycles. Then rest, or continue with the next technique.

When practicing:

Learn to divide the breath without relating it to corresponding parts of the body.

Divide the inhalations into five, by subdividing the chest: from the diaphragm to below the breast; from below the breast to the upper rib cage; and from the upper ribs to the collarbones.

Refinement of the Technique

- Keep the volume and pace of the breath equal in each division. In the pauses, observe the action of the breath in the relevant part of the body.
- Take care not to become tense.

2: *Interrupted Exhalation, Long Inhalation*

Lie for Prāṇāyāma (see p. 156). Close the eyes and relax for a few minutes. Take two or three normal breaths, finishing with an exhalation.

▷Inhale completely, drawing the breath in from the pubis to the collarbones. The lift of the chest must be maintained while doing so.

1 Exhale partially, from the collarbones to the diaphragm. Pause for a few seconds. Observe the diaphragm and keep it still.

2 Exhale partially, from the diaphragm to the pelvic rim. Pause. Deflate the abdomen.

3 Exhale completely, from the pelvic rim to the pubis. Pause. Take two or three normal breaths to rest the lungs.◁

Repeat from ▷to◁ for six or more cycles. Then relax in Śavāsana or continue with the next technique.

Refinement of the Technique

- Follow the exhalation mentally and still the mind at each pause.

Focus *Relaxing the brain while breathing*

The intake of breath should not activate the brain. To release tension, relax the brain while exhaling. Learn to recognize where breathing is taking place, and see that the motions of breathing remain in the lungs. Feel the breath entering and leaving the lungs through the throat.

विलोम प्राणायाम

Viloma Prāṇāyāma (sitting)

DURING THE pauses, the breath is made to spread within the lungs, bringing a feeling of freshness.♦♦♦

1: INTERRUPTED INHALATION, LONG EXHALATION

Sit for Prāṇāyāma (see p. 157). Close the eyes and lower the head. Take a few normal breaths, ending with an exhalation.

▷Divide the trunk and the breath into three:

1 Inhale partially, as if from the pubis to the pelvic rim. Pause for a few seconds. Keep a very slight grip on the lower abdomen and lift it.

2 Inhale partially, as if from the pelvic rim to the diaphragm, then pause. Maintain a lift of that area.

3 Inhale fully, as if from the diaphragm to the collarbones, then pause. Lift up from the base of the chest.

Exhale slowly, controlling the outflow of the breath. Take two or three normal breaths in order to rest the lungs.◁

Repeat from ▷to◁ for six or more cycles. Raise the head and sit quietly for a few moments. Then either lie down and relax or continue with the next breathing technique.

Refinement of the Technique

- Do not strain in the pauses. Stay still and do not allow the breath to shake the body.

Focus *Lifting the trunk when sitting*

The trunk and the spine should stretch up from the base and should feel light. Adjust the height of the blankets according to whether the spine can lift or not. If it does not stretch up, use three or four blankets. Keep the folded edges to the front. Support the tops of the thighs as well as the buttocks, so that the trunk does not tilt forward. Move the buttock bones away from each other and keep them in line.

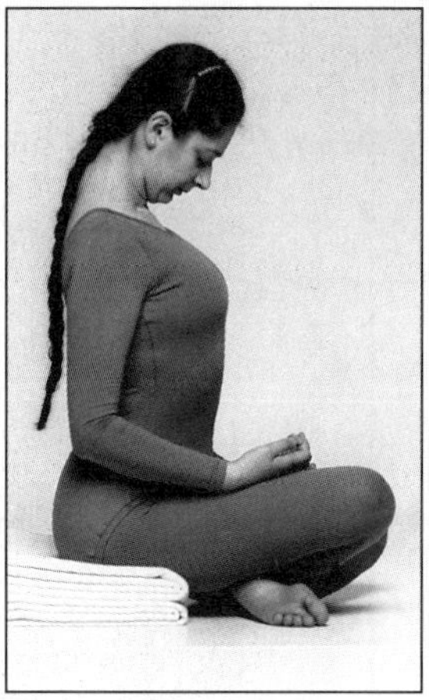

Maintain a firm posture throughout, with the spine and chest lifting. This allows the bodily energy to rise and be distributed, otherwise concentration is lost.

2: INTERRUPTED EXHALATION, LONG INHALATION

Sit for Prāṇāyāma (see p. 157). Close the eyes and lower the head. Take a few normal breaths, ending with an exhalation.

▷Take a long, deep inhalation. Pause to establish the lift of the chest.

Keep the same divisions of the trunk and breath as before (see left).

1 Exhale partially, as if from the collarbones to the diaphragm, then pause. Do not collapse the rib cage.

2 Exhale partially, as if from the diaphragm to the pelvic rim, then pause. Do not allow any breath to enter the area.

3 Exhale completely, as if from the pelvic rim to the pubis. Pause, keeping the mind and body still. Take two or three normal breaths to rest the lungs.◁

Repeat from ▷to◁ for six or more cycles. Raise the head and sit quietly for a few moments. Then lie down in Śavāsana.

When practicing, divide the trunk and breathe into four, five, or more sections.

Refinement of the Technique

- Keep the interrupted exhalations smooth.
- Observe the different parts of the body as the breath is suspended.

Reflection

Prāṇāyāmá is a subtle, precious gift. Although difficult, it is attainable through practice. It is like playing a musical instrument with delicate fingers or painting a picture with a fine brush. Each separate breath flows smoothly into the next, making an undulating pattern of rising inhalations and falling exhalations. The rhythm becomes part of the body and the mind savors its beauty. Through Prāṇāyāma, energy is drawn from the external atmosphere; the individual mingles with the universal, with awareness.

प्रत्याहार

Pratyāhāra

Be so silent that you hear the sound within. Not even the ticking of the clock should disturb.

B.K.S. IYENGAR

Although the senses are quietened during Prāṇāyāma, Pratyāhāra is a separate discipline which draws them to a standstill. It is a period of suspension of activity. This rests the nervous system and collects the mind.

Pratyāhāra is a preparation for concentration and meditation.

It is difficult to achieve and the following technique, Saṇmukhī Mudrā, is helpful. The light touch of the fingers on the eyes, ears, nose, and lips shuts off the disturbance of the external world.

Guidelines for Practice

Saṇmukhī Mudrā should be practiced only when some experience is gained in Prāṇāyāma.

It need be done only occasionally.

It is useful as a means to recover from exhaustion or tension, as it is refreshing.

It can be done either sitting or lying down.

Cautions

Do not press the eyeballs.
Do not close the ears if suffering from an ear infection.
Do not practice this if suffering from depression.

Technique for Saṇmukhī Mudrā

Sit as for Prāṇāyāma (see p. 157), with the trunk erect and the head straight. Close the eyes. Stay quietly for a few moments.

Raise the hands to the face with the elbows spread to the sides, upper arms at shoulder level. Lightly place the index fingers below the eyebrows, the middle fingers on the centers of the eyelids just above the eyelashes, the ring fingers on the depressions just above the base of the nostrils, and the little fingers on the upper lips near the corners. Place the thumbs on the flaps over the earholes.

Gently widen the space between the index and middle fingers, drawing the upper eyelids down. Do not press hard with the fingers or disturb the eyes.

Gently narrow the nostrils with the ring fingers evenly on both sides; do not let the breath hit the fingers. Let the little fingers feel the light touch of the breath. Let the volume of breath lessen.

With the thumbs cover and close the ears, exerting minimum pressure to avoid strain. Keep the pressure even in both ears. Stay for two minutes or longer, without disturbing any part of the body.

Keep the fingers sensitive. Keep the eyes soft, the muscles of the ears relaxed, and the nostrils and corners of the lips passive.

Experience the stillness that comes to the senses. Experience the coolness in the eyes.

Then lower the arms, release the hands, and lie down. Hold onto the stillness for as long as possible.

Reflection

It is sometimes essential to withdraw from everyday activities in order to revive the body, mind, and spirit. One way is to go on vacation and take a break from the pressures of life. Strength returns for continuing work afresh. The Yogi's way is to disengage the senses from the outside world and retreat into an internal world where spiritual resources abound.

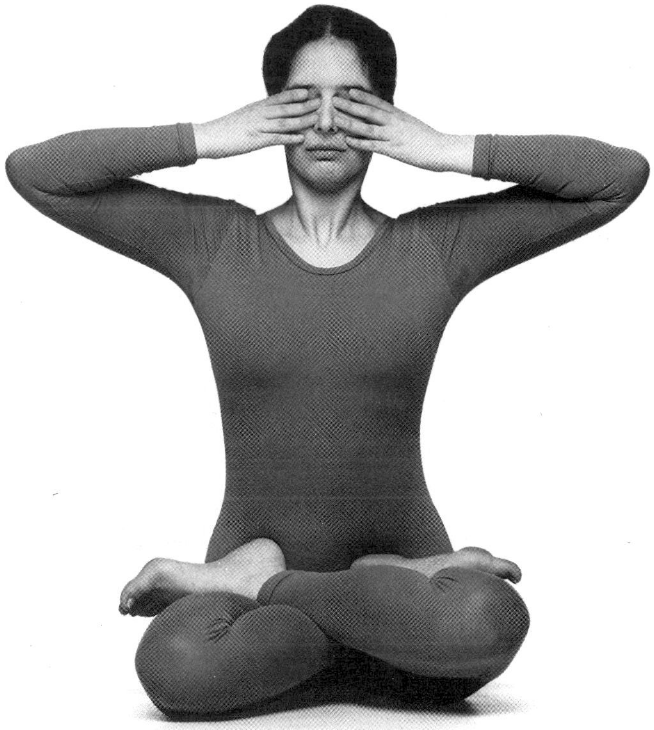

Saṇmukhī Mudrā

The Philosophy of Yoga

"On studying all the philosophies, I have come to the conclusion that none is so worthy of study as the Yoga philosophy."

ŚIVA SAṀHITĀ, I.17

Yoga is a unique blend of theoretical knowledge and practical application. For this reason alone it is worth studying. The practice of the fourth limb (*prāṇāyāma)* gives an awareness that a philosophical journey has already begun.

Yoga deals with the most profound of mysteries, the essential nature of the human being in relation to the universe. The meaning of Yoga is union or yoking, from the Sanskrit root *yuj,* to unite. In the context of Yoga philosophy, the union is between the individual soul and the universal soul. The individual has to search for the divine within, and Yoga provides the systematic steps to achieve this, ensuring that progress can be measured.

Yoga philosophy has appealed to great thinkers over the centuries and its practice has been extolled for its benefits. In modern times Yoga has spread to all corners of the world and has helped countless people. For all these reasons, the teachings of Yoga should be approached with an open mind. As with any new subject, the concepts may at first seem difficult to grasp, but once they are understood they give a profound insight into human existence.

YOGA TEXTS

References to Yoga are found throughout Indian scriptures in the form of explanations, definitions, and eulogies.

The most ancient scriptures rank among the oldest in the world. The earliest are the *Vedas,* the root of all subsequent teachings. They are considered to be revealed by God at the beginning of time and to contain eternal truth. They consist of sacred hymns, ritualistic rules and formulae, philosophical speculation, and ancient lore.

In the West, the best known part of the *Vedas* are the *Upaniṣads* – philosophical and mystical treatises and poems exploring the nature of the universal soul. The *Kaṭha Upaniṣad* speaks of the stilling of the mind and control of the senses, and the *Śvetāśvatara Upaniṣad* describes the practice and beneficial results of Yoga.

There is a set of specialist Yoga *Upaniṣads* of varying antiquity that deal with the revelation of the soul by means of meditation. The sacred syllable "aum" is given as the best object of meditation.

Other ancient works are the *Purāṇas,* dealing with cosmology and the world order. Usually meditation and the stilling of the mind are discussed but a significant reference is made in a principal *Purāṇa* – *Śrīmad Bhāgavatam* – to the therapeutic aspect of Yoga *āsanas.*

One of the earliest references to Yoga is in a ritualistic manual, *Ahirbudhnya Saṁhitā,* considered to be at least 3,000 years old. This defines Yoga as the union of the individual self with the highest Self. It outlines Yoga theory and practice, including the eight limbs enumerated by Patañjali (see p. 169). It states that two texts of Yoga were revealed in the beginning, one being "mind-restraining Yoga," and the second the "Yoga of action." These works are now lost.

In a separate category are the great epic histories, the *Rāmāyana* and *Mahābhārata,* which narrate stories of the incarnations of God. Interspersed with the narrative are discourses on moral and philosophical topics. The *Mahābhārata* is an important source of knowledge about Yoga. In the story itself the characters invariably resort to Yoga and meditation to collect their minds before any important undertaking. There are long discourses on Yoga philosophy.

The *Bhagavad Gītā (Song of the Lord)* is a great Yoga text which is still read and recited every day by millions of people in India. It forms the scriptural portion of the *Mahābhārata,* being a dialogue between God (Lord Krishna) and his devotee, Arjuna, on the eve of battle. It consists of eighteen chapters, discussing different aspects of Yoga. Among them are the Yoga of action (*karma yoga*), the Yoga of knowledge (*jñāna yoga*) and the Yoga of devotion (*bhakti yoga*). Stilling the mind by meditation is also described. Various subjects are covered: religious duty, ethical living, selfless action, stability of mind, eradication of desires, and renunciation. It deals broadly with the nature of the universe and creation, and with the glory of the soul and Divinity.

From these bodies of literature a philosophical compilation was made which brought together the entire sum of knowledge about Yoga. This is the *Yoga Sūtra* of Patañjali, also known as the *Yoga of Eight*

Limbs (Aṣṭāṅga Yoga). Its date is estimated variously to be between 200 and 800 years BC, although traditional accounts place it earlier. Patañjali's *Yoga Sūtra* is the authoritative text, recognized by all schools of Yoga, and is the source for all subsequent works.

Parallel with Yoga, five other classical systems arose, dealing with different ways of perceiving the universal truth. One of them, *Sāṁkhya* ("enumeration"), is paired with Yoga and together they provide a complete conceptual framework of the evolution and nature of the universe, and the place of man and God within it. God, the soul, and primordial matter are given as the three principles coexisting eternally.

Various Types of Yoga

After Patañjali, many other authors wrote on the subject, laying stress on one or another aspect and founding schools on their theories. Some authors interpreted and wrote commentaries on the *Yoga Sūtra,* and others specialized in the various branches of Yoga that are mentioned in the texts: *Rāja, Haṭha, Mantra,* and *Laya* Yoga (*Yoga Upaniṣads* and *Haṭha Yoga* texts) or *Bhakti, Karma,* and *Jñāna* Yoga (*Bhagavad Gītā*). These are distinct aspects of Yoga which can be followed according to individual disposition or sectarian tradition. They presuppose a certain mastery of the subject as a whole.

Rāja Yoga is the union of the mind with the soul in the transcendent state of *samādhi*. *Rāja* means mastery of the mind and senses. Patañjali's Yoga is sometimes classified as *Rāja* Yoga because it has these aims.

Haṭha Yoga (the Yoga of willpower) aims to attain liberation through the grace of the divine power (*Kuṇḍalinī*) which lies dormant in each individual. This power is aroused by means of various practices that clear the paths and centers of energy in the body. These include *āsanas;* special internal cleansing processes using water and cloth (*kriyās*); *prāṇāyāmas* designed to channel and maintain the flow of energy; and closing actions (*bandhas*), preventing the loss of energy. *Haṭha* Yoga is described in various medieval works, the most important of which are the *Haṭha Yoga Pradīpikā* of *Svātmārāma* (possibly 15th century), and the *Gheraṇḍa* and *Śiva Saṁhitās*.

In *Mantra* Yoga, perfection is attained through the recitation of sacred syllables (*mantra*). It is considered useful for those of weak intellect (*Yogatattva* and *Varāha Upaniṣads*).

In *Laya* Yoga perfection is attained through absorption (*laya*) in God (*Yogatattva* and *Varāha Upaniṣads*). This is a desireless state where sensory objects are forgotten in the experience of the ultimate bliss.

PATAÑJALI

Patañjali holds a unique position in the line of great Indian sages and benefactors of mankind. He is venerated in Indian tradition as the author of classical treatises on medicine, grammar, and Yoga. These three sciences effect the purification of the human body, speech, and mind.

He is said to be an incarnation of the serpent Ananta (meaning "The Infinite One") on whom Lord Vishnu, the preserver of the world, rests in slumber before the beginning of creation.

Patañjali was born to a saintly woman called Goṇikā who had spent her life in spiritual pursuits. He fell into her cupped hands in the form of a tiny snake as she was offering an oblation of water to the Sun. Hence he was named Patañjali, from *pata,* meaning snake or fallen, and *añjali,* meaning hands folded in prayer. He is depicted iconographically with a man's torso and the coiled tail of a serpent.

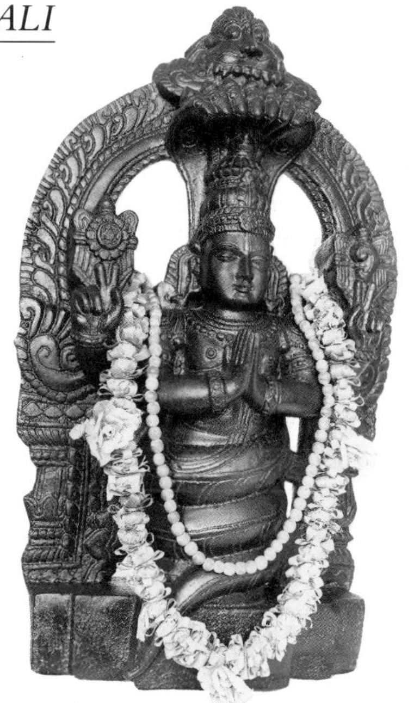

All these types of Yoga are grounded in the eight limbs of Yoga and are interconnected.

Patañjali's Yoga Sūtra

Patañjali's *Yoga Sūtra* is divided into four chapters, dealing with absorption in the universal principle (*samādhi*), practice (*sādhana*), accomplishments (*vibhūti*), and spiritual liberation (*kaivalya*). These topics are condensed into 196 aphorisms (*sūtras*).

Patañjali's work embraces all the branches of Yoga. He shows it to be a complete and internally consistent science. It has a vocabulary of carefully defined and classified technical terms and a framework of concepts, premises, practical observations, and instructions, woven together by reasoned argument and the attestation of experience. The result is a detailed delineation of the path of Yoga from beginning to end, including motivation for undertaking it, obstacles that may be met, distractions on the way, and arrival at the final goal. The goal is to clear the clouding of the intelligence, and from this enlightenment to gain liberation.

The first chapter, *Samādhi Pāda,* presents Yoga as the stilling of the fluctuations of the mind. It describes the various states of the mind and modes of consciousness from the unpredictable, changeable states which hold sway in everyday life to the sublime states of superconsciousness and deep meditation.

The second chapter, *Sādhanā Pāda,* gives the means for transforming the mind from its customary scattered state to a concentrated one that leads to the sublime. These are the eight limbs of Yoga. The first five constitute practices (*sādhanā*): ethical behavior, personal disciplines, practice of postures, breathing techniques, and control of the senses. The effects of these practices lead to the last three limbs: concentration, meditation, and the transcendent state of *samādhi*.

The third chapter, *Vibhūti Pāda,* enumerates the various powers and extrasensory perceptions which come to an accomplished Yogi. These can be a trap for the practitioner. Attachment to them can cause a break in practice and loss of previous achievements. One must progress beyond their range towards the higher goal.

The fourth chapter, *Kaivalya Pāda,* describes the final journey of the soul toward emancipation. The Yogi realizes the ultimate spiritual reality of the universe. This experienced knowledge shines forth and he is liberated from all ties to the material world.

The *Sūtras* are difficult to understand. This is partly because of their subject matter and partly because present-day life and ways of thinking seem far removed from those of ancient times. They presuppose familiarity with a host of philosophical concepts; for example, about the nature and purpose of the universe and about human psychology. They also presume a background of practical experience of Yoga.

Like other Indian classical teachings, they belong to an oral tradition where knowledge was imparted from master to disciple at first hand. Only students capable of understanding were allowed to receive instruction. This had the double benefit of maintaining a high standard and keeping the teaching pure. Although the essential doctrines have been preserved, the schools which promulgated them no longer exist and the base of understanding has largely been lost.

Commentaries on Yoga Sūtras

The *Yoga Sūtras* are the subject of a number of important explanatory commentaries. The primary and most ancient of these is by Vyāsa; it is often read together with the text itself. Other important ones span the 8th to the 18th centuries, AD. The commentaries expand, clarify and interpret the *Sūtras*.

Modern scholars have also translated and interpreted the *Yoga Sūtras,* as have sectarian schools, stressing particular aspects of Yoga. Not all write with the benefit of practice of Patañjali's Yoga to give insight into the subtle realms of Yoga.

Amongst these commentators, B.K.S. Iyengar is exceptional in having explored the various aspects of classical Yoga. Following in the tradition of Patañjali, he considers Yoga as one unified subject. All the eight limbs are made to play their part in the spiritual development of the individual. He clarifies the *Yoga Sūtras* in the light of experienced knowledge. His insights have uncovered meanings and threads of reasoning hitherto obscure in theoretical study. His interpretation is both logical and relevant to Yoga practice.

The outline of Yoga philosophy, based on explanations by B.K.S. Iyengar and his son Prashant, is taken from the following *Yoga Sūtras* of Patañjali: Chapter I, Sūtras 2, 6-15, 19, 20, 24-26, 33-39, 51; Chapter II, Sūtras 1, 6, 13, 16, 23, 30, 32, 34, 46, 49-52, 54; Chapter III, Sūtras 1-3, 7, 8, 51, 56; Chapter IV, Sūtras 10, 12, 18, 19, 24, 29, 34.

The Mystery of the Universe

Yoga is closely allied to another philosophical system called *Sāṁkhya*. *Sāṁkhya* systematizes Vedic concepts about the nature of the universe and creation. These concepts form the background to Yoga philosophy.

The universe consists of two distinct principles: matter (*prakṛti*) and spirit (*puruṣa*).

The diversity of creation is traced back on a metaphysical level to a single source. (This is a similar process to that of modern physics: here all substances are analyzed into combinations of over 100 elements which are in turn traced back to a limited number of atomic and subatomic particles. A common aim is to find the unifying principle which underlies all substances.)

The substance of the material world (*prakṛti*) is indestructible and eternal. It has three qualities (*guṇas*), which together in various combinations are present in the entire created world. They are: *sattva,* the quality of light and intelligence; *rajas,* the quality of energy and motivation; and *tamas,* the quality of mass and material substance. *Prakṛti* ranges from undifferentiated matter to phenomenal creation, the latter being definable and perceptible, and consisting of objects, senses, mind, and organs. All are pervaded by the three qualities or *guṇas.*

The spiritual entity (*puruṣa*) is the principle or essence of consciousness (*citta*) and is pure. It is indestructible and eternal. It is also known as the *ātman,* the soul or inner self of all beings. There are an infinite number of *puruṣas.*

The interaction of *prakṛti* and *puruṣa* results in creation. As matter and spirit are eternal, creation does not occur once out of nothing but follows a repeated cycle of manifestation and dissolution.

Only *Īśvara,* the Lord or Divine Principle, is unconditioned by time and the law of cause and effect. He is the fount of the universe and of all knowledge, and is the greatest of teachers. In the Yoga system he is considered a "special" or exalted *puruṣa.*

Saṁkhyā enumerates 24 constituents of creation which unfold during the evolution of the universe.

The first to evolve from primeval matter is the cosmic principle of intelligence (*mahat*). This has a high proportion of *sattva* and small quantities of *rajas* and *tamas.* It is intelligence in its seed form; it cannot be perceived but is inferred because of the existence of intelligent life in the universe. Next to evolve is the cosmic principle of ego (*ahaṁkāra*), which accounts for the fact that the created forms of the universe are individual entities. It is at this stage that name and form can be distinguished.

From the cosmic principle of ego, creation evolves into two distinct kinds: living and nonliving. The former is characterized by psychosensory features and a high proportion of the principles of intelligence, ego, and mind. These all fall under the category of *sattva.* Living creation is also distinguished according to the *guṇas,* human beings having more *sattva* in their make-up than animals and plants.

Psychosensory creation begins with the mind (*manas*). From this evolve the five cognitive senses of eyes, ears, nose, tongue, and skin, and the five organs of action, arms, legs, speech, generative organ, and excretory organ. The mind consists of four faculties: the gathering mind, also called *manas;* consciousness (*citta*); intelligence (*buddhi*); and ego or the principle of individual identity (*ahaṁkāra*). These are the instruments through which the individual is able to function intellectually, emotionally, and physically.

In Indian philosophy the mind is classified as matter, not as spirit. Spirit is unchanging in its essential nature, whereas mind and matter are changeable, subject to the *guṇas,* and characterized by waves and fluctuations. Again, it is interesting to note here that in modern physics there is an essential equivalence between energy and matter.

Matter forms the covering for the spiritual entities. It constitutes both the external world and the means to perceive it. The conjunction of the material with the spiritual gives rise to experience.

The second kind of creation is nonsentient. It begins with the infra-atomic structure of the elemental principles of earth, water, fire, air, and ether. These then evolve into the five gross elements. The gross elements are not the physical substances of earth, water, and so on, but the principles inherent in them. By the term "earth" should be understood the principles of solidity, heaviness, and smell; by "water," liquidity, coolness, and taste; by "fire," luminosity, heat, and form; by "air," gaseousness, motion, and touch; and by "ether," sound, space, and the property of contraction and expansion.

The various combinations and proportions of elements, senses, and organs, with different permutations of the three *guṇas,* account for the diversity of created forms in the universe.

It is important for a Yogi to know the stages of evolution of the universe, since the goal is identification with the ultimate principle. To achieve this, Yoga reverses the process of evolution, tracing it back from the senses and mind to the inner self. The essential identity of the soul with the ultimate principle of existence, the substratum of the universe, is realized. At the gross level, the body and mind, through a gradual progression, become more *sattvic.* The Yogi proceeds, through the discipline of the eight stages of Yoga, towards identification with the Infinite.

The Nature of Experience

The purpose of creation is to serve the individual being. The material world gives experience. When the experiences of life are drawn on to gain spiritual wisdom, this leads the soul towards liberation. Yoga philosophy deals in detail with the nature of experience and the need for a positive outlook.

Experience is of three types: pleasurable, painful, and delusive. The first two categories relate to rational action, in search of pleasure and avoidance of pain. In delusive experience the intelligence is clouded, and actions are impulsive, without regard to the result.

Yoga philosophy observes that living in the world is bound up with pain and suffering, and takes the view that all suffering – whether physical, mental, or spiritual – is unwelcome. It teaches that it is desirable and possible to be liberated from it. Patañjali says, "*heyham duhkham anāgatam*" (II.16) – "avoid the sorrows which are to come": an injunction to practice Yoga for strength to meet possible future misfortunes.

Pleasure is desired by all, but it is linked to pain. When it comes to an end, it may bring a sense of loss. Thus, in the ultimate analysis pleasure, too, is unwelcome and one should strive to be free from attachment to it. This requires the cultivation of a dispassionate frame of mind.

The experiences and situations of life are determined by past actions. Attachments and aversions cause one to act, and, according to the universal law of cause and effect, each action has repercussions. These reactions again prompt further actions and one is caught up in the wheel of life. In this way, embodied souls assume incarnation over and over again.

The Nature of Consciousness

Consciousness fluctuates between five states (*vṛttis*), meaning literally "versions." The first is real perception or correct knowledge (*pramāṇa*) which must be based on direct perception, inference, or reliable testimony, such as that of the scriptures. The second is illusion (*viparyaya*), based on false perception. The third state is imagination (*vikalpa*), where ideas have no substance and do not correspond to actuality. The fourth state is sleep (*nidrā*), where consciousness is inactive. The fifth state is memory (*smṛti*), whereby experiences are stored in the mind.

There are five types of human afflictions (*kleśas*): lack of spiritual wisdom; egoism or individualism; attachment to pleasure; aversion to pain; and holding onto life.

These afflictions form part of the infrastructure that shapes the conscious mind. The infrastructure also consists of subliminal impressions (*saṁskāras*), gained from past experiences, giving the mind its particular dispositions and propensities. These two together – *kleśas* and *saṁskāras* – form the subtle body of each individual, which is not destroyed at death but transmigrates from birth to birth and accounts for the diversity of characters and experiences in the world.

Consciousness has two modes – negative and positive – which incline the mind toward mundane ends or toward spiritual and religious goals. The former mode is called "painful," as it generates the *kleśas* through attachment to the experiences of the world. The latter is "non-painful," as it eradicates the *kleśas.*

The removal of the afflictions brings about a state of absolute tranquillity called *citta prasādanam.* This peace of mind does not come easily but has to be cultivated. There are various ways of doing this, according to one's temperament and inclination.

In order to avoid emotional disturbance, it is important to know how to react to people and circumstances. Where there is happinesss, one should be friendly; where there is misery, one should be compassionate; where there is virtue, one should rejoice; and where there is wickedness, one should be indifferent. Any other kind of reaction – for example, jealousy, anger, indignation, or resentment – does not engender peace.

Thoughts, emotions, and deeds that go against ethical precepts result in pain and ignorance. They are caused by greed, anger, or delusion. These negative states of mind lead to unpleasant consequences, which unsettle the mind further. They need to be checked by the practice of Yoga.

The mind can be quietened through breathing practices, and a particular *prāṇāyāma* of retaining the breath after exhalation is mentioned. Meditation also stills the mind. Consciousness is brought to bear on a sublime, uplifting object or experience, such as the exemplary life of a saint, or religious worship.

In these ways the obstacles that disturb the calmness of mind are overcome. The serene state attained is *citta vṛtti nirodhaḥ,* the restraint of the fluctuations of consciousness, which Patañjali gives as the definition of Yoga at the very beginning of the *Yoga Sūtra* (I.2). This is *samādhi,* where consciousness becomes pure and can be used as an instrument to reveal the ultimate truth of existence. Here the body is under complete control and is at one with mind and soul. The identity of the soul with the universal spirit is realized.

THE EIGHT LIMBS OF YOGA

Yoga is classically divided into eight aspects or limbs, *aṣṭāṅga*. The limbs are interlinked; each has numerous facets that are revealed through study of the texts and by practice. They lead progressively to the highest stages of awareness and to spiritual life. Their disciplines become more and more internal.

The limbs are as follows:

(i) *Yama*

This consists of the ethical precepts of nonviolence (*ahiṁsā*), truthfulness (*satya*), nonstealing (*asteya*), chastity (*brahmacarya*), and finally, noncovetousness (*aparigraha*).

These principles of right living are universal and form the foundation of Yoga. The essence of *Yama* is not to harm any living creature in either thought, word, or deed.

The translation of concepts here is only approximate. Each has a range of meanings and applications that vary according to one's own circumstances and stage of progress.

(ii) *Niyama*

These are personal practices to be observed. They are cleanliness of mind and body (*śauca*), contentment (*santoṣa*), fervor for the subject (*tapas*), study of the self (*svādhyāya*), and surrender of all thoughts and actions to God (*Īśvarapraṇidhāna*).

Niyama establishes discipline in daily life.

(iii) *Āsanas*

These are the Yoga postures. *Āsanas* are described as having the properties of being steady (*sthira*), and joyful (*sukham*). Long continued efforts are necessary to attain mastery and perfection. Body and mind move in harmony and become absorbed in the infinite. All dualities of mind cease.

Patañjali does not mention any *āsanas* by name, but a tradition of *āsana* practice is implied. Some postures are given in the various commentaries on his work and in other Yoga texts. Traditionally there are said to be 840,000 *āsanas,* corresponding to the full potential of human movement. Systematic, precise practice of *āsanas* died out in India after Patañjali's time. In recent years the range and depth of the *āsanas* are becoming known again, through the work of B.K.S. Iyengar.

(iv) *Prāṇāyāma*

This is the art of Yoga breathing, consisting of the regulation and refinement of the inhalation, exhalation, and retention of breath. Learning to control and channel the life breath induces an introspective attitude and opens the gateway to spiritual knowledge.

Prāṇāyāma should be learned only after a degree of proficiency has been gained in the *āsanas.*

Breath consists of the gross element of air and *prāṇa,* the life force pervading the universe. *Prāṇa* is the communicating link between the human organism and the cosmos. As it consists of energy, strong warnings are given in all traditional Yoga texts against the practice of *prāṇāyāma* without supervision, and before a student is ready.

(v) *Pratyāhāra*

This is the drawing in of the senses from the external world into the interior self. External disturbances and distractions are unable to cross the threshold of the inner world.

(vi) *Dhāraṇā*

This is uninterrupted concentration, with the mind focused steadily on a particular point or object. Constant practice is needed to achieve this.

(vii) ***Dhyāna***

This is meditation. The span of concentration is increased so that the whole mind encompasses the object and contemplates it unwaveringly. Subject and object draw near each other.

(viii) ***Samādhi***

This is a transcending state beyond meditation where the psychological process stops as consciousness becomes totally absorbed in the soul. It is a state of truth and bliss.

Samādhi is the culmination of Yoga practice and is rarely attained. It is divided into a number of levels of spiritual evolution relating to more and more subtle realms. The pinnacle is described as "*samādhi* without seed" where there are no imprints of actions and desires in the mind. This is also known as *kaivalya* or the isolation of the soul from matter. The Yogi has completed the involutionary journey toward the source and substratum of creation and is liberated.

The first five limbs, *yama, niyama, āsana, prāṇāyāma,* and *pratyāhāra,* are known as the disciplines (*sādhanā*) of Yoga. They are to be undertaken with undiminished efforts and a spirit of detachment from the attractions of the world.

They still the mind and senses, and prepare the ground for *dhāraṇā, dhyāna,* and *samādhi.* These three are classed as attainments of Yoga.

The heightened states of consciousness engendered by *dhāraṇā, dhyāna,* and *samādhi* result in spiritual wisdom. They also bring various supernormal attainments (*siddhis*), according to the object of meditation. Some are within the range of human experience, such as clairvoyance, clairaudience, and the ability to read minds. Others seem more extraordinary, such as the conquest of hunger and thirst or the ability to become light or heavy, small or large.

The *siddhis* are an indication that the Yogi is on the right path. He develops nonattachment toward them as they do not fulfil his ultimate aim.

When the soul is free from the entanglement with nature, it can revert to its original, pure state. The Yogi has eradicated the imprints and desires that are deeply embedded in the consciousness. He has broken the chain of cause and effect, and thus of time. Past and future having no relevance for him, he exists in the eternal present.

He is able to differentiate between consciousness and the soul. He realizes that consciousness acts in conjunction with the mind, intellect, and senses to enable him to function in the world.

Meditation is focused on the self and there ensues the highest religious experience, where virtue and enlightenment pour forth. The true self is revealed in its shining purity. This unwavering state is known as the ultimate liberation (*kaivalya*).

PART III
THE SOUL

DHYĀNA & SURRENDER

"When the sun has set, and the moon has set, and the fire has gone out, and speech has stopped, what light does a person here have?" "The soul, indeed, is his light," said he, "for with the soul, indeed, as the light, one sits, moves about, does one's work, and returns."

BṚHADĀRAṆYAKA UPANIṢAD, IV.3.6.

Surrender of the Self

The mind is drawn to surrender to the Infinite One. This surrender, by breaking the chain of distracting thoughts, increases the intensity of one's concentration.

B.K.S. IYENGAR

The third cornerstone of the practice of Yoga is *Īśvarapraṇidhāna*. It involves surrendering oneself to God, in order to reveal the soul. It leads to inner peace, answering the deepest need of mankind, and brings fulfilment of the soul.

Experiencing Inner Peace

Inner peace is the absence of internal and external conflict. The conscience is clear and there is strength to sustain others. The mind is undisturbed by mundane desires; neither is it and is not shaken by circumstances. There is harmony in the soul as it rests in the divine.

In Indian philosophy the soul is analyzed, pictured, and located. Situated in the spiritual heart at the base of the center of the chest cavity, its light is hidden for the majority of people, but shines in saints and Yogis. It is subtle yet powerful. It is linked to the universal spirit, God, who is considered to be within as well as outside oneself.

Everyone has a soul, and through Yoga the soul can be unveiled.

The practice of Yoga has up till now brought the aspirant a great deal of knowledge. At the same time it is realized that the individual is insignificant in the face of the Supreme. By letting go of personal pride, the experience of Yoga is carried into a deeper dimension, where God becomes the guide.

God can be understood as a personal deity or as the abstract principle of Truth and Perfection. According to Indian philosophy, there are six primary divine qualities. These are true knowledge, strength, mastery of the body, mind and self, unshakeable firmness, the power to break limitations, and energy. As the Yogi proceeds on his journey toward the ultimate goal, he strives to make them manifest in himself. The perfect Yogi is endowed with beauty, grace, strength, and luster, which Patañjali calls the "wealth of the body."

The grace of God is necessary to gain a glimpse of the soul. *Īśvarapraṇidhāna* is a devotional act. It involves humility and love.

Surrender of the self means giving up egotism, the sense of the "I" – the smaller or selfish self. The subjective involvement in "I see," "I want," "I do" must be shed so that actions do not disturb the inner being.

In this way Yoga is a philosophy within a religious framework. The individual is not required to believe in any religious dogma and there are no prescribed modes of worship. According to Patañjali, the practitioner can be of any religious persuasion and, true to this, many people find that their personal belief is strengthened through their practice.

The interpretation of how Yoga philosophy relates to practice is based on the following *Yoga Sūtras* of Patañjali: Chapter I, Sūtras 2, 20-22, 24-26, 28, 33-39, 49; Chapter II, Sūtra 48; Chapter III: Sūtra 47; Chapter IV: Sūtras 25-26.

Synthesis of the Limbs of Yoga

All the limbs of Yoga play their part in achieving this state of harmony. *Yama* gives a basis of moral behavior. *Niyama* develops a self-disciplined and contented mind. *Āsana* builds a healthy, strong body; this has a direct impact on the state of the mind. *Prāṇāyāma* and *pratyāhāra* develop tranquillity, which forms a receptive base for meditative practices. *Dhāraṇā* and *dhyāna* enhance the state of inner peace, preparing the soul for immersion in the bliss of *samādhi*, the union of the soul with the divine.

Āsana is the first conscious step on the path of Yoga. From then on all the limbs are integrated to some extent. *Āsana* practice involves being ethical and disciplined, extending the breath, and drawing the senses away from the exterior world. Concentration and meditation bring about complete absorption in it.

In order to channel effort in the right direction and lay the foundation for success, five positive qualities are necessary. These are faith (*śraddhā*), vigor (*vīrya*), memory (*smṛti*), absorption (*samādhi*), and wisdom (*prajñā*).

Faith is based on subjective experience; it is not just idealistic or blind belief. Vigor relates to the amount of mental and physical effort put into practice. Memory involves assimilating knowledge and recalling experience. It spurs the intelligence. Absorption is keeping the attention within the framework of the subject. Wisdom results from this absorption. Based on sure self-knowledge, it broadens to an understanding of others.

Three steps are required to reach the state of absorption: repetition, understanding, and sincerity of purpose. Progress will be more rapid if these are borne in mind. The steps apply to all aspects of Yoga, but here the *āsanas* are taken, by way of example.

The first step is to become familiar with the object desired. In the case of an *āsana,* the name and meaning of the *āsana* should be known as they symbolize its inner essence. Its form should be studied in order to perfect the minute details which define it. Repetition molds the body into its shape and imprints the subtle aspect of its name into the consciousness.

The second step involves total attention, giving body, mind, and heart to the *āsana.* One has to reflect while performing it, in order to realize its full potential. An attitude of humility and receptivity is essential to catch any light of knowledge that comes.

The third step is intensely personal, where knowledge and commitment deepen. The Yoga practice becomes more important than the person performing it, so that the ego is subdued. Practice becomes necessary to life. The *āsana* becomes a friend to turn to in time of need. Finally one surrenders completely and becomes immersed in the *āsana.*

In this way the practice of Yoga becomes an act of devotion. The spirit in which the sacred syllable "aum," or any prayer, is repeated to achieve meditation permeates all actions.

Meditation in Action

When the self, mind, intelligence, and consciousness extend together with the inner organs and the outer body, the self and its vehicle, the body, become one. Then there are no dualities. This unified state gives a taste of *citta vṛtti nirodhaḥ,* the state where the fluctuations of the mind cease.

When the *āsanas* are performed in this way, this is dynamic meditation. The mind is alert and active; it moves with every action of the body and penetrates every remote cell.

Thus, in order to keep the knee straight, attention is focused on the knee. This is concentration. Then, holding the attention there, the mind moves to the next focus – thigh, hip, waist, and so on – and from there to another part of the body, and another, until attention is diffused all over the body without any lessening of intensity. This is meditation.

The intensity of involvement should not be greater in one area than another. When it is even, there is no oscillation in the mind. It does not move to the past or future but dwells in the present.

At this time the analytical part of the brain remains passive and the meditative brain observes the body from within. There is a feeling of internal peace. This experience is indescribable. It spurs the practitioner to continue the search for the soul.

B.K.S. Iyengar describes this as meditation in action, where the inner being expresses itself on the surface during the performance of the *āsanas.* This is distinguished from passive meditation, where one sits in a meditative pose, drawing the senses inward and communing with the deity within.

The Expression of the Soul

When the body is mastered through *āsana,* the mind controlled through *prāṇāyāma* and the senses subdued through *pratyāhāra,* the fruit of Yoga practice is experienced. Consciousness is focused on the spiritual center, to make contact with the soul.

Knowledge of the soul goes beyond sensory perception and rational thought, as all these belong to the realm of nature (*prakṛti*). In meditation on gross objects, such as on a rose or flame, the psychological faculty is being used, since these objects can be apprehended by the senses. This is not Yoga meditation.

In Yoga, the mind must be disengaged from gross objects and from the senses and focused on higher, subtler realms. Thus the highest knowledge is gained through revelation or intuition. Yoga is a training to develop the intuitive faculty and bring about the sublimation of the senses and mind.

When the senses and mind are transcended, experience is of the soul alone. The physical, physiological, and mental functions are at peace and there is absolute stillness of the consciousness (*citta vṛtti nirodhaḥ*).

Consciousness is in its pure, pristine state. It is compared to a flawless crystal that reflects objects in their true form. Similarly, consciousness reveals the essential, intangible core of all objects. This intuitive vision of the Truth is the highest wisdom. It can penetrate the mystery of the universe and the reality of existence. It is the acme of human experience. It is the expression of the soul.

ध्यान

Dhyāna

Meditation does not make the mind dull. Rather, in meditation the mind is still but razor sharp, silent but vibrant with energy. But this state cannot be achieved without a firm, stable sitting posture, where the spine ascends and the mind descends and dissolves in the consciousness of the heart, where the true Self reveals itself.

B.K.S. IYENGAR

Meditation is a state of timelessness where everyday concerns have no relevance. It is beyond psychological time and space. It connects the spiritual core of the individual consciously with the infinite universe. Meditation gives the experience of bliss.

GUIDELINES FOR PRACTICE

Meditation is not for beginners.

It is practiced after a regular routine of prāṇāyāma has become established. Prāṇāyāma trains the body to be steady and the mind to concentrate.

It may be practiced after prāṇāyāma or by itself.

It is not easy to do meditation, as the mind does not stay still long and reverts to mundane thoughts. Honest practice is essential: if the mind refuses to concentrate, it is better to accept this and try again another day.

Though the technique of sitting in meditation should be followed, meditation itself is a state of being which cannot be learned. Practice alone is not a guarantee of attaining it, or of recapturing it when once experienced. The experience comes when one is ready for it.

Caution

Do not do meditation if suffering from depression or from a nervous breakdown.

TECHNIQUE FOR DHYĀNA

Sit in Padmāsana (p. 54), or any posture used in meditation. Keep the spine erect and the head straight. Compose the body and mind. Draw the upper lids down to close the eyes.

Raise the arms and lightly join the palms in front of the chest; point the thumbs toward the base of the sternum, and the fingers away from the chest. Bring the chest slightly forward and take the elbows down and back toward the waist. Extend the palms toward the fingertips; lightly tuck in the skin of the backs of the hands and knuckles toward the bones. Relax the wrists.

STAGE 1

Withdraw the gaze of the eyes from the lids and relax the eyeballs. Withdraw the hearing from the openings of the ears. Withdraw the breath from contact with the nostrils, keeping it as fine and subtle as possible. Withdraw sensation from the front of the tongue.

At a very subtle level, withdraw the flesh of the body from the skin. Withdraw the skull from the scalp and the brain from the skull. Be more aware in the back brain at the base of the skull than in the front brain near the forehead.

Let the eyes exist in the eyes, the ears in the ears, the nose in the nose, and the tongue in the tongue; let the skin of the body rest in itself. Experience the silence that comes.

Experience the refinement of the consciousness.

STAGE 2

Draw the sight and hearing, and the sensation in the tongue, inward. Let them descend and meet at the site of the soul behind the sternum at the base.

Let the thumbs salute and merge in the soul; let the fingers salute and merge in the universal.

AUM

At the end of the practice, carefully release the hands and lie down. Slowly open the eyes and come to normal, before getting up.

Remain quiet for some time without communicating with others.

Courses

The courses on the following pages have been designed to enable students to practice systematically. Course I is for beginners; Course II is for students at a general level of practice; Course III is for those at intermediate level; and Course IV is for advanced students. Postures marked with one diamond in the *Āsana* section are found in Course I, those with two diamonds in Course II, and so on. Sometimes the intermediate stage of a more difficult posture is introduced in an earlier course.

The *āsanas* are introduced in their appropriate context and their progression is structured. Most of the postures may be repeated two or three times, except for Śīrṣāsana and Sarvāṅgāsana. The courses include repetition and consolidation.

Guidance is given on how to evaluate progress, and when to proceed further. This depends on the frequency and duration of practice and on natural aptitude.

Course I introduces the basic *āsanas*. The succeeding courses build on this original foundation. In Courses II to IV the lessons are grouped into monthly cycles, with a different emphasis of postures each week of the month. This results in a variety of lessons.

There is, however, an underlying unity. Each lesson starts with postures that extend the body or collect the mind, then intensifies, and ends with postures that stabilize the practice.

Inverted postures are normally done every time. Relaxation should not be neglected.

During menstruation the sequence of lessons should not be continued. Suitable *āsanas* are given on p. 187.

COURSE I

This course consists of 12 lessons. It contains the āsanas that can safely be done by beginners. First their shape should be studied and gradually details incorporated to make the postures more correct.

The emphasis is on learning the standing poses, through which the body gains strength and coordination. Other postures are given to widen the scope of learning, to develop agility, and to relax.

Together with the physical aspect of the postures, glimpses come of a meditative, silent quality. In this way the postures are both exhilarating and relaxing.

It is beneficial to practice for a short time every day, rather than a longer session once a week. If practicing every day, spend two days a week doing sitting poses, inverted poses, and relaxation, omitting the standing poses.

Those who practice less often will take longer to gain a basic knowledge of the postures contained in the course.

Caution *Take particular care of the knees. Learn to straighten and extend them without straining.*

SUGGESTED SCHEME OF PRACTICE

Alternate lessons 1 and 2 in the first week, then lessons 2 and 3 in the second week, and so on until by week 12 all lessons have been done twice. Finally, consolidate practice by repeating all the lessons once more.

Lesson 1

Sukhāsana (p. 53) and Parvatāsana (p. 51); Tāḍāsana (p. 18); Ūrdhva Hastāsana (p. 19); Vṛkṣāsana (p. 21); Utthita Trikoṇāsana (p. 22); Utthita Pārśvakoṇāsana (p. 24); Vīrabhadrāsana II (p. 28); Pārśvottānāsana on ledge (p. 40); Uttānāsana I (p. 44), hands on ledge; Sukhāsana; Sarvāṅgāsana (p. 108); Ardha Halāsana (p. 110); lying, legs bent over abdomen (p. 85); Śavāsana I (p. 150).

☐ Do Uttānāsana I between standing poses or after 2 poses, to rest. If back aches, place hands on ledge. Repeat standing poses twice each. Learn to adjust height of blankets in Sarvāṅgāsana. If Sarvāṅgāsana is difficult, lie with legs up against a wall (p. 80).

Lesson 2

Sukhāsana and Parvatāsana (p. 53); Utthita Hasta Pādāṅguṣṭhāsana I and II (p. 20); Tāḍāsana (p. 18); Vṛkṣāsana (p. 21); Trikoṇāsana (p. 22); Pārśvakoṇāsana (p. 24); Vīrabhadrāsana I (p. 26), hands on waist; Vīrabhadrāsana II (p. 28); Pārṣvottānāsana (p. 40), catching the elbows; Uttānāsana I (p. 44), hands on ledge; Vīrāsana and Vīrāsana forward bend (pp. 50-51); Gomukhāsana (p. 56), arms only; Sarvāṅgāsana (p. 108); Ardha Halāsana (p. 110); Śavāsana I (p. 150).

☐ Rest in Uttānāsana I after Vīrabhadrāsana I. Before doing Sarvāṅgāsana, lie down and stretch. In Śavāsana, learn to lie straight.

Lesson 3

Vīrāsana (p. 50); Utthita Hasta Pādāṅguṣṭhāsana I and II (p. 20); Uttānāsana I (p. 44), hands on ledge; Trikoṇāsana (p. 22); Pārśvakoṇāsana (p. 24); Vīrabhadrāsana I (p. 26); Uttānāsana I (p. 44); Vīrabhadrāsana II (p. 28); Pārśvottānāsana (p. 40); Prasārita Pādottānāsana (p. 42); Vīrāsana and Vīrāsana forward bend (pp. 50-51); Sukhāsana (p. 53); Gomukhāsana (p. 56), arms only; Sarvāṅgāsana (p. 108); Halāsana or Ardha Halāsana (p. 110); Śavāsana I (p. 150).

☐ Keep arms up in Vīrabhadrāsana I. Trikoṇāsana, Pārśvakoṇāsana, Vīrabhadrāsana I, Vīrabhadrāsana II, and Pārśvottānāsana are the five basic standing poses.

Lesson 4

Vīrāsana (p. 50); Adho Mukha Śvānāsana (p. 90); Vīrāsana forward bend (p. 51); Tāḍāsana (p. 18); Trikoṇāsana (p. 22); Pārśvakoṇāsana (p. 24); Vīrabhadrāsana I (p. 26); Uttānāsana I (p. 44); Vīrabhadrāsana II (p. 28); Pārśvottānāsana (p. 40); Garuḍāsana (p. 46); Utkaṭāsana (p. 47); Adho Mukha Śvānāsana (p. 90); Parvatāsana in Vīrāsana (p. 51); Vīrāsana forward bend (p. 51); Sarvāṅgāsana (p. 108); Ardha Halāsana or Halāsana (p. 110); Śavāsana I (p. 150).

□ Do Adho Mukha Śvānāsana by walking back from Uttānāsana. Do standing poses with back against wall.

Lesson 5

Tāḍāsana (p. 18); Trikoṇāsana (p. 22); Pārśva Koṇāsana (p. 24); Vīrabhadrāsana I (p. 26); Uttānāsana I (p. 44); Vīrabhadrāsana II (p. 28); Pārśvottānāsana (p. 40); Marīcyāsana, standing (p. 70); Bharadvājāsana on chair (p. 71); Vīrāsana and forward bend (pp. 50-51); Sarvāṅgāsana (p. 108); Halāsana (p. 110); Jaṭhara Parivartanāsana variation (p. 85) with legs bent; Śavāsana I (p. 150).

□ Do standing poses with one foot against wall. Lie down and stretch before doing Sarvāṅgāsana.

Lesson 6

Lying on cross bolsters (p. 80); Uttānāsana I (p. 44); Adho Mukha Śvānāsana (p. 90); Vīrāsana and Parvatāsana (pp. 50-51); Sukhāsana and Parvatāsana (p. 53); Triaṅg Mukhaikapāda Paścimottānāsana (p. 61); Paścimottānāsana (p. 64); Sarvāṅgāsana (p. 108); Halāsana (p. 110); Viparīta Karaṇī (p. 122).

□ In Vīrāsana pay attention to line of bent legs and to understanding whether knees are relaxed or strained. In Triaṅg Mukhaikapāda Paścimottānāsana and Paścimottānāsana use a belt to get a concave action of back.

Lesson 7

Utthita Hasta Pādāṅguṣṭhāsana I and II (pp. 20-21); Tāḍāsana (p. 18); Vṛkṣāsana (p. 21); Trikoṇāsana (p. 22); Pārśva Koṇāsana (p. 24); Vīrabhadrāsana I (p. 26); Vīrabhadrāsana II (p. 28); Ardha Candrāsana (p. 30); Vīrabhadrāsana III (p. 32), hands on ledge; Pārśvottānāsana (p. 40); Prasārita Pādottānāsana I (p. 42); Vīrāsana and forward bend (pp. 50-51); Daṇḍāsana (p. 52); Paripūrṇa Nāvāsana (p. 58); Jānuśīrṣāsana (p. 59), head up; Triaṅg Mukhaikapāda Paścimottānāsana (p. 61); Paścimottānāsana (p. 64); Sarvāṅgāsana (p. 108); Halāsana (p. 110); Śavāsana I (p. 150).

□ Bend forward in Uttānāsana I after Vīrabhadrāsana I if necessary. Do Ardha Candrāsana against a wall. Use a belt and keep head up for Jānuśīrṣāsana, Triaṅg Mukhaikapāda Paścimottānāsana, and Paścimottānāsana.

Lesson 8

Adho Mukha Śvānāsana (p. 90); Uttānāsana I (p. 44); Tāḍāsana (p. 18); Trikoṇāsana (p. 22); Pārśva Koṇāsana (p. 24); Vīrabhadrāsana I (p. 26); Vīrabhadrāsana II (p. 28); Ardha Candrāsana (p. 30); Pārśvottānāsana (p. 40); Vīrāsana (p. 50); Sukhāsana (p. 53); Baddha Koṇāsana (p. 57); Sarvāṅgāsana (p. 108); Halāsana (p. 110); Sarvāṅgāsana (p. 108); Eka Pāda Sarvāṅgāsana (p. 111); Pārśvaikapāda Sarvāṅgāsana (p. 111); Supta Baddha Koṇāsana (p. 81), without bolster; Śavāsana I (p. 150).

□ In Pārśvottānāsana, practice alternative method, keeping head down while going to other side through center.

Lesson 9

Lying with the legs up (p. 80); Adho Mukha Śvānāsana (p. 90); Tāḍāsana (p. 18); Trikoṇāsana (p. 22); Pārśva Koṇāsana (p. 24); Vīrabhadrāsana I (p. 26); Vīrabhadrāsana II (p. 28); Ardha Candrāsana (p. 30); Vīrabhadrāsana III (p. 32), hands on ledge; Pārśvottānāsana (p. 40); Parīghāsana (p. 48); Uṣṭrāsana (p. 134); Ūrdhva Mukha Śvānāsana (p. 91); Adho Mukha Śvānāsana (p. 90); Sarvāṅgāsana (p. 108); Halāsana (p. 110); Śavāsana I (p. 150).

□ Do Uṣṭrāsana with support if preferred.

Lesson 10

Tāḍāsana (p. 18); Vṛkṣāsana (p. 21); Garuḍāsana (p. 46); Utkaṭāsana (p. 47); Parīghāsana (p. 48); Sukhāsana and Parvātāsana (p. 53); Sukhāsana forward bend (p. 53); Vīrāsana (p. 50); Baddha Koṇāsana (p. 57); Bharadvājāsana I (p. 72); Sarvāṅgāsana (p. 108); Halāsana (p. 110); Eka Pāda Sarvāṅgāsana (p. 111); Pārśvaikapāda Sarvāṅgāsana (p. 111); Ūrdhva Prasārita Pādāsana (p. 84), step 4 only; Śavāsana I (p. 150).

□ In Bharadvājāsana I, do not complete the posture but work in intermediate stage with the hands on the floor. In Ūrdhva Prasārita Pādāsana, bend the knees over the abdomen and then stretch the legs up.

Lesson 11

Marīcyāsana, standing (p. 70); Bharadvājāsana on chair (p. 71); Tāḍāsana (p. 18); Trikoṇāsana (p. 22); Pārśva Koṇāsana (p. 24); Vīrabhadrāsana I (p. 26); Vīrabhadrāsana II (p. 28); Ardha Candrāsana (p. 30); Pārśvottānāsana (p. 40); Prasārita Pādottānāsana (p. 42); Sarvāṅgāsana (p. 108); Halāsana (p. 110); Śavāsana I (p. 150).

□ Start to increase timings in Sarvāṅgāsana and Halāsana.

Lesson 12

Uttānāsana I (p. 44); Adho Mukha Śvānāsana (p. 90); Ūrdhva Mukha Śvānāsana (p. 91); Adho Mukha Śvānāsana (p. 90); Vīrāsana (p. 50); Daṇḍāsana (p. 52); Paripūrṇa Nāvāsana (p. 58); Jānu Śīrṣāsana (p. 59); Triaṅg Mukhaikapāda Paścimottānāsana (p. 61); Paścimottānāsana (p. 64); Baddha Koṇāsana (p. 57); Upaviṣṭa Koṇāsana (p. 65), step 1; Bharadvājāsana I (p. 72); Sarvāṅgāsana (p. 108); Halāsana (p. 110); Śavāsana I (p. 150).

□ Repeat sitting poses twice. In Bharadvājāsana I, remain in intermediate stage.

COURSE II

This course contains 36 lessons. It gives a general background consisting of sitting poses, twists, and prone, supine, and inverted poses. As stability is gained in the practice of these postures, simple backbends and prāṇāyāma are also introduced.

Practice can be structured by concentrating on different parts of the body in each lesson. For instance, in one lesson, the theme can be the extension of the feet; in another, the line of the legs; in another, the turn of the hips, and so on.

Here the details given in "Work in the posture" and in the focuses will be found helpful.

One posture a day can be chosen for doing more thoroughly and thoughtfully. In this way the quality of practice will improve.

The lessons are classified into four groups, according to which particular group of postures predominates:
A: Standing Poses, B: Sitting Poses, C: Miscellaneous Poses or Backbends, and D: Relaxation and Prāṇāyāma. These may be done every month in rotation.

SUGGESTED SCHEME OF PRACTICE

The following is a suggested course for daily practice. With time spent consolidating, it takes about 18 months to complete. Lessons A, B, C, and D relate to each week of practice. In the first month, alternate lessons 1A and 2A, 1B and 2B, 1C and 2C, and 1D and 2D. Then repeat the first month. In the third month, alternate lessons 2A and 3A and repeat 1A; 2B and 3B and repeat 1B; 2C and 3C and repeat 1C; and 2D and 3D and repeat 1D. In the fourth month, consolidate practice so far. Repeat this scheme of practice through lessons 4 to 9, consolidating practice after lessons 3, 6, and 9 by repeating the previous 3 months' lessons. Finally, after lesson 9, spend six months consolidating all the lessons: 1-9, A-D.

Lesson 1A (Standing)

Utthita Hasta Pādāṅguṣṭhāsana I and II (pp. 20-21); Tāḍāsana (p.18); Trikoṇāsana (p. 22); Pārśva Koṇāsana (p. 24); Vīrabhadrāsana I (p. 26); Vīrabhadrāsana II (p. 28); Ardha Candrāsana (p. 30); Vīrabhadrāsana III (p. 32); Parivṛtta Trikoṇāsana (p. 34); Pārśvottānāsana (p. 40); Prasārita Pādottānāsana I (p. 42); Uttānāsana II (p. 45); Vīrāsana forward bend (p. 51); Supta Pādāṅguṣṭhāsana (p. 88), steps 2 and 3 only; Ardha Halāsana (p. 110); Śavāsana I (p.150).

☐ Do Parivṛtta Trikoṇāsana with back foot against a wall and keep hand on a brick. In Pārśvottānāsana, do alternative method. Do not jump feet together at end but spread them, release hands and go into Prasārita Pādottānāsana I.

Lesson 1B (Sitting)

Uttānāsana I (p. 44); Adho Mukha Śvānāsana (p. 90); Daṇḍāsana (p. 52); Jānu Śīrṣāsana (p. 59); Ardha Baddha Padma Paścimottānāsana (p. 60); Triaṅg Mukhaikapāda Paścimottānāsana (p. 61); Marīcyāsana I (p. 63); Paścimottānāsana (p. 64); Bharadvājāsana I (p. 72); Marīcyāsana III (p. 73); Sarvāṅgāsana (p. 108); Halāsana (p. 110); Supta Koṇāsana (p. 113); Karṇapīḍāsana (p. 112); Halāsana (p. 110); Śavāsana I (p. 150).

☐ Jānu Śīrṣāsana, Ardha Baddha Padma Paścimottānāsana, Triaṅg Mukhaikapāda Paścimottānāsana, Marīcyāsana I, and Paścimottānāsana are the five basic forward bends. Repeat each twice. In Marīcyāsana I, first bend forward only; then repeat pose and turn. In twists, do intermediate stages only.

Lesson 1C (Miscellaneous)

Tāḍāsana (p. 18); Trikoṇāsana (p. 22); Pārśva Koṇāsana (p. 24); Vīrabhadrāsana I (p. 26); Uttānāsana I (p. 44); Vīrabhadrāsana II (p. 28); Ardha Candrāsana (p. 30); Parivṛtta Trikoṇāsana (p. 34); Parivṛtta Pārśva Koṇāsana (p. 36); Parivṛtta Ardha Candrāsana (p. 38); Pārśvottānāsana (p. 40); Vīrāsana forward bend (p. 51); Ūrdhva Prasārita Pādāsana (p. 84); Sarvāṅgāsana (p. 108); Halāsana (p. 110); Śavāsana I (p. 150).

☐ In Ūrdhva Prasārita Pādāsana, bend legs to go up, then come down with straight legs.

Lesson 1D (Relaxation)

Supta Baddha Koṇāsana (p. 81); Adho Mukha Śvānāsana (p. 90); Daṇḍāsana (p. 52); Jānu Śīrṣāsana (p. 59); Paścimottānāsana (p. 64); Sarvāṅgāsana on chair (p. 118); Ardha Halāsana (p. 110); Setu Bandha Sarvāṅgāsana on bench (p. 120); Śavāsana II (p. 152), 15 mins.

☐ This lesson teaches how to use props for supported *āsanas*. In Adho Mukha Śvānāsana, rest head on bolster or folded blanket.

Lesson 2A (Standing)

Tāḍāsana (p. 18); Vṛkṣāsana (p. 21); Trikoṇāsana (p. 22); Pārśva Koṇāsana (p. 24); Vīrabhadrāsana I (p. 26); Vīrabhadrāsana II (p. 28); Ardha Candrāsana (p. 30); Vīrabhadrāsana III (p. 32); Pārśvottānāsana (p. 40); Parīghāsana (p. 48); Vīrāsana forward bend (p. 51); Sarvāṅgāsana (p. 108); Halāsana (p. 110); Setu Bandha Sarvāṅgāsana variation (p. 116), catching ankles; Śavāsana I (p. 150).

☐ Keep arms up between each side of postures.

Lesson 2B (Sitting)

Vīrāsana (p. 50); Gomukhāsana (p. 56); Baddha Koṇāsana (p. 57); Upaviṣtha Koṇāsana (p. 65), step 1; Paripūrṇa Nāvāsana (p. 58); Ardha Nāvāsana (p. 58); Jānu Śīrṣāsana (p. 59); Triaṅg Mukhaikapāda Paścimottānāsana (p. 61); Ardha Baddha Padma Paścimottānāsana (p.60); Marīcyāsana I

p. 63); Paścimottānāsana (p. 64); Bharadvājāsana I (p. 72); Marīcyāsana III (p. 73); Sarvāṅgāsana (p. 108); Halāsana (p. 110); Eka Pāda Sarvāṅgāsana (p. 111); Pārśvaikapāda Sarvāṅgāsana (p. 111); Supta Koṇāsana (p. 113); Pārśva Halāsana (p. 112); Śavāsana I (p. 150).

□ Press hands against a wall or a ledge when practicing Marīcyāsana III.

Lesson 2C (Miscellaneous)

Adho Mukha Śvānāsana (p. 90); Ūrdhva Mukha Śvānasana (p.91); Caturaṅga Daṇḍāsana (p. 89); repeat this sequence a few times; Trikoṇāsana (p. 22); Pārśva Koṇāsana (p. 24); Vīrabhadrāsana II (p. 28); Vīrabhadrāsana I (p. 26); Pārśvottānāsana (p. 40); Vṛkṣāsana (p. 21); Garuḍāsana (p. 46); Utkaṭāsana (p. 47); Supta Vīrāsana (p. 82); Sarvāṅgāsana (p. 108); Halāsana (p. 110); Śavāsana I (p. 150).

□ Do Supta Vīrāsana with support (with high arrangement of blankets or bolsters if necessary).

Lesson 2D (Relaxation)

Lying on cross bolsters (p. 80); Supta Baddha Koṇāsana (p. 81); Supta Vīrāsana (p. 82), supported; Vīrāsana forward bend (p. 51); Adho Mukha Śvānāsana (p. 90), head supported; Sarvāṅgāsana on chair (p. 118); Ardha Halāsana (p. 110); Setu Bandha Sarvāṅgāsana on bench (p. 120); Śavāsana II (p. 152).

□ Observe breathing becoming deeper through supported *āsanas*.

Lesson 3A (Standing)

Tāḍāsana (p. 18); Trikoṇāsana (p. 22); Pārśva Koṇāsana (p. 24); Vīrabhadrāsana I (p. 26); Vīrabhadrāsana II (p. 28); Parivṛtta Trikoṇāsana (p. 34); Parivṛtta Pārsvakoṇāsana (p. 36); Pārśvottānāsana (p. 41); Jānu Śīrṣāsana (p. 59); Triaṅg Mukhaikapāda Paścimottānāsana (p. 61); Ardha Baddha Padma Paścimottānāsana (p. 60); Marīcyāsana I (p. 63); Paścimottānāsana (p. 64); Sarvāṅgāsana (p. 108); Halāsana (p. 110); Śavāsana I (p. 150).

□ Spend time on Tāḍāsana. Understand focuses given for standing postures.

Lesson 3B (Sitting)

Uttānāsana I (p. 44); Adho Mukha Śvānāsana (p. 90), hands against a wall; Uttānāsana II (p. 45); Daṇḍāsana (p. 54); Marīcyāsana III (p. 73); Ardha Matsyendrāsana I (p. 74); Pāśāsana (p. 76); Paścimottānāsana (p. 64), 3 mins; Sarvāṅgāsana (p. 108), 5 mins; Halāsana (p. 110), 3 mins; Halāsana-Paścimottānāsana sequence, × 6-8; Śavāsana I (p. 150).

□ In Uttānāsana II keep feet apart if back is stiff. Pay attention to Daṇḍāsana. Do twists near a wall or with back hand on ledge and repeat several times.

Lesson 3C (Backbends)

Tāḍāsana (p. 18); Trikoṇāsana (p. 22); Pārśvakoṇāsana (p. 24); Vīrabhadrāsana I (p. 26); Vīrabhadrāsana II (p. 28); Pārśvottānāsana (p. 40); Uṣṭrāsana (p. 134); Śalabhāsana I (p. 92); Dhanurāsana (p. 94); Ūrdhva Mukha Śvānāsana (p. 91); Adho Mukha Śvānāsana (p. 90); Ardha Halāsana (p. 110); Sarvāṅgāsana (p. 108); Śavāsana I (p. 150).

□ Do Uṣṭrāsana with help of a chair.

Lesson 3D (Relaxation)

Vīrāsana (p. 21); Jānu Śīrṣāsana (p. 59), head supported, × 2; Triaṅg Mukahikapāda Paścimottānāsana (p. 61), head supported, × 2; Paścimottānāsana (p. 64), head supported; Marīcyāsana III (p. 73), intermediate stage only; Sarvāṅgāsana on chair (p. 118); Ardha Halāsana (p. 110); Setu Bandha Sarvāṅgāsana on bench (p. 120) or lying on cross bolsters (p. 80); Śavāsana II (p. 152).

□ In forward bends keep timings of 2 mins for each side; 3 mins for Paścimottānāsana.

Lesson 4A (Standing)

Tāḍāsana (p. 18); Trikoṇāsana (p. 22); Pārśva Koṇāsana (p. 24); Vīrabhadrāsana I (p. 26); Vīrabhadrāsana II (p. 28); Ardha Candrāsana (p. 30); Vīrabhadrāsana III (p. 32); Pārśvottānāsana (p. 40); Prasārita Pādottānāsana I (p. 42); Uttānāsana (p. 44); Adho Mukha Śvānāsana (p. 90); Vīrāsana forward bend (p. 51); Śīrṣāsana I (p. 100); Sarvāṅgāsana (p. 108); Halāsana (p. 110); Paścimottānāsana (p. 64); Śavāsana I (p. 150).

□ Learn to stay in Prasārita Pādottānāsana as preparation for head-balance, placing head on bolster or equivalent if it does not reach the floor. Start practicing Śīrṣāsana against a wall or in a corner.

Lesson 4B (Sitting)

Utthita Hasta Pādānguṣṭhāsana I and II (pp. 20-21); Supta Pādānguṣṭhāsana (p. 88), steps 2 and 3; Jānu Śīrṣāsana (p. 59); Triaṅg Mukhaikapāda Paścimottānāsana (p. 61); Ardha Baddha Padma Paścimottānāsana (p. 60); Marīcyāsana I (p. 63); Paścimottānāsana (p. 64); Marīcyāsana III (p. 73); Śīrṣāsana (p. 100); Sarvāṅgāsana (p. 108); Halāsana (p. 110); Eka Pāda Sarvāṅgāsana (p. 111); Pārśvaikapāda Sarvāṅgāsana (p. 111); Śavāsana II (p. 152).

□ Compare Utthita Hasta Pādānguṣṭhāsana with Supta Pādāṅguṣṭhāsana and the two Sarvāṅgāsana variations. Continue Śīrṣāsana against a wall.

Lesson 4C (Miscellaneous)

Parvatāsana in Sukhāsana (p. 53); Parvatāsana in Vīrāsana (p. 51); Padmāsana (p. 54); Uttānāsana I (p. 44); Adho Mukha Śvānāsana (p. 90); Paścimottānāsana (p. 64); Śīrṣāsana (p. 100); Adho Mukha Śvānāsana (p. 90); Uttānāsana I (p. 44); Paścimottānāsana (p. 64); Ūrdhva Prasārita Pādāsana, (p. 84) × 2; Sarvāṅgāsana (p. 108); Halāsana (p. 110); Setu Bandha Sarvāṅgāsana (p. 116); Śavāsana I (p. 150).

□ Be careful of knees in Padmāsana; practice several times with one leg on top and other underneath. Sequence before and after Śīrṣāsana is to keep head relaxed. Go into Setu Bandha Sarvāṅgāsana from floor.

Lesson 4D (Relaxation and Prāṇāyama)

Supta Vīrāsana (p. 82); Supta Baddha Koṇāsana (p. 81); Vīrāsana forward bend (p. 51); Śīrṣāsana (p. 100); Sarvāṅgāsana on chair (p. 118); Ardha Halāsana (p. 110); Setu Bandha Sarvāṅgāsana on bench (p. 120); Śavāsana II (p. 152); normal breathing, lying down (p. 156) 10 mins.

□ Vīrāsana forward bend is to prepare head for Śīrṣāsana. Be comfortable and relaxed before beginning breathing practice.

Lesson 5A (Standing)

Adho Mukha Śvānāsana (p. 90), × 3; Tāḍāsana (p. 18); Trikoṇāsana (p. 22); Pārśva Koṇāsana (p. 24); Vīrabhadrāsana I (p. 26); Vīrabhadrāsana II (p. 28); Vīrabhadrāsana III (p. 32); Ardha Candrāsana (p. 30); Pārśvottānāsana (p. 64); Garuḍāsana (p. 46); Utkaṭāsana (p. 47); Vīrāsana forward bend (p. 51); Śīrṣāsana (p. 100); Sarvāṅgāsana (p. 108); Halāsana (p. 110); Jānu Śīrṣāsana (p. 59); Paścimottānāsana (p. 64); Śavāsana I (p. 150).

□ Do Adho Mukha Śvānāsana first with hands against wall, then feet, then again hands. Do standing poses with back against wall, except for Vīrabhadrāsana I and Pārśvottānāsana: here keep back heel against wall. Recapitulate alignment. Do Pārśvottānāsana with hands down.

Lesson 5B (Sitting)

Vīrāsana (p. 50); Parvatāsana in Vīrāsana (p. 51); Adho Mukha Śvānāsana (p. 90); Uttānāsana (p. 44); Śīrṣāsana (p. 100); Jānu Śīrṣāsana (p. 59); Ardha Baddha Padma Paścimottānāsana (p. 60); Triaṅg Mukhaikapāda Paścimottānāsana (p. 61); Marīcyāsana I (p. 63); Paścimottānāsana (p. 64); Paripūrṇa Nāvāsana (p. 58); Ardha Nāvāsana (p. 58); Gomukhāsana (p. 56); Baddha Koṇāsana (p. 57); Upaviṣṭa Koṇāsana (p. 65), step 1; Padmāsana (p. 54); Vīrāsana (p. 50); Sarvāṅgāsana (p. 108); Ardha Halāsana (p. 110); Śavāsana I (p. 150).

□ If back feels strained after forward bends, do one or two twists.

Lesson 5C (Miscellaneous)

Tāḍāsana (p. 18); Ūrdhva Hastāsana (p. 19); Uttānāsana II (p. 45); Adho Mukha Śvānāsana (p. 90); Ūrdhva Mukha Śvānāsana (p. 91); Caturaṅga Daṇḍāsana (p. 89); repeat this sequence × 3; Uttānāsana I (p. 44); Śīrṣāsana (p. 100); Viparīta Daṇḍāsana on chair (p. 136), step 3 × 3; Bharadvājāsana on chair (p. 71); Paścimottānāsana (p. 64), using chair; Sarvāṅgāsana (p. 108); Halāsana (p. 110); Pārśva Halāsana (p. 112); Śavāsana I (p. 150).

□ In Viparīta Daṇḍāsana on chair, learn to adjust blankets and neck.

Lesson 5D (Relaxation and Prāṇāyāma)

Uttānāsana I (p.44); Adho Mukha Śvānāsana (p. 90); head supported; Vīrāsana forward bend (p. 51); Śīrṣāsana (p. 100); Jānu Śīrṣāsana (p. 59), head supported; Paścimottānāsana (p. 64), head supported; Sarvāṅgāsana on chair (p. 118); Ardha Halāsana (p. 110); Sarvāṅgāsana on chair (p. 118); Śavāsana II (p. 152); normal breathing, lying down (p. 156), 10-15 mins.

□ For Sarvāṅgāsana on chair and Halāsana prepare chair and stool so you can go from one to other without coming down.

Lesson 6A (Standing)

Tāḍāsana (p. 18); Vṛkṣāsana (p. 21); Trikoṇāsana (p. 22); Pārśva Koṇāsana (p. 24); Vīrabhadrāsana I (p. 26); Vīrabhadrāsana II (p. 28); Trikoṇāsana (p. 22); Pārśva Koṇāsana (p. 24); Parivṛtta Ardha Candrāsana (p. 38); Pārśvottānāsana (p. 40); Prasārita Pādottānāsana (p. 42); Vīrāsana forward bend (p. 51); Vīrāsana and Parvatāsana (p. 51); Śīrṣāsana (p. 100); Sarvāṅgāsana (p. 108); Halāsana (p. 110); Karṇapīḍāsana (p. 144); Śavāsana I (p. 150).

□ As before, rest forward in Uttānāsana between standing poses if necessary.

Lesson 6B (Sitting)

Supta Vīrāsana (p. 82); Adho Mukha Śvānāsana (p. 90); Uttānāsana I and II (p. 44); Śīrṣāsana (p. 100); Jānu Śīrṣāsana (p. 59); Bharadvājāsana I (p. 72); Triaṅg Mukhaikapāda Paścimottānāsana (p. 61); Bharadvājāsana II (p. 77); Paścimottānāsana (p. 64); Pāśāsana (p. 76); Sarvāṅgāsana – forward bend sequence (p. 148); Śavāsana I (p. 150).

□ In Sarvāṅgāsana – forward bend sequence, learn to coordinate actions of limbs while body is in motion.

Lesson 6C (Backbends)

Tāḍāsana (p. 18); Trikoṇāsana (p. 22); Pārśva Koṇāsana (p. 24); Vīrabhadrāsana I (p. 26); Vīrabhadrāsana II (p. 28); Pārśvottānāsana (p. 40); Śīrṣāsana (p. 100); Ūrdhva Mukha Śvānāsana (p. 91); Śalabhāsana I (p. 92); Śalabhāsana II (p. 93); Dhanurāsana (p. 94); Ardha Halāsana (p. 110); Sarvāṅgāsana (p. 108); Halāsana (p. 110); Pārśva Halāsana (p. 112); Śavāsana I (p. 150).

□ In backbends, pay attention to keeping sacrum and pubis down.

Lesson 6D (Relaxation and Prāṇāyāma)

Sukhāsana (p. 100); Vīrāsana (p. 50); Padmāsana (p. 54); Vīrāsana (p. 50); Adho Mukha Śvānāsana (p. 90); Śīrṣāsana (p. 100); Sarvāṅgāsana on chair (p. 118); Ardha Halāsana (p. 110); Setu Bandha Sarvāṅgāsana on bench (p. 120); Śavāsana II (p. 152); normal breathing, lying down (p. 156); Ujjāyī Prāṇāyāma I and II (pp. 158-9); Śavāsana I (p. 150).

□ Do sitting poses against wall, in order to learn to sit straight.

Lesson 7A (Standing)

Utthita Hasta Pādāṅguṣṭhāsana I and II (p. 20); Tāḍāsana (p. 18); Trikoṇāsana (p. 22); Pārśva Koṇāsana (p. 24); Vīrabhadrāsana I (p. 26); Vīrabhadrāsana II (p. 28); Ardha Candrāsana (p. 30); Vīrabhadrāsana III (p. 32); Trikoṇāsana (p. 22); Pārśvottānāsana (p. 40); Viparīta Daṇḍāsana on chair (p. 142); Śīrṣāsana (p. 100); Jānu Śīrṣāsana (p. 59); Triaṅg Mukhaikapāda Paścimottānāsana (p. 61); Ardha Baddha Padma Paścimottānāsana (p. 60); Paścimottānāsana (p. 64); Sarvāṅgāsana (p. 108); Halāsana (p. 110); Śavāsana I (p. 150).

□ Concentrate on one of the standing poses and use all the methods for it. Do Śīrṣāsana a few inches from the wall to gain confidence. Once stable and straight, do in center of room.

Lesson 7B (Sitting)

Baddha Koṇāsana (p. 57), against wall, 5 mins; Upaviṣṭa Koṇāsana (p. 65), against wall, 5 mins; Baddha Koṇāsana (p. 57); Jānu Śīrṣāsana (p. 59); Ardha Baddha Padma Paścimottānāsana (p. 60); Triaṅg Mukhaikapāda Paścimottānāsana (p. 61); Marīcyāsana I (p. 63); Paścimottānāsana (p. 64); Pārśva Upaviṣṭa Koṇāsana (p. 66); Supta Baddha Koṇāsana (p. 81); Setu Bandha Sarvāṅgāsana on bench (p. 120); Śavāsana II (p. 152); normal breathing, lying down (p. 156), 10 mins.

□ Repeat forward bends twice each. As inverted postures have been omitted, this lesson may be practiced during menstruation.

Lesson 7C (Miscellaneous)

Supta Vīrāsana (p. 82), Bhekāsana (p. 86); Padmāsana (p. 54); Vīrāsana (p. 50); Śīrṣāsana (p. 100); Supta Pādānguṣṭāsana (p. 88), steps 2 and 3 only; Anantāsana (p. 87); Ūrdhva Prasārita Pādāsana (p. 84); Jaṭhara Parivartanāsana (p. 85); Sarvāṅgāsana (p. 108); Halāsana (p. 110); Eka Pāda Sarvāṅgāsana (p. 111); Pārśvaika Pāda Sarvāṅgāsana (p. 111); Karṇapīḍāsana (p. 112); Supta Koṇāsana (p. 113); Pārśva Halāsana (p. 112); Setu Bandha Sarvāṅgāsana (p. 116); Śavāsana I (p. 150).

□ Do Bhekāsana one leg at a time, then both together. In Jaṭhara Parivartanāsana go halfway, or as far as possible without losing control. Do Setu Bandha Sarvāṅgāsana from floor.

Lesson 7D (Relaxation and Prāṇāyāma)

Viparīta Karaṇī (p. 122); Supta Vīrāsana (p. 82); Uttānāsana I (p. 44); Adho Mukha Śvānāsana (p. 90); Śīrṣāsana (p. 100); Sarvāṅgāsana on chair (p. 118); Setu Bandha Sarvāṅgāsana on bench (p. 120); Śavāsana II (p. 152); Ujjāyī Prāṇāyāma II, lying down (p. 159); Śavāsana I (p. 150).

□ Increase timings in āsanas so that chest opens more and relaxation becomes deeper. This prepares body and mind for Prāṇāyāma.

Lesson 8A (Standing)

Tāḍāsana (p. 18); Ūrdhva Hastāsana (p. 19); Trikoṇāsana (p. 22); Pārśva Koṇāsana (p. 24); Vīrabhadrāsana I (p. 26) going into Vīrabhadrāsana III (p. 32); Uttānāsana I (p. 44); Vīrabhadrāsana II (p. 28); Ardha Candrāsana (p. 30); Trikoṇāsana (p. 22); Pārśvottānāsana (p. 40); Prasārita Pādottānasana I (p. 42); Adho Mukha Śvānāsana (p. 90); Śīrṣāsana (p. 100); Sukhāsana with Parvatāsana and forward bend (p. 53); Vīrāsana (p. 50); Gomukhāsana (p. 56); Sarvāṅgāsana (p. 108); Halāsana (p. 110); Śavāsana II (p. 152).

□ Bear rhythm in mind in standing poses. Synchronize movements with breathing.

Lesson 8B (Sitting)

Sukhāsana and Parvatāsana (p. 53); Vīrāsana and Parvatāsana (p. 50); Adho Mukha Śvānāsana (p. 90), using wall; Śīrṣāsana (p. 100); Pārśva Śīrṣāsana (p. 102); Jānu Śīrṣāsana (p. 59); Ardha Baddha Padma Paścimottānāsana (p. 60); Triaṅg Mukhaikapāda Paścimottānāsana (p. 61); Krauñcāsana (p. 62), step 2; Marīcyāsana I (p. 63); Paścimottānāsana (p. 64); Pārśva Upaviṣṭa Koṇāsana (p. 66); Baddha Koṇāsana (p. 57); Sarvāṅgāsana (p. 108); Halāsana variation (p. 110), clasping hands behind back; Paścimottānāsana (p. 64); Śavāsana II (p. 152).

□ Do Pārśva Śīrṣāsana against wall, paying attention to line and to keeping neck extended. Do not attempt it if Śīrṣāsana is not strong.

Lesson 8C (Backbends)

Supta Vīrāsana (p. 82); Uttānāsana (p. 44); Adho Mukha Śvānāsana (p. 90); Trikoṇāsana (p. 22); Pārśva Koṇāsana (p. 24); Vīrabhadrāsana I (p. 26); Vīrabhadrāsana II (p. 28); Pārśvottānāsana (p. 40); Śīrṣāsana (p. 100); Viparīta Daṇḍāsana on chair (p. 136), × 3; Ūrdhva Dhanurāsana (p. 138), × 3; Marīcyāsana III (p. 73); Ardha Matsyendrāsana I (p. 74); Pāśāsana (p. 76); Ardha Halāsana (p. 110); Śavāsana I (p. 150).

□ Do standing poses with back foot against wall. In Viparīta Daṇḍāsana on chair, take arms over head when doing it the third time. Repeat twists twice each, remaining in intermediate stage.

Lesson 8D (Relaxation and Prāṇāyāma)

Sukhāsana (p. 100); Vīrāsana (p. 50); Padmāsana (p. 54); Vīrāsana (p. 50); Adho Mukha Śvānāsana (p. 90); Śīrṣāsana (p. 100); Sarvāṅgāsana on chair (p. 118); Ardha Halāsana (p. 110); Setu Bandha Sarvāṅgāsana on bench (p. 120); Śavāsana II (p. 152); normal breathing, lying down (p. 156); Ujjāyī Prāṇāyāma I and II (p. 158-9); Śavāsana I (p. 150).

☐ Do sitting poses against wall, in order to learn to sit straight.

Lesson 9A (Standing)

Sūrya Namaskār variation (p. 148); jumping into standing poses (p. 17); Uttānāsana I (p. 44); Supta Vīrāsana (p. 82); Śīrṣāsana (p. 100); Pārśva Śīrṣāsana (p. 102); Daṇḍāsana (p. 52); Jānu Śīrṣāsana (p. 59); Triaṅg Mukhaikapāda Paścimottānāsana (p. 61); Ardha Baddha Padma Paścimottānāsana (p. 60); Paścimottānāsana (p. 64); Bharadvājāsana I (p. 72); Bharadvājāsana II (p. 77); Sarvāṅgāsana (p. 108); Halāsana (p. 110); Setu Bandha Sarvāṅgāsana (p. 116); Śavāsana I (p. 150).

☐ Do as many jumpings as possible without becoming tired. Do Setu Bandha Sarvāṅgāsana from floor.

Lesson 9B (Sitting)

Adho Mukha Śvānāsana (p. 90); Uttānāsana I (p. 44); Vīrāsana (p. 50); Baddha Koṇāsana (p. 57); Upaviṣṭa Koṇāsana (p. 65), step 1; Baddha Koṇāsana (p. 57); Śīrṣāsana (p. 100); Baddha Koṇāsana in Śīrṣāsana (p. 104); Upaviṣṭa Koṇāsana in Śīrṣāsana (p. 105); Jānu Śīrṣāsana (p. 59); Ardha Baddha Padma Paścimottānāsana (p. 60); Triaṅg Mukhaikapāda Paścimottānāsana (p. 61); Krauñcāsana (p. 62), step 2; Paścimottānāsana (p. 64); Pārśva Upaviṣṭa Koṇāsana (p. 66); Marīcyāsana III (p. 73); Ardha Matsyendrāsana I (p. 74); Sarvāṅgāsana (p. 108); Halāsana (p. 110); Eka Pāda Sarvāṅgāsana (p. 111); Pārśvaika Pāda Sarvāṅgāsana (p. 111); Supta Koṇāsana (p. 113); Pārśva Halāsana (p. 112); Śavāsana II (p. 152).

☐ Work on arms, shoulders, and shoulder blades in Adho Mukha Śvānāsana and Śīrṣāsana. Do forward bends with a concave back, using a belt. Repeat twists 3 times, catching last time.

Lesson 9C (Backbends)

Adho Mukha Śvānāsana (p. 90), × 2; Śīrṣāsana (p. 100); Tāḍāsana (p. 18); Trikoṇāsana (p. 22); Pārśva Koṇāsana (p. 24); Vīrabhadrāsana I (p. 26); Vīrabhadrāsana II (p. 28); Vīrabhadrāsana III (p. 32); Ardha Candrāsana (p. 30); Pārśvottānāsana (p. 40); Viparīta Daṇḍāsana on chair (p. 136), × 3; Ūrdhva Dhanurāsana (p. 138), × 3; Marīcyāsana III (p. 73), intermediate stage, × 3; Ardha Halāsana (p. 110); Śavāsana I (p. 150).

☐ In Viparīta Daṇḍāsana on chair, take arms over head at end. In Ūrdhva Dhanurāsana place hands on a height, e.g. on bricks.

Lesson 9D (Relaxation and Prāṇāyāma)

Lying on cross bolsters (p. 80); Supta Vīrāsana (p. 82); Supta Baddha Koṇāsana (p. 81); Śīrṣāsana (p. 100); Sarvāṅgāsana on chair (p. 118); Ardha Halāsana (p. 110); Setu Bandha Sarvāṅgāsana on bench (p. 120); Śavāsana II (p. 152); normal breathing, lying down (p. 156); Ujjāyī Prāṇāyāma I, II and III (pp. 158-160); Śavāsana I (p. 150).

☐ If back aches from bending back, do Bharadvājāsana on chair (p. 71) and Marīcyāsana, standing (p. 70), before lying down.

CONSOLIDATION

Finally, repeat lessons 1 to 9, A to D.

Increase the times taken in Śīrṣāsana and Sarvāṅgāsana to gain balance and confidence. Learn to relax in the postures. Learn to feel the extent to which the body is following the details that have been given in the postures. Spend longer in Śavāsana to improve the quality of relaxation.

Do not proceed to Course III until you can comfortably hold Śīrṣāsana for 5 minutes, Sarvāṅgāsana for 10 minutes and Halāsana for 5 minutes. This usually takes a minimum of 2 years' practice.

COURSE III

This course consists of 16 lessons. It increases the range of sitting and inverted postures and introduces balancings and jumpings.

As the principles and techniques of the postures are absorbed, practice increases in intensity and sensitivity.

SUGGESTED SCHEME OF PRACTICE

Alternate the lessons outlined here with lessons from Course II. After lesson 4, A-D have been practiced, consolidate progress by repeating all the lessons, and then for the next four months, repeat lessons 1 and 2, A-D, 2 and 3 A-D, and so on each month. Finally, spend 3 months consolidating all the lessons so far.

Lesson 1A (Standing)

Tāḍāsana (p. 18); Trikoṇāsana (p. 22); Parivṛtta Trikoṇāsana (p. 34); Pārśva Koṇāsana (p. 24); Parivṛtta Pārśva Koṇāsana (p. 38); Vīrabhadrāsana I (p. 26); Vīrabhadrāsana II (p. 28); Pārśvottānāsana (p.40); Prasārita Pādottānāsana I (p. 42); Prasārita Pādottānāsana II (p. 43); Uttānāsana II (p. 45); Uttānāsana II, variation (p. 45); Śīrṣāsana I (p. 98); Pārśva Śīrṣāsana (p. 102); Sarvāṅgāsana (p. 108); Halāsana (p. 110); Jānu Śīrṣāsana (p. 59); Paścimottānāsana (p. 64); Śavāsana I (p. 150).

☐ Work on detail and accuracy, spending more time on each posture.

Lesson 1B (Sitting)

Vīrāsana (p. 50); Padmāsana (p. 54); Jānu Śīrṣāsana (p. 59); Ardha Baddha Padma Paścimottānāsana (p. 60); Triaṅg Mukhaikapāda Paścimottānāsana (p. 61); Krauñcāsana (p. 62); Marīcyāsana I (p. 63); Paścimottānāsana (p. 64); Pārśva Upaviṣṭa Koṇāsana (p. 66); Upaviṣṭa Koṇāsana (p. 65); Baddha Koṇāsana (p. 57); Baddha Koṇāsana forward bend (p. 57); Śīrṣāsana I (p. 98); Sarvāṅgāsana (p. 108); Nirālamba Sarvāṅgāsana (p. 109); Halāsana (p. 110); Anantāsana (p. 87); Supta Pādāṅguṣṭhāsana (p. 88); Ūrdhva Prasārita Pādāsana (p. 84); Jaṭhara Parivartanāsana (p. 85); Śavāsana I (p. 150).

☐ Stay in Vīrāsana and Padmāsana to establish tranquillity in forward bends that follow.

Lesson 1C (Jumpings and Balancings)

Adho Mukha Śvānāsana (p. 90); Adho Mukha Vṛkṣāsana (p. 96); Uttānāsana I (p. 44); Śīrṣāsana I (p. 98); Sūrya Namaskār (p. 146); Ūrdhva Hastāsana (p. 19); Uttānāsana II (p. 45); Bakāsana (p. 130), × 3; Ūrdhva Hastāsana (p. 19); Uttānāsana II (p. 45); Bhujapīḍāsana (p. 129), × 3; Paścimottānāsana (p. 64); Sarvāṅgāsana (p. 108), 10 mins; Halāsana (p. 110); Setu Bandha Sarvāṅgāsana (p. 116), × 3; Halāsana (p. 110); Śavāsana I (p. 150).

☐ In Adho Mukha Vṛkṣāsana, practice kicking up until you succeed. Do not bend the elbows. Learn to drop back from Sarvāṅgāsana into Setu Bandha Sarvāṅgāsana and jump up again.

Lesson 1D (Relaxation and Prāṇāyāma)

Adho Mukha Śvānāsana (p. 90); Uttānāsana I (p. 44); Śīrṣāsana I (p. 98); Sarvāṅgāsana on chair (p. 118); Ardha Halāsana (p. 110); Setu Bandha Sarvāṅgāsana on bench (p. 120); Śavāsana II (p. 152); normal breathing, lying down (p. 156); Viloma Prāṇāyāma I and II, lying down (p. 161); Śavāsana I (p. 150).

☐ Increase timings in inverted postures.

Lesson 2A (Standing)

Tāḍāsana (p. 18); Parivṛtta Trikoṇāsana (p. 38); Parivṛtta Pārśva Koṇāsana (p. 38); Parivṛtta Ardha Candrāsana (p. 30); Adho Mukha Śvānāsana (p. 90); Śīrṣāsana I (p. 98); Pārsva Śīrṣāsana (p. 102); Parivṛtta Eka Pāda Śīrṣāsana (p. 102); Sarvāṅgāsana (p. 108); Halāsana (p. 110); Eka Pāda Sarvāṅgāsana (p. 111); Pārśvaika Pāda Sarvāṅgāsana (p. 111); Supta Koṇāsana (p. 113); Pārśva Halāsana (p. 112); Karṇapīḍāsana (p. 112); Sarvāṅgāsana (p. 108); Setu Bandha Sarvāṅgāsana (p. 116), dropping back; Halāsana (p. 110); Setu Bandha Sarvāṅgāsana on bench (p. 120); Śavāsana I (p. 150).

☐ Repeat reverse standing poses several times each.

Lesson 2B (Sitting)

Adho Mukha Vṛkṣāsana (p. 96); Uttānāsana I and II (p. 44); Śīrṣāsana I (p. 98); Pārśva Śīrṣāsana (p. 102); Parivṛtta Eka Pāda Śīrṣāsana (p. 102); Parivṛtta Eka Pāda Śīrṣāsana (p. 102); Eka Pāda Śīrṣāsana (p. 103); Pārśvaikapāda Śīrṣāsana (p. 103); Padmāsana (p. 54); Parvatāsana in Padmāsana (p. 55); Vīrāsana (p. 50); Sarvāṅgāsana (p. 108); Halāsana (p. 110); Nirālamba Sarvāṅgāsana (p. 109); Halāsana variation (p. 110); Jānu Śīrṣāsana (p. 59); Ardha Baddha Padma Paścimottānāsana, full posture (p. 60); Triaṅg Mukhaikapāda Paścimottānāsana (p. 61); Marīcyāsana I (p. 63); Paścimottānāsana (p. 64); Pārśva Upaviṣṭa Koṇāsana (p. 66); Parivṛtta Jānu Śīrṣāsana (p. 67); Parivṛtta Upaviṣṭa Koṇāsana (p. 66); Śavāsana II (p. 152), 10-15 min.

☐ Observe breathing in postures. In forward bends, learn to synchronize actions with breath.

Lesson 2C (Backbends)

Supta Vīrāsana (p. 82); Matsyāsana (p. 83); Supta Vīrāsana (p. 82); Bhekāsana (p. 86); Adho Mukha Śvānāsana (p. 90); Uttānāsana II (p. 45); Adho Mukha Vṛkṣāsana (p. 96); Śīrṣāsana I (p. 98); Viparīta Daṇḍāsana on chair (p. 136) × 3; Ūrdhva Dhanurāsana (p. 138) × 6-8; Marīcyāsana III (p. 73); Ardha Matsyendrāsana I (p. 74); Ardha Halāsana (p. 110); Śavāsana I (p. 150).

☐ Press sacrum down well in Bhekāsana. In Ūrdhva Dhanurāsana, pay attention to keeping body centered between arms and legs. In twists, do intermediate stage only.

Lesson 2D (Relaxation and Prāṇāyāma)

Supta Baddha Koṇāsana (p. 81); Supta Vīrāsana (p. 82); Matsyāsana (p. 83); Vīrāsana forward bend (p. 51); Viparīta Daṇḍāsana on chair, head supported (p. 136); Sarvāṅgāsana on chair (p. 118); Ardha Halāsana (p. 110); Setu Bandha Sarvāṅgāsana on bench (p. 120); Śavāsana II (p. 152); normal breathing, lying down (p. 156); Ujjāyī Prāṇāyāma III, lying down (p. 160); Viloma Prāṇāyāma I and II, lying down (p. 161); Śavāsana I (p. 150).

☐ Experiment with height of bolster or blankets in Setu Bandha Sarvāṅgāsana, in case less is needed.

Lesson 3A (Standing)

Uttānāsana I (p. 44); Adho Mukha Śvānāsana (p. 90); Adho Mukha Vṛkṣāsana (p. 96); Śīrṣāsana I (p. 98); Pārśva Vīrāsana in Śīrṣāsana (p. 105); Tāḍāsana (p. 18); Trikoṇāsana (p. 22); Pārśva Koṇāsana (p. 24); Vīrabhadrāsana I (p. 26); Vīrabhadrāsana II (p. 28); Ardha Candrāsana (p. 30); Vīrabhadrāsana III (p. 32); Pārśvottānāsana (p. 40); Prasārita Pādottānāsana (p. 42); Utkaṭāsana (p. 47); Uttānāsana II (p. 45); Lolāsana (p. 124); Eka Hasta Bhujāsana (p. 125); Sarvāṅgāsana (p. 108); Halāsana (p. 110); Eka Pāda Sarvāṇgāsana (p. 111); Pārśvaika Pāda Sarvāṅgāsana (p. 111); Pārśva Halāsana (p.112); Śavāsana I (p. 150).

☐ Observe movements of sacroiliac joints in standing poses.

Lesson 3B (Sitting)

Adho Mukha Śvānāsana (p. 90); Uttānāsana I and II (p. 44); Śīrṣāsana I (p. 98); Marīcyāsana III (p. 73); Ardha Matsyendrāsana I (p. 74); Pāśāsana (p. 76); Bhāradvājāsana II (p. 77); Ardha Matsyendrāsana II (p. 78); Jānu Śīrṣāsana (p. 59); Ardha Baddha Padma Paścimottānāsana (p. 60), full posture; Triaṅg Mukhaikapāda Paścimottānāsana (p. 61); Paścimottānāsana (p. 64); Padmāsana (p. 54); Baddha Padmāsana (p. 55); Sarvāṅgāsana (p. 108); Halāsana (p. 110); Supta Koṇāsana (p. 113); Ūrdhva Padmāsana in Sarvāṅgāsana (p. 114); Śavāsana I (p. 150).

☐ In twists, concentrate on turning hips.

Lesson 3C (Inverted)

Viparīta Daṇḍāsana on chair (p. 136); Śīrṣāsana I (p. 98); Pārśva Śīrṣāsana (p. 102); Parivṛtta Eka Pāda Śīrṣāsana (p. 102); Eka Pāda Śīrṣāsana (p. 103); Pārśvaika Pāda Śīrṣāsana (p. 103); Ūrdhva Daṇḍāsana (p. 105); Sūrya Namaskār with variation (p. 146); Halāsana (p. 110); Sarvāṅgāsana (p. 108); Eka Pāda Sarvāṅgāsana (p. 111); Pārśvaika Pāda Sarvāṅgāsana (p. 111); Pārśva Halāsana (p. 112); Supta Koṇāsana (p. 113), Karṇapīḍāsana (p. 112); Eka Pāda Setu Bandha Sarvāṅgāsana (p. 117); Setu Bandha Sarvāṅgāsana (p. 116); Halāsana (p. 110); Śavāsana I (p. 150).

☐ Learn to drop back with one leg into Eka Pāda Setu Bandha Sarvāṅgāsana from Eka Pāda Sarvāṅgāsana.

Lesson 3D (Relaxation and Prāṇāyāma)

Supta Vīrāsana (p. 82); Viparīta Daṇḍāsana on chair (p. 136), head supported; Śīrṣāsana I (p. 98); Sarvāṇgāsana on chair (p. 118); Ardha Halāsana (p. 110); Setu Bandha Sarvāṅgāsana on bench (p. 120); Śavāsana II (p. 152); Ujjāyī Prāṇāyāma I and II, lying down (pp. 158-9); Viloma Prāṇāyāma I and II, lying down (pp. 161-2); Śavāsana I (p. 150).

☐ Make inhalations and exhalations same length and volume.

Lesson 4A (Standing)

Adho Mukha Vṛkṣāsana (p. 96); Śīrṣāsana II (p. 107); Trikoṇāsana (p. 22); Parivṛtta Trikoṇāsana (p. 34); Pārśva Koṇāsana (p. 24); Parivṛtta Pārśvakoṇāsana (p. 38); Vīrabhadrāsana I (p. 26); Vīrabhadrāsana II (p. 28); Ardha Candrāsana (p. 30); Parivṛtta Ardha Candrāsana (p. 38); Pārśvottānāsana (p. 40); Uttānāsana II (p. 45); Utthita Hasta Padāṅguṣṭhāsana I and II (p. 20), catching foot, without ledge; Uṣṭrāsana (p. 134); Ūrdhva Mukha Śvānāsana (p. 91); Dhanurāsana (p. 94); Bhujaṅgāsana (p. 93); Adho Mukha Śvānāsana (p. 90); Sarvāṅgāsana (p. 108); Halāsana (p. 110); Śavāsana I (p. 150).

☐ In Adho Mukha Vṛkṣāsana, learn to stretch arms vertically up. Pay attention to arms in all other postures.

Lesson 4B (Sitting)

Ūrdhva Mukha Śvānāsana (p. 91); Adho Mukha Śvānāsana (p. 90); Caturaṅga Daṇḍāsana (p. 89); Śīrṣāsana I (p. 98); Baddha Koṇāsana in Śīrṣāsana (p. 104); Upaviṣṭa Koṇāsana in Śīrṣāsana (p. 105); Urdhva Daṇḍāsana (p. 105); Padmāsana (p. 54); Matsyāsana (p. 83); Vīrāsana (p. 50); Supta Vīrāsana (p. 82); Daṇḍāsana (p. 52); Paripūrṇa Nāvāsana (p. 58); Ardha Nāvāsana (p. 58), Jānu Śīrṣāsana (p. 59); Ardha Baddha Padma Paścimottānāsana (p. 60); Triaṅg Mukhaikapāda Paścimottānāsana (p. 61); Krauñcāsana (p. 62); Marīcyāsana I (p. 63); Paścimottānāsana (p. 64); Pārśva Upaviṣṭa Koṇāsana (p. 66); Upaviṣṭa Koṇāsana (p. 65); Sarvāṅgāsana (p. 108); Halāsana (p. 110), Eka Pāda Sarvāṅgāsana (p. 111); Pārśvaika Pāda Sarvāṅgāsana (p. 111); Supta Koṇāsana (p. 113); Karṇapīḍāsana (p. 112); Pārśva Halāsana (p. 112); Setu Bandha Sarvāṅgāsana (p. 116); Ūrdhva Padmāsana in Sarvāṅgāsana (p. 114); Piṇḍāsana in Sarvāṅgāsana (p. 114); Śavāsana I (p. 150).

☐ Do not force knees in Padmāsana or any of its variations.

Lesson 4C (Backbends)

Adho Mukha Vṛkṣāsana (p.96); Piñca Mayūrāsana (p. 97); Śīrṣāsana I (p. 98); Viparīta Daṇḍāsana on chair (p. 136); Ūrdhva Dhanurāsana (p. 94); Dvi Pāda Viparīta Daṇḍāsana, against wall (p. 142); Ūrdhva Dhanurāsana from Śīrṣāsana (p. 140); Vīrāsana forward bend (p. 51); Jānu Śīrṣāsana (p. 59), × 3; Paścimottānāsana (p. 64); Ardha Halāsana (p. 110); Śavāsana I (p. 150).

☐ Do Ūrdhva Dhanurāsana several times in different ways: with hands on bricks and against a wall, and in center of the room. In forward bends, allow back to release gradually without forcing or stretching it.

Lesson 4D (Prāṇāyāma)

Śavāsana II (p. 152); normal breathing, lying down (p. 156); Viloma Prāṇāyāma I and II, lying down (pp. 161-2); normal breathing, sitting (p. 157); Śavāsana I (p. 150).

☐ Be careful not to overstrain. Quality, not quantity, of Prāṇāyāma is important.

Consolidation

Repeat all the lessons.

Absorb the details of the poses and aim for steadiness in them. Understand the purpose of the intermediate stages. Begin to work more on backbends.

Do not go on to Course IV until you have achieved a

steady Śīrṣāsana for 15 minutes, Sarvāṅgāsana for 20 minutes and Halāsana for 10 minutes. In addition, Śīrṣāsana variations should be strong. Adho Mukha Vṛkṣāsana, Piñca Mayūrāsana, Ūrdhva Dhanurāsana and dropping back from Śīrṣāsana should all come with ease. You should also be able to do Padmāsana, to touch the head on the shins in forward bends, keeping the legs straight, and to catch the hands in twists.

COURSE IV

This course consists of 6 lessons, as an example of how to incorporate some of the āsanas of the fourth level of difficulty into practice.

The postures practiced so far will have given a great deal of strength and mobility. Through doing the advanced āsanas, lightness and agility are gained. The ability to discriminate between correct and incorrect actions also increases at this stage.

SUGGESTED SCHEME OF PRACTICE

Practice may be arranged so that each day of the week has a different emphasis, with, for example, standing poses done on one day, sitting poses on the next, then backbends, balancings, twists, inverted poses, and relaxation. Other postures may also be included. Prāṇāyāma may be done after a relaxation program or separately, at a different time of day.

Caution *It is essential first to learn prāṇāyāma under the guidance of a teacher.*

Lesson 1 (Standing and Balancings)

Ūrdhva Hastāsana (p. 19) and Uttānāsana II (p. 45) up and down in quick succession, × 10; Śīrṣāsana II (p. 107); Trikoṇāsana (p. 22); Parivṛtta Trikoṇāsana (p. 34); Pārśva Koṇāsana (p. 24); Parivṛtta Pārśva Koṇāsana (p. 38); Ardha Candrāsana (p. 30); Parivṛtta Ardha Candrāsana (p. 38); Uttānāsana I (p. 44); Bhujapīḍāsana (p. 129); Bakāsana (p. 130); Pārśva Bakāsana (p. 132); Aṣṭa Vakrāsana (p. 128); Sarvāṅgāsana (p. 108); Ardha Halāsana (p. 110); Setu Bandha Sarvāṅgāsana on bench (p. 120); Śavāsana I (p. 150).

Lesson 2 (Sitting)

Sūrya Namaskār (p. 146); Śīrṣāsana I (p. 98); Pārśva Śīrṣāsana (p. 102); Parivṛtta Eka Pāda Śīrṣāsana (p. 102); Eka Pāda Śīrṣāsana (p. 103); Pārśvaika Pāda Śīrṣāsana (p. 103); Ūrdhva Padmāsana in Śīrṣāsana (p. 106); Jānu Śīrṣāsana (p. 59); Ardha Baddha Padma Paścimottānāsana (p. 60); Triaṅg Mukhaikapāda Paścimottānāsana (p. 61); Marīcyāsana I (p. 63); Paścimottānāsana (p. 64); Parivṛtta Jānu Śīrṣāsana (p. 67); Parivṛtta Upaviṣṭa Koṇāsana (p. 66); Sarvāṅgāsana (p. 108); Halāsana (p. 110); Eka Pāda Sarvāṅgāsana (p. 111); Pārśvaika Pāda Sarvāṅgāsana (p. 111); Supta Koṇāsana (p. 113); Pārśva Halāsana (p. 112); Pārśva Sarvāṅgāsana (p. 113); Śavāsana I (p. 150).

Lesson 3 (Backbends)

Supta Vīrāsana (p. 82); Matsyāsana (p. 83); Śīrṣāsana (p. 100); Viparīta Daṇḍāsana on chair (p. 136), × 3; Ūrdhva Dhanurāsana (p. 138), × 3; Ūrdhva Dhanurāsana from Śīrṣāsana (p. 140), × 6; Dvi Pāda Viparita Daṇḍāsana (p. 142), × 3; Adho Mukha Vṛkṣāsana (p. 96); Adho Mukha Śvānāsana (p. 90); Uttānāsana I (p. 44); Ardha Halāsana (p. 110).

Lesson 4 (Balancings and Backbends)

Adho Mukha Vṛkṣāsana (p. 96); Piñca Mayūrāsana (p. 97); Uttānāsana I (p. 44); Śīrṣāsana II (p. 107); Bakāsana from Śīrṣāsana (p. 131), then drop back and lift up into Ūrdhva Dhanurāsana (p. 138), × 6; Vīrāsana forward bend (p. 51); Jānu Śīrṣāsana (p. 59); Paścimottānāsana (p. 64); Ardha Halāsana (p. 110); Śavāsana I (p. 150).

Lesson 5 (Padmāsana)

Vīrāsana (p. 50); Supta Vīrāsana (p. 82); Padmāsana (p. 54); Matsyāsana (p. 83); Parvatāsana in Padmāsana (p. 55); Baddha Padmāsana (p. 55); Śīrṣāsana I (p. 98); Padmāsana in Śīrṣāsana (p. 106); Pārśva Ūrdhva Padmāsana in Śīrṣāsana (p. 115); Piṇḍāsana in Śīrṣāsana (p. 106); Sarvāṅgāsana (p. 108); Ūrdhva Padmāsana in Sarvāṅgāsana (p. 114); Piṇḍāsana and Pārśva Piṇḍāsana in Sarvāṅgāsana (p. 115); Pārśva Ūrdhva Padmāsana in Sarvāṅgāsana (p. 115); Śavāsana I (p. 150).

Lesson 6 (Backbends)

Supta Vīrāsana (p. 82); Bhekāsana (p. 86); Uttānāsana II (p. 45); Adho Mukha Śvānāsana (p. 90); Adho Mukha Vṛkṣāsana (p. 96); Piñca Mayurāsana (p. 97); Ūrdhva Dhanurāsana from Śīrṣāsana (p. 140), × 3; Ūrdhva Dhanurāsana (p. 138), × 3; Dvi Pāda Viparīta Daṇḍāsana (p. 142), × 3; Kapotāsana (p. 144), on chair, × 3; Eka Pāda Rājakapotāsana (p. 143), near wall, using belt; Kapotāsana (p. 144); Vīrāsana forward bend (p. 51); Marīcyāsana III (p. 73), × 3; Ardha Halāsana (p. 110); Śavāsana I (p. 150).

CONSOLIDATION

Make sure that all the different parts of the body are active in all postures. Be firm in your understanding of base and key points of postures. Relate the directions in poses to the directions of Tāḍāsana. Keep the mind and self totally within postures, to experience them to the full.

Remedial Programs

This section gives programs of āsanas to alleviate some medical conditions. Where Prāṇāyāma is included, it should be done lying down and preferably at a different time from the main program.

For remedial purposes, the postures are adapted to suit individual needs. For this reason it is necessary to have the guidance of a suitably qualified teacher.

Programs for serious medical conditions are not given. In such cases, help should be sought from a qualified specialist teacher.

In cases of recent operations or injuries, time should be allowed for the wounds to heal before Yoga practice is undertaken. Here it is best to seek medical advice.

During fever or in acute illness rest is required. Afterward, the recuperation program should be followed.

Where alternative programs have been suggested, the one that gives the most relief, or the postures within it, should be practiced.

When following a program for a particular condition, it is best to continue it until relief is gained before starting on the regular courses.

The programs contain postures of different levels of difficulty (see p. 16). Those who have not done Yoga before should work on beginners' postures within the programs until they progress. Later, more advanced postures from the same group may be added. Prāṇāyāma should not be done by beginners.

Timings in this section are as in the main instructions for the āsanas, unless otherwise specified.

The programs should always end in Śavāsana (p. 150).

Amenorrhea see Gynecological Problems

Anemia

Lying on cross bolsters (p. 80); Supta Vīrāsana (p. 82); Adho Mukha Śvānāsana, head supported (p. 90); Śīrṣāsana and cycle (pp. 98-105); twists (pp. 72-6); Sarvāṅgāsana on chair (p. 118) and Ardha Halāsana (p. 110); Setu Bandha Sarvāṅgāsana on bench (p. 120).

Ujjāyī Prāṇāyāma I (p. 158) and Viloma Prāṇāyāma II (p. 162).

Arthritis and Rheumatic Conditions

1 *Fibrositis and muscular rheumatism*

When not in pain, all postures may be done. Care should be taken not to aggravate a painful condition.

2 *Osteoarthritis (Osteoarthrosis)*

All postures may be done, paying particular attention to working the affected joints.

3 *Rheumatoid Arthritis*

Lying on cross bolsters (p. 80); Bharadvājāsana on chair and Bharadvājāsana I (pp. 71-2), twice each; Parvatāsana in Sukhāsana (p. 53); Jānu Śīrṣāsana and Paścimottānāsana (pp. 59, 64), head supported; Adho Mukha Śvānāsana (p. 90), head supported; Śīrṣāsana (p. 100); Sarvāṅgāsana on chair (p. 118); Ardha Halāsana (p. 110).

When not in pain, all other postures may be done.

4 *Spondylitis*

All standing poses with wall support, particularly Parivṛtta Trikoṇāsana (p. 34); Parivṛtta Pārśvakoṇāsana (p. 36) and Parivṛtta Ardha Candrāsana (p. 28); Pārśvottānāsana (p. 40), hands on ledge; twists (pp. 70-3); Vīrāsana forward bend (p. 50); Śīrṣāsana and Pārśva Śīrṣāsana (pp. 100, 103); Sarvāṅgāsana (p. 110); Halāsana and Pārśva Halāsana (pp. 110, 112); Viparīta Karaṇī (p. 122); Śavāsana II (p. 152).

In the case of cervical spondylitis, Śīrṣāsana and Sarvāṅgāsana should be done only with supervision.

Backache

A Standing Marīcyāsana (p. 70), × 3; Bharadvājāsana on chair (p. 71); × 3; Trikoṇāsana (p. 22); Pārśvakoṇāsana (p. 24); Ardha Candrāsana (p. 30), all twice; Uttānāsana (p. 44), hands on ledge; Jaṭhara Parivartanāsana (p. 85), knees bent; Ardha Halāsana (p. 110); Viparīta Karaṇī (p. 122).

B Utthita Hasta Padāṅguṣṭhāsana I and II (p. 20), twice each; Trikoṇāsana and Parivṛtta Trikoṇāsana (pp. 22, 34); Pārśvakoṇāsana and Parivṛtta Pārśvakoṇāsana (pp. 24, 36), Ardha Candrāsana and Parivṛtta Ardha Candrāsana (pp. 30, 38); Supta Padāṅguṣṭhāsana (p. 88), with belt or against column, twice; Ardha Halāsana (p. 110); Śavāsana I (p. 150), legs bent on chair.

Concentration, lack of

A Adho Mukha Śvānāsana (p. 90); Ūrdhva Śvānāsana (p. 91); Śīrṣāsana and cycle (pp. 98-106); Sarvāṅgāsana and cycle (pp. 108-115); Setu Bandha Sarvāṅgāsana (p. 116); Śavāsana II (p. 152).

B Adho Mukha Vṛkṣāsana (p. 96); Pīnca Mayūrāsana (p. 97); Viparīta Daṇḍāsana on chair (p. 136); Ūrdhva Dhanurāsana (p. 138); Ardha Halāsana (p. 110).

Constipation

A Trikoṇāsana (p. 22); Pārśvakoṇāsana (p. 24), Vīrabhadrāsana I and II (pp. 26, 28); Parivṛtta Trikoṇāsana (p. 34) and Parivṛtta Pārśvakoṇāsana (p. 36); Pārśvottānāsana (p. 40); twists (pp. 70-78); Sarvāṅgāsana and cycle (pp. 108-115).

B (For those in regular practice) Śīrṣāsana and cycle (pp. 98-106), especially Piṇḍāsana (p. 106); Sarvāṅgāsana and cycle (pp. 108-115), especially Piṇḍāsana (p. 114) and Pārśva Piṇḍāsana (p. 116).

Cramp

If cramp occurs during Yoga practice, relax the affected part and do deep breathing until it disappears.

Depression

A Adho Mukha Vṛkṣāsana (p. 96); Pīnca Mayūrāsana (p. 97); Śīrṣāsana (p. 98); Viparīta Daṇḍāsana on chair (p. 136); Sarvāṅgāsana on chair (p. 118); Setu Bandha Sarvāṅgāsana on bench (p. 120); Ūrdhva Dhanurāsana (p. 138), × 3; Śavāsana II (p. 152).

B Sarvāṅgāsana and forward bend sequence (p. 148); six sequences done in quick succession.

Diarrhea
Śīrṣāsana (p. 100); Sarvāṅgāsana on chair (p. 118); Ardha Halāsana (p. 110); Setu Bandha Sarvāṅgāsana on bench (p. 120); Viparīta Karaṇī (p. 122).

Ears
1 Ear Pressure when doing inverted postures
See Cautions in Śīrṣāsana (p. 98) and Sarvāṅgāsana (p. 108).

2 Tinnitus and Fluid in Ears
Adho Mukha Śvānāsana (p. 90); Śīrṣāsana (p. 100); Viparīta Daṇḍāsana on chair (p. 136); Sarvāṅgāsana (p. 108); Ardha Halāsana (p. 110); Jānu Śīrṣāsana (p. 59), head supported; Paścimottānāsana (p. 64), head supported; lying on cross bolsters (p. 80). The head and the ears have to be adjusted carefully.

Eye Strain
For the following programs tie an elastic bandage around the forehead with one part lightly covering the eyes (p. 151). Uncover the eyes between postures, if necessary. *Remove contact lenses.*
A Adho Mukha Śvānāsana (p. 90); Śīrṣāsana (p. 98); Sarvāṅgāsana (p. 108) or Sarvāṅgāsana on chair (p. 118); Ardha Halāsana (p. 110) or Halāsana (p. 110); forward bends, head supported (pp. 59, 60, 61, 63, 66); Viparīta Karaṇī (p. 122); normal breathing, lying down (p. 156).

Śīrṣāsana and Sarvāṅgāsana should be done only if they relieve the eye strain.

B Ṣaṇmukhī Mudrā (p. 163).

Fatigue
A Viparīta Karaṇī (p. 122); Supta Baddha Koṇāsana (p. 81); Supta Vīrāsana (p. 82); Adho Mukha Śvānāsana (p. 90); Śīrṣāsana (p. 98); Sarvāṅgāsana on chair (p. 118); Ardha Halāsana (p. 110); Setu Bandha Sarvāṅgāsana on bench (p. 120); Śavāsana I or II (p. 150 or 152).
(If the back aches as a result of the back-bending movements, do Standing Marīcyāsana [p. 70] and Bharadvājāsana on chair [p. 71] before Śavāsana.)

B Uttānāsana (p. 44); Adho Mukha Śvānāsana (p. 90); Vīrāsana forward bend (p. 51); Sarvāṅgāsana and forward bend sequence, simple variation (p. 148), several times; Halāsana (p. 110), for 3 mins; Sarvāṅgāsana (p. 108), for 5 mins; Paścimottānāsana (p. 64), for 1 min; Śavāsana I (p. 150).

Fibrositis see Arthritis and Rheumatic Conditions

Giddiness
A Forward bends (pp. 59, 60, 61, 64, 66), head supported.

B Śavāsana II (p. 152).

Gynecological Problems
1 Amenorrhea
Supta Baddha Koṇāsana (p. 81); Baddha Koṇāsana (p. 57); Upaviṣṭa Koṇāsana (p. 65), sitting up; Adho Mukha Śvānāsana (p. 90); Śīrṣāsana (p. 98); Baddha Koṇāsana and Upaviṣṭa Koṇāsana in Śīrṣāsana (p. 104); forward bends (pp. 59, 60, 61, 64, 66); Sarvāṅgāsana on chair (p. 118); Ardha Halāsana (p. 110); Setu Bandha Sarvāṅgāsana on bench (p. 120).

2 Premenstrual Tension
Baddha Koṇāsana (p. 57) and Supta Baddha Koṇāsana (p. 81); Supta Vīrāsana (p. 82); Adho Mukha Śvānāsana (p. 90); Śīrṣāsana (p. 98) and Pārśva Śīrṣāsana (p. 103); Sarvāṅgāsana on chair (p. 118); Ardha Halāsana (p. 110); Setu Bandha Sarvāṅgāsana on bench (p. 120).

Ujjāyī Prāṇāyāma I and II (pp. 158-9).

3 Uterus, Prolapsed
Lying on cross bolsters (p. 80); Supta Baddha Koṇāsana (p. 57); Adho Mukha Śvānāsana (p. 90); Śīrṣāsana (p. 98); Baddha Koṇāsana and Upaviṣṭa Koṇāsana in Śīrṣāsana (p. 104); Sarvāṅgāsana on chair (p. 118); Ardha Halāsana (p. 110); Setu Bandha Sarvāṅgāsana on bench (p. 120); Viparīta Karaṇī (p. 122).

For other menstrual and gynecological problems, see *Yoga: A Gem for Women*, by Geeta S. Iyengar.

Headache
A Lying on cross bolsters (p. 80); Bharadvājāsana on chair (p. 71); standing Marīcyāsana (p. 80); Bharadvājāsana I (p. 72); Marīcyāsana I, twisting (p. 63); Marīcyāsana III (p. 73); Ardha Matsyendrāsana I (p. 74); Supta Vīrāsana (p. 82); Supta Baddha Koṇāsana (p. 81); Śavāsana II (p. 152).

B Jānu Śīrṣāsana (p. 59) and other forward bends (pp. 60, 61, 64), head bandaged and supported.

Ujjāyī Prāṇāyāma II (p. 159); Viloma Prāṇāyāma II (p. 162).

Inverted postures, especially Ardha Halāsana (p. 110), often give relief.

Hernia
1 Hiatus
Vīrāsana and Parvatāsana (p. 50); Supta Vīrāsana (p. 82), supported; Matsyāsana (p. 83), supported; Viparīta Daṇḍāsana on chair (p. 136); Uṣṭrāsana (p. 135), supported; Bharadvājāsana I (p. 72), twice; Śavāsana II (p. 152).

2 Inguinal
Vīrāsana (p. 50); Śīrṣāsana (p. 100); Ardha Nāvāsana and Paripūrṇa Nāvāsana (p. 58), using a belt or resting the feet on a chair; Sarvāṅgāsana (p. 108); Halāsana (p. 110); Supta Koṇāsana (p. 113); Karṇapīḍāsana (p. 112); Viparīta Karaṇī (p. 122); Ujjāyī Prāṇāyāma I (p. 158).

Indigestion
Supta Vīrāsana (p. 82); Matsyāsana (p. 83); Supta Baddha Koṇāsana (p. 81).

Insomnia
A Adho Mukha Śvānāsana (p. 90); Viparīta Daṇḍāsana on chair (p. 136); Śīrṣāsana (p. 98); Sarvāṅgāsana on chair (p. 118); Ardha Halāsana (p. 110); Setu Bandha Sarvāṅgāsana on bench (p. 120); Ujjāyī Prāṇāyāma I and II (pp. 158-9).

B Vīrāsana and forward bend (p. 50); Jānu Śīrṣāsana (p. 59), head supported; Ardha Baddha Padma Paścimottānāsana (p. 60); Triaṅg Mukhaikapāda Paścimottānāsana (p. 61); Paścimottānāsana (p. 64); Ardha Halāsana (p. 110); Supta Baddha Koṇāsana (p. 81).

***Knee** Cartilage Problems*
Śīrṣāsana (p. 98); Sarvāṅgāsana (p. 108) and Ardha Halāsana (p. 110) should be done to rest the knees. Standing poses should be done with particular attention to the alignment of the knees, to avoid strain. In sitting poses careful adjustment

of the bent leg may be needed so that there is no pain (see ways of practicing and focuses, pp. 50 and 54).

If the pain is acute, avoid bent leg postures and seek advice.

Leg ache
Vīrāsana (p. 50); Supta Vīrāsana (p. 82); Bhekāsana (p. 86); Padmāsana (p. 54); Baddha Koṇāsana (p. 57); Adho Mukha Śvānāsana (p. 90); Śīrṣāsana (p. 98); Sarvāṅgāsana and cycle (p. 108-115); Ardha Halāsana (p. 110), Viparīta Karaṇī (p. 122).

Menstruation
Baddha Koṇāsana (p. 57) and Upaviṣṭa Koṇāsana (p. 65), against a wall, 5 mins each; forward bends (pp. 59, 60, 61), 3 mins each side; Paścimottānāsana (p. 64), 5 mins; Supta Baddha Koṇāsana (p. 81); Setu Bandha Sarvāṅgāsana on bench (p. 120).

Ujjāyī Prāṇāyāma I, II and III (pp. 158-9).

Migraine see Headache

Osteoarthritis see Arthritis and Rheumatic Conditions

Pregnancy
If you are pregnant, advise your Yoga teacher of any previous miscarriages or medical history. Medical advice may also be required. Without a teacher, it is not advisable to start Yoga in pregnancy.

The following program will need to be adapted from week to week. It should not be done during weeks 11 to 13, when exertion is to be avoided.

In all postures the abdomen should be well extended to create space for the baby. There should be no discomfort or strain.

In inverted postures it is best to have a helper so as not to jerk the body while going up.

A Viparīta Karaṇī (p. 122); Baddha Koṇāsana (p. 57) and Upaviṣṭa Koṇāsana (p. 65), against a wall; Vīrāsana (p. 50); Śīrṣāsana (p. 100; if already practiced); Sarvāṅgāsana with chair (p. 118); Ardha Halāsana (p. 110); Śavāsana II (p. 152) on stepped arrangement of blankets, legs in Baddha Koṇāsana.

Ujjāyī Prāṇāyāma I and II (pp. 158-9).

B Viparīta Karaṇī (p. 122); Supta Vīrāsana (p. 82) supported; Jānu Śīrṣāsana (p. 59), Triaṅg Mukhaikapāda Paścimottānāsana (p. 61), Ardha Baddha Padma Paścimottānāsana (p. 60) and Paścimottānāsana (p. 64), all with concave back, using a belt; Setu Bandha Sarvāṅgāsana on bench (p. 120) or lying on cross bolsters (p. 80); Śavāsana II (p. 152), on stepped arrangement of several blankets, with the legs in Baddha Koṇāsana; Śavāsana II.

Premenstrual Tension see Gynecological Problems

Recuperation
Lying on cross bolsters (p. 80); Supta Vīrāsana (p. 82), supported; Jānu Śīrṣāsana (p. 59) and Paścimottānāsana (p. 64), head supported; Setu Bandha Sarvāṅgāsana on bench (p. 120), Viparīta Karaṇī (p. 122); Śavāsana I or II (p. 150 or 152).

Normal breathing, lying down (p. 156).

Rheumatism see Arthritis and Rheumatic Conditions

Sciatica
Do not jump into the standing poses.

Utthita Hasta Pādāṅguṣṭhāsana I and II (p. 20); standing poses (pp. 22-42), with the front leg turned 10-20° more than usual; Uttānāsana I (p. 44), hands on ledge, standing with the toes turned in and the heels turned out; Vīrāsana (p. 50); Śīrṣāsana (p. 100), with the toes in and the heels out; Supta Pādāṅguṣṭhāsana (p. 88), especially with the leg supported; Ardha Halāsana (p. 110) or Supta Koṇāsana (p. 113), with the thighs supported on two stools.

Scoliosis
Parvatāsana in Sukhāsana or Vīrāsana (p. 50 or 53); all standing poses (pp. 22-42); Adho Mukha Śvānāsana (p. 90); Śīrṣāsana and Pārśva Śīrṣāsana (p. 100, 102), twists (pp. 72-6), near a wall or ledge; Sarvāṅgāsana (p. 108) and Halāsana (p. 110).

Spondylitis see Arthritis and Rheumatic Conditions

Stress
Adho Mukha Śvānāsana (p. 90), head supported; Viparīta Daṇḍāsana on chair (p. 136), head supported; Sarvāṅgāsana on chair (p. 118); Ardha Halāsana (p. 110); Jānu Śīrṣāsana (p. 59) and Paścimottānāsana (p. 64), eyes bandaged and head supported, up to 5 min each; Viparīta Karaṇī (p. 122).

Viloma Prāṇāyāma II (p. 162).

Tinnitus see Ears

Uterus, Prolapsed see Gynecological Problems

Varicose Veins
Vīrāsana (p. 50); Supta Vīrāsana (p. 82); Bhekāsana (p. 86); Śīrṣāsana and cycle (pp. 98-106); Sarvāṅgāsana and cycle (pp. 108-115); forward bends (pp. 59-63).

Vertigo see Giddiness

Whiplash
A Standing poses (pp. 22-40), against a wall, especially Ardha Candrāsana (p. 30) and Parivṛtta Ardha Candrāsana (p. 30), paying attention to making the thoracic spine concave; twists (pp. 70-77):

B Adho Mukha Śvānāsana (p. 90); Adho Mukha Vṛkṣāsana (p. 96); Pīnca Mayūrāsana (p. 97); Viparīta Daṇḍāsana on chair (p. 136); Ūrdhva Dhanurāsana (p. 138); Marīcyāsana III (p. 73); Ardha Halāsana (p. 110).

Śīrṣāsana (p. 100) should be done on the front of the head, near the forehead.

Index

Page numbers for the main postures are in **bold**.

Further Reading

B. K. S. Iyengar *Light on Yoga* (Schocken); The Concise Light on Yoga (Schocken); *Light on Prāṇāyāma* (Crossroad); *The Art of Yoga* (Unwin Hyman); *The Tree of Yoga* (Shambhala); *Yoga Sutra of Patañjali* (Ramamani Iyengar Memorial Yoga Institute, India)

About B. K. S. Iyengar: *Body The Shrine, Yoga Thy Light* (Light on Yoga Research Trust, India); *The Life and Work of B. K. S. Iyengar* (Timeless Books, Canada)

Geeta S. Iyengar *Yoga: A Gem for Women* (Allied Pubs., India/Timeless Books, Canada)

YOGA PHILOSOPHY

Bhagavad Gītā (any edition)
Selections from the Upaniṣads (any edition)
Yoga Sūtras (any edition)
Haṭha Yoga Pradīpika (Theosophical Society, India)
Gheraṇḍa Saṁhitā (Munshiram Manoharlal, India/AMS Press, New York)
Śiva Saṁhitā (Munshiram Manoharlal, India/AMS Press, New York)
Yoga Upaniṣads (Theosophical Society, India)

Authors' Acknowledgments

First and foremost our grateful thanks to our Guru, Yogācharya Sri B. K. S. Iyengar, who has taught us all we know about Yoga, and with whose encouragement we undertook this book. He has given us unstinting support and advice throughout, and has also read the manuscript.

Thanks also to his son, Prashant, who patiently clarified the Yoga philosophy for us and also checked the manuscript; and to his daughter, Geeta, for her explanations of Yoga practice.

We are indebted to Dorling Kindersley for bringing out this book, and are grateful to all their staff for their kindness and hard work, especially Daphne Razazan, Susan Berry, Steven Wooster, Claudine Meissner, and Claire le Bas; to typesetters Vic Chambers and Tony Wallace; and to photographer Jeff Veitch.

We owe much to Shyam's beloved wife, Rukmini, for her support and understanding and to our friend Eugenie Hammond for her help and advice throughout. We are grateful to Mr Tendulkar for typing the first manuscript and to Mr Madan Arora for permission to use the photograph of B. K. S. Iyengar in Naṭarājāsana. We would like to thank Noelle Perez-Christiaens for permission to use quotations by Mr Iyengar from her collection, *Sparks of Divinity*.

Finally, we must thank our colleagues and students at the Iyengar Yoga Institute for their support and interest.

Dorling Kindersley would like to thank Tina Vaughan for art directing the photography and for her help with the design; Claire le Bas and Carolyn Ryden for their editorial help; Mrs Rosemary Grossman for the Sanskrit calligraphy; Hilary Bird for the index; Sue Sian for doing the makeup, and Beverley of "Splitz" for the leotards.

Headline setting
Airedale Graphics

Typesetting
Chambers Wallace, London

Reproduction
Fotographics Ltd